W9-CBT-628

TAKE CHARGE OF TYPE 2 DIABETES WITH…

- A diet designed to improve insulin sensitivity

- The right dietary balance of carbohydrates, protein, and fat

- Exercise that clears the blood of glucose, contributes to weight loss, improves blood flow, and strengthens the heart

- Nutritional supplement suggestions such as fish oil, vitamins, minerals, and herbs

- Additional therapies for diabetic complications including topical ointments, chelation, and hyperbaric oxygen.

REVERSING DIABETES

Now completely revised and updated, this bestselling guide will arm you with safer—and equally effective—ways of treating diabetes than the popular drugs that have become first-line therapy. Through a sensible diet, exercise, and specific nutritional supplement suggestions, you can dramatically improve blood sugar control…reduce—if not eliminate—reliance on medication…and decrease your risk of the complications and other diseases associated with diabetes.

Also by Julian Whitaker, M.D.

Reversing Hypertension
Reversing Heart Disease

REVERSING DIABETES

Revised and Updated

JULIAN WHITAKER, M.D.

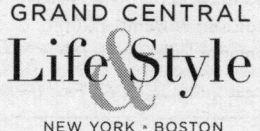

GRAND CENTRAL
Life & Style

NEW YORK · BOSTON

Grand Central Life & Style
Hachette Book Group
1290 Avenue of the Americas
New York, NY 10104

www.GrandCentralLifeandStyle.com

Grand Central Life & Style is an imprint of Grand Central Publishing. The Grand Central Life & Style name and logo are trademarks of Hachette Book Group, Inc.

The Hachette Speakers Bureau provides a wide range of authors for speaking events. To find out more, go to www.hachettespeakersbureau.com or call (866) 376-6591.

The publisher is not responsible for websites (or their content) that are not owned by the publisher.

Printed in the United States of America

Originally published in hardcover by Hachette Book Group
First mass market edition: November 2009
First oversize mass market edition: October 2014

10 9 8 7 6 5 4 3 2
OPM

I would like to dedicate this book to all the diabetic patients who read it, put it to use, and benefit from it.

Acknowledgments

As with any project that tries to cover a lot of bases, this book is the result of the efforts of many. To start with, I would like to acknowledge all of the physicians, both research scientists and clinicians, who went through the effort to publish the work that forms the basis of the material contained in this volume.

Second, I would like to acknowledge the editorial staff at Warner Books, especially my editor, Diana Baroni, as well as Lillian Rodberg, copy editor, who worked very hard at improving sections of the original manuscript, and Roland Ottewell, copy editor for the second edition.

For reviewing sections of the original manuscript and offering critical suggestions, I would like to acknowledge James W. Anderson, M.D., chief of the Metabolic Research Group and professor of medicine and clinical nutrition, Veterans Affairs Medical Center, University of Kentucky; Thaddeus E. Prout, M.D., F.A.C.P., associate professor emeritus, Department of Medicine, the Johns Hopkins School of Medicine in Baltimore; and John K. Davidson, M.D., Ph.D., emeritus professor of medicine, Emory University School of Medicine, and founding director of the Diabetes Unit, Grady Memorial Hospital in Atlanta.

Special thanks to Peggy Dace for her research and edits in updating this book, Kelly Griffin for her proofreading, and Elena Granofsky for keeping things on track. Mark Wettler of Wettler Information Services, who undertook the time-consuming food and recipe analysis, and Patricia Mercado and Valerie Close, who assisted in typing and retyping the original manuscript, also deserve recognition. I would also like to acknowledge Diane Lara, nutritionist at the Whitaker Wellness Institute, who put together the all-important diet regiment of this book. Their time and efforts were substantial. A final thanks goes to my wife, Connie—for everything.

Contents

Preface

In 1979, I opened the Whitaker Wellness Institute. My goal was to provide patients who have diabetes, heart disease, and high blood pressure with a training ground where they could get the education and motivation needed to put what may be the most powerful therapeutic tools to work for them: diet, vigorous exercise, and targeted nutritional supplements.

By the time I founded the Institute, I had concluded that most physicians were ignoring the appropriate use of nutrition and exercise in treating diabetes and other degenerative conditions. This was happening despite the fact that for decades researchers and medical publications had made it clear that simple lifestyle changes were exceptionally effective therapies for patients with these diseases.

Somewhere along the line, we in the medical profession seem to have dropped the ball. We keep looking for "the answer," that single technological breakthrough that will make everything all right for our patients. And with the current explosion of technology, we stand convinced that the answer is just around the corner.

While we are waiting, however, our patients continue to suffer, not because the breakthrough is yet to come, but because we ignore what is the only "answer" necessary for many of them: a disciplined program of diet, exercise, and targeted nutritional supplementation that the *patient* views as the most important part of his or her treatment.

Diabetic patients are suffering because we are not doing nearly enough to help them with the simpler, less dramatic tools that are available today. Why wait for some yet-to-be discovered "miracle cure" when a solution is already available for helping millions of diabetics in this country to become drug free and healthier in every measurable respect? They simply need education and motivation to follow the proper diet, to exercise, and to lose weight.

For more than twenty-two years now my clinic has been treating patients suffering from serious diseases with the primary tools of nutrition, exercise, and nutritional supplementation. Drugs and invasive techniques are used only to supplement the lifestyle program, *not the other way around*. Our results are impressive. With this shift in emphasis, the degree of improvement and the amount of medication that can be eliminated are startling.

From day one I have specialized in the treatment of diabetes. My experience with thousands of diabetic patients has shown me what works and what doesn't work, what lifestyle changes patients are willing to make and what they are not. The result is the program we currently utilize at the Whitaker Wellness Institute. I sincerely wish that every patient with diabetes could come to my Institute or work with another physician or clinic that approaches diabetes in a similar way.

Since that is impossible, I have written this book to

guide patients through the Whitaker Wellness Institute program for reversing diabetes. Its purpose is to show you that there are safer, less invasive, yet equally effective ways of treating diabetes than the popular drugs that have become first-line therapy. I'll show you how, by utilizing "low-tech" exercise and nutritional therapies, you can dramatically improve blood sugar control, reduce—if not eliminate—reliance on medication, and decrease your risk of the complications and other diseases associated with diabetes.

What Is Diabetes?

CHAPTER 1

What to Expect If You Have Diabetes

There are 16 million diabetics in this country, and many more have a "pre-diabetic" condition known as impaired glucose tolerance, meaning they're on the road toward developing diabetes. With diabetes now affecting close to 6 percent of the U.S. population and more than 18 percent of those over sixty-five, the incidence of this condition is growing by leaps and bounds. Worldwide it has more than tripled in the last thirty-five years and is expected to double again within the next quarter century, affecting a total of 300 million people.[1]

This is tragic. Diabetes is the sixth leading cause of death by disease in our country and a chief contributor to blindness, kidney disease, memory loss, lower extremity amputations, and premature death from heart disease.

But a diagnosis of diabetes needn't be a sentence of death and disability. This condition can be treated and complications can be prevented. I have worked with thousands of diabetic patients at the Whitaker Wellness Institute over the past twenty-two years and have put together a treatment program that approaches diabetes from an alternative angle. Rather than relying on life-long drug regimens, we instruct our patients in dietary measures that naturally keep their blood sugar under control. They learn how exercise improves the diabetic condition and what nutritional supplements lower blood sugar as effectively as drugs. At the same time we teach our patients how to protect themselves from the complications that plague so many diabetics.

The purpose of this book is to share with you the program of diet, exercise, and nutritional supplementation that so many of my patients have utilized to effectively reverse diabetes.

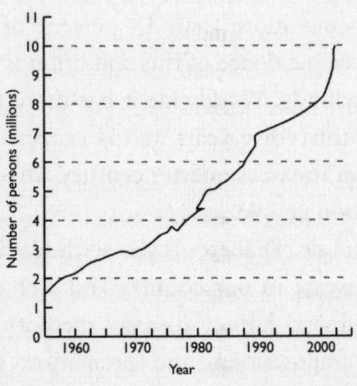

Figure 1. Rising rates of diabetes in the U.S.
Source: National Institutes of Health and Centers for Disease Control and Prevention.

What Is Diabetes?

Medical dictionaries actually list many forms of diabetes, but when we talk about diabetes we are generally referring to *diabetes mellitus*, sometimes called sugar diabetes. "Diabetes" comes from the Greek word for "to go through"—and indeed, frequent urination is a major symptom of this disease. "Mellitus" comes from the Greek word for honey, a reference to the glucose or sugar lost in the urine.

Diabetes mellitus is a disorder of the body's means of utilizing glucose, a simple sugar that is the basic fuel that energizes our cells. Before the food we eat can be used as fuel by our muscles and other tissues, it must first be converted into glucose. Then the glucose must enter the individual cells, where it is metabolized, or "burned," to provide energy for the cells' functions. The hormone insulin, which is produced in the pancreas, is essential for this process, as it ushers glucose into the cells.

There are two basic kinds of diabetes mellitus, type 1 and type 2. Type 1 diabetes used to be called juvenile diabetes because its symptoms often become apparent in childhood or infancy. Type 2 diabetes usually, though not always, shows up in middle age or later and was once called maturity- or adult-onset diabetes. Type 1 diabetes, which arises from a lack of insulin in the body, always requires supplemental insulin and is also known as *insulin-dependent diabetes mellitus* (IDDM). Type 2 diabetes does not reflect a lack of insulin but rather the inability of the body to use it effectively. It is sometimes referred to as *non-insulin-dependent diabetes mellitus* (NIDDM). These two types of diabetes differ in many respects and are in fact considered to be two separate entities. In order to understand these differences, you must first understand how insulin functions in your body.

What Is Insulin?

Insulin is a hormone produced in patches of specialized cells scattered throughout the pancreas, a large gland located in the back of the abdominal cavity. These "islands," which contain insulin-producing beta cells, were named the islets of Langerhans in honor of the German pathologist Paul Langerhans, who first described them in 1869. He had no idea that they produced insulin or had anything to do with the diabetic condition; insulin was to be discovered half a century later.

Insulin is required for glucose circulating in the bloodstream to enter the cells, where it is used in the energy-producing chemical reactions that drive the heart, the brain, and every cell in your body. Insulin works like a key, opening the cell door and allowing glucose to enter. It does this by signaling proteins that reside within the cell to rise to the cell's surface and usher in glucose. There are exceptions to this general rule. Insulin is not necessary for glucose to enter the cells of the brain or the kidneys. Red blood cells are also able to utilize sugar without the assistance of insulin. Furthermore, when you are exercising, the muscle cells can extract glucose from the blood without insulin.

For the most part, however, if insulin is not present, or if *its action is blocked*—a concept that is very important in this book—glucose is not removed from the bloodstream, the blood glucose level rises, and the diabetic condition results. If blood glucose elevates markedly, metabolism is thrown off completely, and the blood becomes more acidic, a condition called diabetic ketoacidosis. A patient in this state may go into a diabetic coma and die.

Clearly, insulin serves a vital function. Whenever there is an inadequate supply of this hormone (type 1 diabetes) or an inability for insulin to do its job (type 2 diabetes), serious problems can occur.

The Costs of Diabetes

The growing incidence of diabetes is exerting a tremendous financial toll on our country. In 1997, the most recent year of available statistics, direct health care costs for the treatment of diabetes were $44.1 billion. Add to that $54 billion in indirect costs such as lost wages, and diabetes is costing us upwards of $100 billion per year.

The human costs are even more significant. The life expectancy of a middle-aged person with type 2 diabetes is five to ten years less than that of the general population. Furthermore, his or her risk of suffering from heart disease, blindness, kidney disease, nerve and circulatory problems, and a host of other medical problems is dramatically increased.

Type 1: Insulin-Dependent Diabetes Mellitus

Type 1 diabetes occurs when the pancreas loses its ability to produce insulin, leading to an acute "key shortage." This type of diabetes, which usually occurs at an early age, is marked by four classic symptoms:

- Frequent and excessive urination (polyuria)

- Excessive thirst and urge to drink large amounts of fluids (polydipsia) to replace the water lost through excessive urination

- Ravenous hunger and excessive eating (polyphagia) in an attempt to feed the body's starving cells

- Weight loss, despite excessive food intake, because the cells cannot utilize glucose

These four symptoms are all related to elevated levels of glucose in the blood and the body's inability to clear it from the bloodstream and use it for energy. When blood glucose levels are normal, the kidneys "conserve" glucose, and there is none in the urine. With diabetes, however, the high levels of glucose in the blood overwhelm the kidneys' conservation ability, and large volumes of glucose-containing urine are excreted.

Thirst and excessive water drinking develop not only because the type 1 diabetic loses copious amounts of water in the urine, but also because the high level of glucose in the blood makes the blood thicker and more concentrated. This sets off the body's thirst sensors, giving the diabetic an unrelenting desire for fluids.

The combination of weight loss with excessive food intake is also characteristic of the early stages of type 1 diabetes. Because the glucose in the blood cannot enter the cells and be used, the cells are starving—in an ocean of plenty—and weight loss rapidly occurs. As with thirst, so with hunger: The diabetic is ravenous and eats much more, but to no avail, as the energy contained in the food, which has been converted to glucose, simply passes through the body and is lost in the urine.

Often type 1 diabetics are first diagnosed in a hospital emergency room when they appear with very high blood sugar levels, usually in the range of 350 to 750 milligrams per deciliter (mg/dl) of blood. (Normal blood sugar levels range between 80 and 110 mg/dl.) Sometimes the patient is in a diabetic coma, a life-threatening condition that must be treated with insulin to correct the basic problem and fluids to replace those that are lost.

Individuals with type 1 diabetes will almost always require insulin injections, but the amount of insulin can usually be reduced by following the principles in this book. Furthermore, by carefully monitoring blood glucose levels and keeping them as close to normal as possible, many of the devastating complications associated with diabetes can be delayed or avoided. Type 1 diabetes is the more serious form of the disease, but also the less common, accounting for only 5 to 10 percent of all cases.

Type 1 Diabetes: What Causes It?

In type 1 diabetes, the cells that produce insulin have been damaged or destroyed and can no longer make enough insulin to regulate blood glucose. Although we do not know exactly what causes type 1 diabetes, it seems to result from the interaction of three factors: (1) an inherited vulnerability, plus (2) acute injury to the beta cells, which (3) stimulates the body's immune system to attack these cells, severely damaging them or destroying them altogether.

An Inherited Tendency

It is well established that a *susceptibility* to type 1 diabetes is inherited. If you are a sibling or offspring of someone with this type of diabetes, you have a one-in-twenty chance of developing the condition, compared with the typical person's one-in-three-hundred chance. Studies of twins are often used to determine whether a condition is inherited, because the genetic makeup of identical twins is the same. In various studies of twins in which one of the pair had type 1 diabetes, the disease also developed in the second twin 25 to 50 percent—but not 100 percent—of the time. This means that it is not diabetes itself that is inherited but something that increases a person's risk of developing it.

This is not to say that type 1 diabetes only appears within certain families. Severe type 1 diabetes can develop in people with *no* family history of the condition. In fact, 85 percent of all patients with type 1 diabetes have *no* family history of diabetes.[2]

Acute Damage to the Beta Cells

Type 1 diabetes doesn't just develop out of the blue. An environmental insult of some kind that causes inflammation of the pancreas, a condition known as insulitis, sets into motion the destruction of the insulin-producing cells that results in type 1 diabetes. Acute damage to the beta cells can stem from a variety of environmental factors. First on the list are viral infections. Dr. J. W. Yoon reported a case in the *New England Journal of Medicine* of a boy of ten who developed severe type 1 diabetes after having the flu. The virus that had caused the boy's illness was isolated and injected into an experimental animal. It destroyed the animal's pancreatic cells, and the animal developed diabetes.[3]

Mumps, measles, chicken pox, and other viral diseases are often reported as antecedents to the development of type 1 diabetes. There are also reports of the disease following exposure to various pesticides and other chemicals found in our environment. Some studies suggest a possible link between pancreatic damage and nitrosamines, harmful chemicals that are formed after ingesting nitrates in smoked meats and other cured foods. These environmental factors may either destroy beta cells outright or initiate an autoimmune reaction, which we will discuss below.

Another proposed culprit is the early introduction of cow's milk to genetically susceptible infants. Several epidemiological studies, which examine the relationship between disease and environmental factors, have found that when children are given cow's milk before three months of age, they are at increased risk of developing type 1 diabetes. Cow's milk contains a specific protein that may trigger the autoimmune response that destroys insulin-producing cells in the pancreas.[4]

Stress may also be a factor. Some of my patients who have type 1 diabetes report that a very stressful life event occurred six months to a year before they developed diabetes. Some had lost a close family member, others had moved abruptly, still others had gone through a particularly stressful time at work or school. Recent studies confirm that stress can indeed alter the immune system, providing support for the hypothesis that stress may be the initiating event, particularly in someone with an inherited vulnerability.

An Out-of-Control Immune Response

The ultimate cause of type 1 diabetes in most cases is an autoimmune reaction, in which the body's immune system attacks its own tissues. One of the ways your immune system keeps you from harm is by producing antibodies, specialized cells that help the body ward off bacteria, viruses, and other foreign or threatening substances. Type 1 diabetes develops when antibodies are created that attack the body's own damaged beta cells. For some as yet unknown reason, the immune system looks upon these damaged cells as foreign and begins producing antibodies against them, which finish them off. The isolation of antibodies to insulin-producing cells in patients with type 1 diabetes is well documented in the medical literature. Indeed, antibodies to pancreatic cells are present in about 75 percent of all type 1 diabetics but in less than 2 percent of people without this condition.[5]

The presence of such antibodies, indicating some degree of autoimmune disease going on in the pancreas, is a distinct risk factor—an early warning sign, if you will—for type 1 diabetes, particularly in younger people with a genetic susceptibility to the disease. Dr.

S. Srikanta of the Joslin Diabetes Center in Boston studied a set of twins and a set of triplets; one child in each set had developed diabetes, indicating a high probability that it would develop in the others. Diabetes did develop in one of the triplets and in the second twin. But years before the condition surfaced in these children, Dr. Srikanta's team found antibodies to islet cells in their bloodstream. These antibodies were *not* found in the triplet who did not develop diabetes.[6]

Can Type 1 Diabetes Be Reversed?

Type 1 diabetes has long been viewed as an unfortunate, irreversible twist of fate—it strikes without warning and there's nothing you can do to prevent it. Contrary to popular belief, however, you don't just wake up one day with type 1 diabetes. As the twin and triplet study discussed above illustrates, slow destruction of the beta cells precedes the development of clinical symptoms by months or years.

There is mounting evidence that if type 1 diabetes can be detected in its earliest stages, while some beta-cell function is still intact, further progression may be prevented. Scientists have determined that specific genes on the sixth chromosome are responsible for the susceptibility to type 1 diabetes, and tests for the presence or absence of these genes have been developed. Tests for pancreatic autoimmune activity such as islet-cell or beta-cell antibodies, which may be detected years before full-blown diabetes arises, are also available. So early detection is possible.

Interventions are currently being explored to stop the progression of beta-cell destruction in at-risk individuals. Intensive insulin therapy early on, before symptoms appear, retards the course of type 1 diabetes in some people. Nicotinamide (also called niacinamide), a form of vitamin B_3, when administered to recent-onset type 1 diabetics, has been observed to reverse the condition by preserving beta-cell function. (More on this in chapter 9.) Immunosuppressive drugs slow down beta-cell death but, so far, provide only brief remission. And islet-cell transplantation and regeneration hold promise, as do vaccinations that modify the immune system's response to insulin.

If you are newly diagnosed with type 1 diabetes you should certainly look into some of these options. In addition, by following the recommendations outlined in part III of this book and utilizing intensive insulin therapy to keep blood glucose levels close to normal, it is possible to avoid complete beta-cell burnout. This cannot only reduce your insulin requirements and make blood glucose control easier, but may also fend off the complications commonly associated with the condition.

Even if you have had type 1 diabetes for years, you will find that blood glucose control will be much easier if you eat right and exercise regularly. Furthermore, by following the nutritional supplement recommendations in chapter 9, you'll give your body additional tools for avoiding heart disease, circulation problems, and nerve and eye damage.

Is It Type I or Type 2?

Whether a patient has type I or type 2 diabetes is generally—although not always—clear to a physician. When in doubt, a C-peptide test can usually provide the answer. C-peptide is an insulin-like protein that is released during the production of insulin. Although it has no known biologic activity, its level in the blood is a useful indicator of insulin secretion by the pancreas. Patients with type 2 diabetes often have high-normal or elevated levels, while those with type I have low or even undetectable levels, indicating little insulin production. I also use the C-peptide test in my clinic to follow patients with type 2 diabetes. Normalization of C-peptide indicates improvement in insulin sensitivity. However, below-normal levels suggest potential exhaustion of insulin-producing islet cells.

Type 2 Diabetes: Non-Insulin-Dependent Diabetes Mellitus

By far the larger percentage (at least 90 percent) of diabetics have type 2 diabetes, which in many respects is a different condition altogether. Rarely does a person with type 2 diabetes present with the classic symptoms of diabetes. Instead, the disease is usually discovered when a routine laboratory exam reveals an elevated blood sugar level, often in the 150–300 mg/dl range. Sure, there are some hints: The typical newly diagnosed type 2 diabetic is middle-aged, overweight, and inactive. But there are few overt signs of early-stage type 2 diabetes.

The type 2 diabetic usually has no defect in insulin production. In fact, while a healthy individual produces about 31 units of insulin per day, the type 2 diabetic may secrete as much as 114 units![7] We are obviously not looking at an insulin shortage here. Instead, there is some kind of block in the cells' ability to utilize the insulin that is produced. There are plenty of insulin "keys" that could open the cells to let in glucose, but the "keyholes" are jammed. This form of diabetes, which stems from an underlying condition known as *insulin resistance*, is highly responsive to treatment methods designed to increase the cells' sensitivity to insulin, which we will discuss in part III.

Causes of Insulin Resistance

The concept of insulin resistance is as important for the 90 percent of diabetics with type 2 diabetes as the concept of insulin deficiency is for the 10 percent with type 1: It is the underlying cause of the condition. Several factors, which we will discuss in detail in chapter 2, contribute to the development of insulin resistance.

- **Obesity,** or too high a proportion of fat in body tissues, is associated with marked insulin resistance. In obese people, type 2 diabetes is as common as a 42-inch waist. Where this excess weight is carried is also a factor, with distribution in the abdominal area conferring greater risk. It is important to realize the effect that obesity has on the cells' sensitivity to insulin, because it means that even if insulin is injected—as it sometimes is in type 2 diabetics—it will not work as it should, and larger and larger doses are often required.

- **Inappropriate diet** is a major contributor to insulin resistance and weight gain and is thus a significant cause of diabetes. Excess fat and refined carbohydrates such as sugar and white flour are the culprits here. Modification of dietary factors that influence insulin sensitivity is particularly important in type 2 diabetes.

- **Inactivity** or a very low level of activity contributes to insulin resistance and may bring on type 2 diabetes in some people. In addition, inactivity often leads to obesity, which compounds the risk. An exercise program dramatically increases insulin sensitivity and improves the diabetic condition.

- **Deficiencies of certain vitamins and minerals** may contribute to insulin resistance, and targeted nutritional supplements are a powerful therapy for the treatment of the condition.

The association between insulin resistance and diabetes was demonstrated more than seventy years ago, and treatment methods to improve insulin sensitivity were identified at that time. Insulin resistance is currently a hot topic of research. It is now known to be associated not only with type 2 diabetes, but also with hypertension, low HDL cholesterol and high triglyceride levels, and increased risk of cardiovascular disease, a cluster of conditions known as *Syndrome X*.

It is important for patients with type 2 diabetes to understand the "big picture" of insulin resistance and Syndrome X, for these individuals often concurrently develop one or more of these other conditions.

Although there is a solid and growing body of research on the role of lifestyle factors in the development and treatment of insulin resistance and type 2 diabetes, physicians for the most part ignore it. Instead of working on ways to improve insulin sensitivity through lifestyle changes, they rely almost exclusively on oral drugs and insulin injections. This is a mistake. In fact, it is the reason for this book.

Diabetes's Youngest Victims

Ten years ago type 2 diabetes was virtually unheard of in children. Today it is approaching epidemic proportions in children and adolescents. The dramatic increase in the incidence of diabetes in this age group directly coincides with rising rates of obesity in kids: 25 percent of American children are overweight. Unless we are able to reverse this trend by helping our children improve their diet and activity level, we are asking for serious trouble.

Making the Diagnosis

Because type 2 diabetes can easily sneak up on you, it often goes undetected for several years after its onset. By the time it is diagnosed, chronically elevated blood glucose and insulin levels may have already damaged the blood vessels, nerves, eyes, kidneys, and other organs. The American Diabetes Association now recommends that all Americans forty-five years of age and older be screened for diabetes every three years. Screening should begin earlier if you have any additional risk factors, such as obesity, a history of gestational diabetes during pregnancy, or a family history of diabetes, or if you belong to one of the high-risk ethnic groups, which include African Americans, Hispanics, Native Americans, and Asians. Overweight children, especially if they have a family history of type 2 diabetes, high cholesterol, or other risk factors, should be screened by age ten. In addition, individuals with hypertension, high triglycerides, and low HDL cholesterol, accompanying factors that we will discuss in greater detail in the next chapter, should be tested for diabetes on a more frequent basis.

There are several types of screening tests. The most common and least expensive test, and the one currently endorsed by the American Diabetes Association, is the fasting glucose test. You fast overnight, then have a small amount of blood drawn and tested for concentration of glucose. Readings of 126 mg/dl or greater on two different days suggest a diagnosis of diabetes. This is the most widely accepted test in determining the presence of diabetes, and the one we rely on at my clinic.

Another screening tool, which used to be a diagnostic standard but was dropped by the American Diabetes Association several years ago (although it is still recommended by the World Health Organization), is the two-hour oral glucose tolerance test. You drink a sugary liquid, wait two hours (during which time you are not allowed to eat, drink, or exercise), then give a blood sample. A reading of 200 mg/dl or greater is indicative of diabetes. We do not routinely utilize this test at the Whitaker Wellness Institute. One reason is because I am not convinced that it is very accurate. Many studies have shown dramatic variations in glucose levels when the test is repeated in the same individuals.

Several factors can affect the outcome of the glucose tolerance test. One is diet, as Dr. J. Shirley Sweeney demonstrated years ago. He rounded up twenty-three young, healthy male medical students and divided them into four groups. Each group was fed a different diet for two days prior to being administered a dextrose tolerance test. (Dextrose is another form of sugar; this is a variation of the glucose tolerance test.)

- ◉ Group 1: High-fat diet; consumed only olive oil, butter, mayonnaise made with egg yolk, and 20 percent cream.

- ◉ Group 2: High-protein diet; received only lean meat and egg whites.

- ◉ Group 3: High-carbohydrate diet; ate only sugar, candy, pastry, white bread, baked potatoes, syrup, bananas, rice, and oatmeal.

- ◉ Group 4: Starvation diet; went without food for two days.

Dr. Sweeney found that volunteers on the high-fat, high-protein, and starvation diets all had diabetes, as determined by the dextrose tolerance test. Only the students on the high-carbohydrate diet tested normal. He then switched the volunteers around and found that when those who had blood sugar levels indicative of diabetes while on their initial high-fat or high-protein diet were put on the high-carbohydrate diet, the test returned to normal. Likewise, when the students who had normal blood sugar levels while on the high-carbohydrate diet were put on any of the other three diets, they immediately developed diabetes as demonstrated by the dextrose tolerance test.

Sweeney concluded that it was "plain from the foregoing experiments that the dextrose tolerance test may be significantly affected by the character of food taken prior to the test."[8] (Dr. Sweeney's research also serves as part of the foundation for a therapeutic high-carbohydrate diet in the treatment of diabetes, which we will discuss in part III.)

Dr. Marvin Siperstein, professor of medicine at the Veterans Administration Medical Center in San Francisco, spoke out against the glucose tolerance test as a tool for diagnosing diabetes at a conference sponsored by the University of California School of Medicine in San Francisco. He pointed out that only 17 percent of a group of nine- to twenty-five-year-olds with abnormal tests had gone on to develop true diabetes by the time they were fifty to sixty years old. And in another group of subjects over age twenty-six, the test was 100 percent inaccurate as a predictor of diabetes in later years. Dr. Siperstein stated quite bluntly:

Thus, whether glucose tolerance is high or low [on the GTT], it has no value. The test is wrong

80–90% of the time, resulting in a grossly absurd
number of patients who are misdiagnosed and
wrongly tagged with the label "diabetic" for
the rest of their lives. Many of these nondiabetic
patients are inappropriately treated with oral
agents and even insulin. Other disadvantages of
inaccurately being labeled as diabetic include a
doubling of life insurance rates, job discrimina-
tion, and problems in retaining a driver's license.[9]

We will return to the glucose tolerance test in the next chapter, for although it is not particularly accurate in diagnosing diabetes, it may be useful, when used appropriately, to determine the presence of insulin resistance.

Uncontrolled Diabetes Leads to Serious Complications

As you can see, I am strongly opposed to burdening patients with inappropriate diagnoses, but I am also acutely aware of the serious complications and physical deterioration that may be caused by diabetes. If you have been diagnosed with diabetes, don't take it lightly. It can be a fearsome disorder, as excess glucose in the bloodstream is extremely damaging to the body. High concentrations of glucose can lead to the cellular accumulation of sorbitol, a by-product of glucose metabolism. The buildup of sorbitol within cells causes them to swell and damage tissues. Sorbitol accumulation has been most strongly linked to complications of the eyes and nerves.

Another destructive mechanism at work in patients with diabetes is glycosylation (or glycation). Glycosylation occurs when glucose binds to, chemically alters, and damages proteins. These altered proteins are called advanced glycation endproducts. (They have the apt acronym of AGE proteins or AGEs.) Over time, AGE proteins may accumulate in the cells and interfere with their normal functioning. Although this process affects everyone to some degree, especially as we age, it is accelerated in people with diabetes. Diabetic complications of the eyes, kidneys, and circulatory system are associated with AGE proteins.

Elevated levels of glucose also increase the production of free radicals. Although free radicals are natural by-products of normal cellular metabolism, they have a dark side. Free-radical damage has been linked to heart disease, cancer, and dozens of other degenerative disorders. This increase in free-radical activity is a dominant reason why diabetics suffer so many complications.

Uncontrolled diabetes takes a tremendous toll. Take a look at these statistics from the American Diabetes Association:

- **Blindness.** The number one cause of blindness in people ages twenty to seventy-four is diabetic retinopathy. Every year, up to 24,000 Americans lose their sight because of vascular complications caused by diabetes. Glaucoma and cataracts are also more common in individuals with diabetes.

- **Kidney failure.** Diabetes is the leading cause of kidney failure and is responsible for 40 percent of all new cases. More than 28,000 diabetics begin treatment each year for end-stage renal disease brought on by diabetes, and at least 100,000 diabetics are currently undergoing dialysis or have received kidney transplants.

- **Nerve damage.** Diabetic neuropathy affects 60 to 70 percent of all diabetics. Symptoms may range from mild loss of sensation in the feet to constant pain in various parts of the body. Nerve damage may also impair digestion and sexual function, particularly in men, and cause a number of other complications.

- **Amputations.** More than 56,000 amputations are performed every year on patients with diabetes, making this condition the leading cause of nontraumatic amputations. If you have diabetes, your risk of leg amputation is up to forty times greater than that of a person with normal blood glucose.

- **Cardiovascular disease.** Elevated blood glucose damages the blood vessels and alters blood lipid levels. High triglyceride levels are common in diabetics, as are low levels of protective HDL cholesterol. In addition, hypertension affects almost 60 percent of individuals with type 2 diabetes. People who have diabetes are two to four times more likely to develop heart disease or have a stroke than nondiabetics, and three-fourths of all diabetics (more than 77,000 annually) ultimately die from heart disease.

- ◉ **Infections.** Impaired circulation and damaged nerves increase the risk of infection. Wounds heal more slowly in diabetics and require more intensive treatment. Areas often affected include the feet, legs, and urinary tract.

- ◉ **Other complications.** Most people are unaware that diabetes also contributes to memory loss, dementia, and periodontal or gum disease.[10]

Pretty scary list, isn't it? But let me stress again: A diagnosis of diabetes doesn't have to mean a lifetime of suffering and premature death. This condition is definitely treatable, even reversible, and complications can be avoided. By maintaining "tight control" (keeping blood glucose levels as close to normal as possible)— which I will show you how to do without resorting to drugs—and replacing the important nutrients lost as a result of the diabetic condition, you can live a long and active life. Let me tell you about my patient R.K.

This Patient Reversed His Diabetes

R.K. arrived at the Whitaker Wellness Institute with a diagnosis of type 2 diabetes, hypertension, and cardiac arrhythmia. He was taking a number of drugs for his blood pressure and heart condition, and he was also on insulin. We immediately put him on a low-fat, high-fiber diet, targeted nutritional supplementation, and a daily exercise program. Knowing this regimen would lower his insulin requirements (it almost always does), we cut his insulin dose in half on the first day to avoid hypoglycemic reactions. On the second day, with his blood sugar in the normal range, we discontinued his insulin altogether while closely monitoring his blood glucose levels.

Remarkably, this patient's blood sugar never went back up. His blood pressure also normalized, and within twelve days he was able to discontinue the diuretics he was taking for his hypertension. Since his arrhythmia had not occurred during his stay at the Institute, the drugs he was taking to control that condition were also stopped on a trial basis as we continued to monitor him closely.

Six months later R.K. was still taking no medications for diabetes or high blood pressure. His heart arrhythmia had recurred, so he resumed one of the drugs. One year later, his fasting blood glucose was a normal 91, his blood pressure a youthful 117/80, and his total cholesterol level a respectable 159.

This patient's diabetes and high blood pressure had disappeared—a miracle cure! But this was done without transplanted pancreas cells, the latest drugs, an insulin pump, or any of the other "technology breakthroughs" that are so much a part of modern medicine. Ironically, if you could credit R.K.'s success to a pill or a machine, it would be heralded as the greatest medical breakthrough since computerized billing. But since it came from something as simple as a doctor and patient sitting down and finally getting serious about what the patient puts into his mouth, the cure has no pizzazz. After all, most physicians have been telling their patients to "diet" for years.

R.K.'s story demonstrates not only the often futile act of chasing symptoms with drugs, but also the power nutrition and exercise can have in the treatment of diabetes and other degenerative conditions. There are many things you can do to improve diabetes, regardless of which type you have. That is the focus of this book. As you will see in part III, this book gives you a program to enhance your cells' sensitivity to insulin, whether it is produced by your pancreas or is supplied by injection. But first, let's take a closer look at the concept of insulin resistance, which, for the vast majority of diabetics, is the root of the problem.

CHAPTER 2

Type 2 Diabetes and Insulin Resistance

Although insulin resistance is the underlying problem for the vast majority of patients with diabetes, most of them are unfamiliar with the concept. Diabetes and insulin are so closely intertwined that it is often assumed that if you have diabetes, you're not producing enough insulin. The reality is that in 90 percent of all diabetics (those with type 2), the pancreas secretes plenty of insulin, more than enough to escort glucose into the cells. However, the cells resist the efforts of insulin and just won't let the glucose in.

Recent research suggests that the root cause of insulin resistance is a breakdown in intercellular signaling. Insulin is a chemical messenger. It signals proteins called GLUT-4 transporters, which reside within the cell, to rise to the cell's membrane, where they grab on to glucose and take it inside. In patients with insulin resistance, the cells don't get the message. They simply can't hear insulin knocking on the door.

The pancreas responds by churning out more and more insulin, and the "knocking" becomes louder and louder. Levels of both glucose and insulin circulating in the blood rise, sometimes dramatically. In the earlier stages of insulin resistance, the message eventually is heard, and glucose is let in. This is known as *compensated insulin resistance*: The pancreas compensates by producing more insulin, and glucose levels eventually

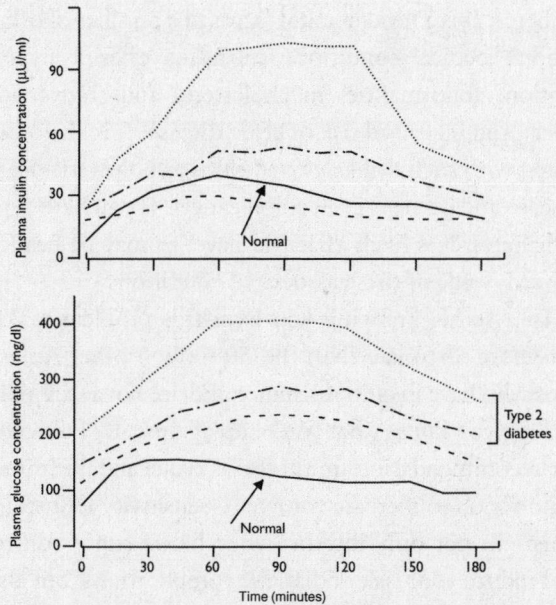

Figure 2. Diagram of glucose and insulin levels after eating, normal and diabetic. Note the exaggerated release of insulin in response to glucose elevations in diabetes—and its failure to adequately lower glucose levels.
From DeFronzo, RA. "Pathophysiology of Type 2 Diabetes: The Role of Insulin Resistance." *Consultant* (suppl.): S10, Nov. 1999.

normalize. However, over time, the stress of excessive insulin production wears out the pancreas, and it cannot keep up this accelerated output. Glucose levels remain elevated for prolonged periods. This is called *uncompensated insulin resistance*, and it is the essence of advanced type 2 diabetes.

Diabetes: The Tip of the Iceberg

Insulin resistance is associated with much more than diabetes. It is a fundamental factor in a number of other serious medical conditions, including obesity, hypertension, abnormalities in cholesterol and triglyceride levels, and increased risk of heart disease. It is also associated with such unlikely conditions as polycystic ovary disease and perhaps even colon cancer. If you have type 2 diabetes, it is likely that you have, or may be headed toward, some of these associated conditions.

In a sense, knowing you have this problem makes you more fortunate than the 60 million other Americans who have insulin resistance and are not aware of it. At least you know what you're up against. By following the recommendations in this book, you can take immediate action to increase your cells' sensitivity to insulin. This will not only improve your blood sugar control and reduce your risk of diabetic complications, but also protect you from the ravages of other very significant health problems.

Unfortunately, few patients with diabetes understand insulin resistance well enough to do something about it. In a survey of more than a thousand type 2 diabetics that was published in *Cardiology Review* in

2000, more than two-thirds of those polled either had no basic understanding of insulin resistance or had never heard of it at all![1]

Physician knowledge and interest lags as well. Most physicians do not regard insulin resistance as a disease, and few attempt to unravel the threads that bind these disparate medical problems together. Medicine has become so specialized that you may see one doctor for your diabetes, another for your hypertension, and yet another for hormonal problems. Given this sort of compartmentalization, it's no wonder that patients often end up being treated with a plethora of drugs, one for each symptom or diagnosis.

One researcher who has done an extraordinary job of tying together the common threads among these seemingly unrelated conditions is Gerald Reaven, M.D., of Stanford University School of Medicine. For more than thirty years Dr. Reaven has been the world's leader in the field of insulin resistance. Dr. Reaven was the first to discover the close link between insulin resistance and hypertension, obesity, blood lipid abnormalities, and glucose intolerance.[2] He coined this clustering of conditions *Syndrome X*. (It is also referred to as the deadly quartet, Reaven's syndrome, metabolic syndrome, and insulin resistance syndrome.) Syndrome X, or insulin resistance syndrome, is a much broader problem than type 2 diabetes. According to Dr. Reaven:

- ◉ Twenty-five to 30 percent of all Americans—60 to 75 million people—are insulin resistant. Only 5 to 10 percent of them will develop type 2 diabetes.

- ⊙ Insulin resistance is as accurate a predictor of heart disease as elevated levels of low-density lipoprotein (LDL) cholesterol. It may account for half of all heart attacks. According to one Canadian study, for each 30 percent rise in insulin levels, there was a corresponding 70 percent increase in risk of heart attack over five years.[3]

- ⊙ Half of all patients with high blood pressure have insulin resistance.

- ⊙ Insulin resistance is closely related to obesity. The fatter you are, the more likely you are to be insulin resistant. However, not every obese person is insulin resistant, nor does being slender guarantee that you are not insulin resistant.[4]

Why Is Insulin Resistance Harmful?

I explained in the previous chapter why elevated levels of glucose are harmful. They result in the accumulation of sorbitol in the cells, which may cause tissue damage, and they also accelerate the binding of sugar to proteins, a process called glycosylation that is involved in diabetic complications. Insulin resistance brings yet another hazard: excess insulin in the bloodstream, a condition called hyperinsulinemia.

In addition to interfering with normal blood sugar regulation, hyperinsulinemia dramatically raises the risk of heart disease by upsetting the normal metabolism of fat in the body. High levels of insulin cue the liver to make more very-low-density lipoprotein (VLDL). VLDL acts as a carrier of fat, or triglycerides, in the blood. The higher your level of VLDL and triglycerides, the more fat you have circulating in your blood. In addition, some VLDL is converted to LDL cholesterol, the "bad" cholesterol that is deposited on artery walls. Even worse, these LDL particles tend to be smaller and denser—and therefore more harmful— than normal LDL. Elevated levels of VLDL also lead to a lowering of the most protective type of cholesterol, high-density lipoprotein (HDL), the "good" cholesterol that escorts cholesterol out of the body.

Hyperinsulinemia is associated with other abnormalities in the blood. It raises levels of fibrinogen, a substance that encourages the formation of blood clots that may contribute to heart attacks, and plasminogen activator inhibitor-1 (PAI-1), which slows down the breakup of these blood clots. In addition, a high insulin level increases the activity of inflammatory compounds such as C-reactive protein that raise the risk of cardiovascular disease.

Is It Diabetes or Is It Syndrome X?

As discussed in the last chapter, the American Diabetes Association's sole diagnostic criterion for diabetes is an elevated blood glucose level on a fasting glucose test. You fast for at least eight hours, have your blood drawn and tested by a lab, and if your blood glucose is 126 mg/dl or higher on two separate readings, you are considered to have diabetes. This threshold was established in 1997, based upon recommendations from the Expert Committee on the Diagnosis and Classification of Diabetes Mellitus, and it has been embraced by the Centers for Disease Control and Prevention and the National Institutes of Health.

Another, less commonly used test for diabetes screening is the oral glucose tolerance test. As I explained in chapter 1, the diagnostic value of this test remains controversial, and I do not routinely utilize it to diagnose diabetes. However, in order to give you "both sides of the story," I must tell you that many experts, including policy makers for the World Health Organization (WHO), recommend that both the fasting glucose test and the two-hour glucose tolerance test be used as screening tools. The rationale for this recommendation is that the fasting glucose test alone will miss many individuals who may not have frank diabetes but do have "pre-diabetes"—impaired glucose tolerance or insulin resistance.

Identifying and treating patients who are well on their way to developing diabetes is important, because insulin resistance begins taking its toll on your body—especially your cardiovascular system—long before it becomes clinically evident. Many experts estimate that the destructive mechanisms associated with insulin resistance are at work for up to fifteen years prior to diagnosis, and the risk of heart disease and other complications is growing all the while.

The Diabetes Epidemiology: Collaborative Analysis of Diagnostic Criteria in Europe (DECODE) is a comprehensive trial that involved more than 25,000 patients followed for an average of 7.3 years. DECODE findings suggest that by the time a patient is diagnosed with type 2 diabetes per the current American Diabetes Association criteria, damage to the cardiovascular system is well under way. Commenting on this in the *Lancet* in 1999, DECODE researchers stated, "Fasting-glucose concentrations alone do not identify individuals at increased risk of death associated with hyperglycaemia. The oral glucose tolerance test provides additional prognostic information and enables detection of individuals with impaired glucose tolerance, who have the greatest attributable risk of death."[5]

This research makes a strong argument for the glucose tolerance test, and indeed, the test, if properly administered, may identify at-risk individuals. If such individuals take this information for what it is worth and begin a lifestyle program like that outlined in part III to improve their insulin sensitivity, then the test could be very valuable. However, I worry about widespread screening resulting in legions of what I call the "worried well." These are patients who are essentially healthy but have been scared by some doctor or test into thinking there's something seriously wrong with them. They become susceptible to needless invasive surgical procedures (in the case of heart disease) or unnecessary drug regimens (in the case of diabetes) that, in my opinion, will only make the situation worse.

Finally, I believe in preventive medicine. Every patient who walks through the doors at the Whitaker Wellness Institute is instructed in a diet, exercise, and nutritional supplement regimen similar to the program for reversing diabetes we will be talking about in part III. Whether or not I know a patient has impaired glucose tolerance, insulin resistance, or "pre-diabetes" doesn't really matter. I will still urge him or her to adopt a healthy lifestyle, which will obviously include measures known to improve insulin resistance, such as weight loss, a low-fat, high-fiber diet, and regular exercise. Unless a diagnosis is the only thing that will motivate the patient to get serious and take action, I rarely run the test.

Should you decide to have a glucose tolerance test, make sure you avoid excess dietary fat and protein for a few days prior to the test. As I showed you in the previous chapter, these dietary factors can skew test results. If your oral glucose tolerance test result is greater than or equal to 200 mg/dl, you meet the diagnostic criteria for diabetes. If it is greater than or equal to 140 mg/dl, you may have insulin resistance. In either case, you should immediately begin the natural therapies discussed in part III.

Do You Have Insulin Resistance?

Dr. Reaven recommends several laboratory tests as indicators of the potential presence of insulin resistance.

- Fasting glucose greater than or equal to 110 mg/dl
- Glucose tolerance test greater than or equal to 140 mg/dl
- Fasting HDL cholesterol less than 35
- Fasting triglycerides greater than 200
- Blood pressure higher than 145/90
- Weight more than 15 pounds over your ideal weight

Genetic Underpinnings of Insulin Resistance

In the past twenty years, the Pima Indians, the majority of whom currently live on a reservation near Phoenix, Arizona, have provided a fertile testing ground for the study of diabetes and insulin resistance. Sixty percent of all Pima Indians over the age of thirty have diabetes. Their average life span is only forty-seven years (their Caucasian neighbors down the street in Phoenix can expect to live about seventy-six years), and the most common causes of death among these people are diabetic kidney disease and heart disease.

It wasn't always this way. According to Jeffrey S. Bland, Ph.D., director of the Institute for Functional Medicine, a physician visiting Indian reservations in the Southwest at the turn of the twentieth century reported only one case of diabetes among the Pimas surveyed. Pioneering physician Dr. Elliott Joslin went to the same area in 1937 and reported twenty-one cases, which was similar to the overall incidence of type 2 diabetes in the U.S. at that time. But by 1954 that number had increased to 283, and by 1965 it had reached an astounding 500![6]

As you might suspect, the Pimas have a genetic susceptibility to insulin resistance and diabetes. This does not mean that these people are somehow weak or flawed. On the contrary. Their genetic inheritance served them well in their traditional lifestyle as warriors traversing long distances aross an inhospitable terrain in the southwestern United States. They were able to survive periods of famine, during which they were forced to go for prolonged periods without food. Indeed, the Pimas thrived under conditions where others perished.

But could this genetic inheritance also explain their current epidemic of diabetes and insulin resistance? According to James V. Neel, of the University of Michigan Medical School, it can and does. As he explains, the Pimas and others with such a genetic susceptibility possess what have been labeled "thrifty genes": They have an exaggerated insulin response to a glucose-rich diet and a tendency to hang on to calories and store them as fat.[7] While this genotype keeps them alive in times of famine, it works to their disadvantage when they are plunked down in the calorie-dense, high-fat environment of modern American culture. This is a dramatic illustration of the interplay between genes and environment. Genetic tendencies are real and they are influential, but so are environmental factors, such as diet and activity level. And until we learn how to turn off certain genetic "switches" (an up-and-coming possibility), the only thing we are able to modify is our own behavior.

Lifestyle Contributors to Diabetes and Insulin Resistance

There are several factors regarding your risk of diabetes and insulin resistance that you just cannot change. For one, you can't trade in your parents. As our discussion of the Pima Indians illustrates, some groups are, based on their genome, more likely to develop these conditions. These include Native Americans, African

Americans, Hispanics, Asians, and Pacific Islanders. Likewise, if you have a family history of diabetes, you yourself are at increased risk.

You also can't turn back the clock. The risk of developing diabetes increases after age forty-five (although, as the discussion above suggests, by the time you're diagnosed with diabetes, you've likely had insulin resistance for many years). Nor can you change how much you weighed at birth: Women who weighed less than five pounds are almost twice as likely to develop type 2 diabetes as women with a birth weight between 7.1 and 8.5 pounds.[8] Other factors beyond your control include your mother's nutritional status during pregnancy and how your own pregnancies fared—your risk increases if you've had gestational diabetes or a baby who weighed more than nine pounds.

But look at this much longer list of modifiable risk factors, all of which are within your control:

Obesity

Since the mid-1980s, the number of Americans who are overweight has more than doubled to 54 percent. Ninety percent of all type 2 diabetics are overweight. Excess fat stored in the cells means excess free fatty acids circulating in the blood. This causes the liver to churn out excessive amounts of glucose, the beta cells to fail to secrete insulin in an appropriate manner, and the cells to be less sensitive to insulin. This is the essence of insulin resistance. There is a circular relationship between excess weight and insulin resistance: Being overweight dramatically increases the risk of insulin resistance, and insulin resistance may cause the body to store more fat and gain weight. While we can debate which comes first, there is a clear consensus that weight loss definitely improves insulin resistance. In fact, adequate weight loss may be curative in a majority of all cases.

Distribution of excess weight is also predictive of insulin resistance. If you carry those extra pounds in a spare tire around your middle, you have what is called abdominal or "apple-shaped" obesity. This puts you at increased risk of insulin resistance, diabetes, and other manifestations of Syndrome X. Fat in this area, as opposed to, say, around the hips, is more metabolically active. It is more easily broken down into free fatty acids that enter the bloodstream, interfere with

Height \ Weight	100	105	110	115	120	125	130	135	140	145	150	155	160	165	170	175	180	185	190	195	200	205
5'0"	20	21	21	22	23	24	25	26	27	28	29	30	31	32	33	34	35	36	37	38	39	40
5'1"	19	20	21	22	23	24	25	26	26	27	28	29	30	31	32	33	34	35	36	37	38	39
5'2"	18	19	20	21	22	23	24	25	26	27	27	28	29	30	31	32	33	34	35	36	37	37
5'3"	18	19	19	20	21	22	23	24	25	26	27	27	28	29	30	31	32	33	34	35	35	36
5'4"	17	18	19	20	21	21	22	23	24	25	26	27	27	28	29	30	31	32	33	33	34	35
5'5"	17	17	18	19	20	21	22	22	23	24	25	26	27	27	28	29	30	31	32	32	33	34
5'6"	16	17	18	19	19	20	21	22	23	23	24	25	26	27	27	28	29	30	31	31	32	33
5'7"	16	16	17	18	19	20	20	21	22	23	23	24	25	26	27	27	28	29	30	31	31	32
5'8"	15	16	17	17	18	19	20	21	21	22	23	24	24	25	26	27	27	28	29	30	30	31
5'9"	15	16	16	17	18	18	19	20	21	21	22	23	24	24	25	26	27	27	28	29	30	30
5'10"	14	15	16	17	17	18	19	19	20	21	22	22	23	24	24	25	26	27	27	28	29	29
5'11"	14	15	15	16	17	17	18	19	20	20	21	22	22	23	24	24	25	26	26	27	28	29
6'0"	14	15	15	16	17	17	18	19	20	20	21	22	22	23	24	24	25	26	26	27	28	29
6'1"	13	14	15	15	16	16	17	18	19	20	20	21	22	22	23	24	24	25	26	26	27	
6'2"	13	13	14	15	15	16	17	17	18	19	19	20	21	21	22	22	23	24	24	25	26	26
6'3"	12	13	14	14	15	16	16	17	18	19	19	20	21	21	22	22	23	24	24	25	26	
6'4"	12	13	13	14	15	15	16	16	17	18	18	19	19	20	21	21	22	23	23	24	24	25

Figure 3. Body Mass Index (BMI). A BMI in the range of 19–25 is healthy; 26 or higher puts you at increased risk of disease.
From Wickelgren, I. "Obesity: How Big a Problem?" *Science* 280(5368): 1364–67, May 29, 1998. Copyright © 1998. American Association for the Advancement of Science. Source: Shape Up America. Used by permission.

the action of insulin, and raise triglyceride and glucose levels.

The most reliable way to determine just how much at risk your weight (and shape) put you is to have your body composition analyzed by a professional. A simple, and pretty accurate, alternative is to use the chart on the next page to figure out your body mass index (BMI). This gives an estimation of your ratio of lean muscle mass to body fat. The healthy range is 19 to 25. A BMI of 26 or higher places you at increased risk.

Another risk factor determinant is hip/waist ratio. Measure the circumference of your waist at its narrowest, just above the hipbones, and your hips at their widest, then divide the measurement of your waist by that of your hips. If your hips are 37 inches and your waist is 28 inches, you have a healthy hip/waist ratio of 0.75. If, however, your hips are 36 inches and your waist is 37 inches, your ratio is a much less desirable 1.03. If you are a woman, a healthy hip/waist ratio is less than 0.8; if you are a man, aim for less than 0.95. The diet and exercise recommendations in part III will help you achieve your optimal weight.

Inactivity

You must get moving if you want to stay healthy. Inactivity and insulin resistance go hand in hand. Studies dating back to the 1970s clearly show that people who exercise regularly have lower fasting glucose levels. As I will explain in detail in chapter 8, exercise enables glucose to enter the cells, particularly those of the muscles, even when insulin is not present. It does so, just as insulin does, by signaling the GLUT-4 transporters inside the cell to rise to the surface and usher in glucose. It also increases the number of these transporters, so that muscle cells are more sensitive to insulin even at rest.

Everyone knows exercise is a healthy habit. Unfortunately, few people make the effort required to exercise regularly. This is an obvious cause of our current epidemic of diabetes, insulin resistance, and the conditions that comprise Syndrome X. Although more intense physical activity is most significantly related to higher insulin sensitivity, even less vigorous activity such as regular walking results in improvements in the action of insulin and reduced risk of insulin resistance.[9] A 1999 study of more than 70,000 female nurses, ages forty to sixty-five, demonstrated that women who engaged in brisk walking had a lower risk of type 2 diabetes than their inactive counterparts.[10]

Poor Diet and Nutritional Deficiencies

What we eat in this country bears little resemblance to what our species has eaten for most of our history. *Homo sapiens sapiens* appeared about 40,000 years ago, and our genetic makeup has changed little since then. Up until about 10,000 years ago, our ancestors were hunter-gatherers. With the emergence of agriculture, grains and dairy were added, but as you can see, these foods were a relatively late addition to the traditional diet of the species. In a compelling article in the *New England Journal of Medicine* entitled "Paleolithic Nutrition," S. Boyd Eaton, M.D., and Melvin Konner, Ph.D., write that the diet that natural selection prepared our species for was low in fat and high in fiber- and nutrient-rich native plant foods and lean protein from wild animals.

Our ancestors ate about the same amount of carbohydrates that we eat today, but these carbohydrates differed dramatically from modern favorites. There was no bread or cereal or sugar, only fresh fruits, nuts, seeds, roots, tubers, and beans. Compared to today's average fiber intake of 10 to 15 grams per day, our ancestors ate more than 45 grams. Their diet was much lower in fat: Wild game contains less than 4 percent fat compared to 30 percent fat in today's livestock. And the type of fat was different—less saturated fat, more essential fatty acids, and no harmful trans fatty acids. Our ancestors got twice as much calcium and almost five times as much vitamin C as we get, and their sodium intake was a scant 10 percent of what most Americans consume today. Chromium, magnesium, folic acid, and other B-complex vitamins—all the vitamins and minerals that are deficient in processed foods—were consumed in abundance.

According to Drs. Eaton and Konner, the disparity between our modern diet and that of our ancestors may be at the root of the most significant health challenges of the twenty-first century. The authors state:

> *Differences between the dietary patterns of our remote ancestors and the patterns now prevalent in industrialized countries appear to have important implications for health, and the specific pattern of nutritional disease is a function of the*

*stage of civilization. Physicians and nutritionists
are increasingly convinced that the dietary habits
adopted by Western society over the past 100 years
make an important etiologic contribution to coronary heart disease, hypertension, diabetes, and
some types of cancer. These conditions have emerged
as dominant health problems only in the past century and are virtually unknown among the few
surviving hunter-gatherer populations whose way
of life and eating habits most closely resemble those
of preagricultural human beings.[11]*

In chapters 6 and 7 we will continue our discussion
of the effects of diet on health and particularly on the
diabetic condition. As you will see, dietary changes are
a powerful and important tool in the treatment of insulin resistance and diabetes.

CHAPTER 3

What to Expect of This Book

Now that the intricacies of the human genome have been unraveled, there are high hopes that we are on the verge of a brave new world of medicine. Without a doubt, an understanding of the genetic influences on disease will have a dramatic impact on some aspects of medicine. On the other hand, although genetic tinkering may be able to eradicate certain diseases, no discovery or breakthrough will ever replace the need for proper care and maintenance of the human body.

Like any machine with working parts, wear and tear is inevitable. Even the most expensive, finely engineered Ferrari will wear out and break down over time. But regardless of how much (or how little) expense and precision went into a car's initial engineering, if you take care of it, keep it oiled and lubed, use the right kind of fuel, and drive it with care, it will last longer and perform better than it would if it did not receive proper maintenance.

Your body is no different, and that's what this book is all about. It is a how-to book that outlines the diabetes treatment program I have developed and refined over the past twenty-five years. As you will see, it is a low-tech approach. Don't expect to read about cutting-edge drugs or pancreatic cell transplants that are "just around the corner." You are looking for solutions today!

Important Note: Work with Your Doctor

Although this is primarily a lifestyle program, involving things you do on your own every day, it is important that you let your physician know what you're doing, particularly if you are taking any medications for diabetes. *You must be under the care of a physician because your medication requirements are likely to change rapidly.* You may see dramatic changes in blood glucose levels within days of starting this program, and the prognosis for long-term diabetes control is equally dramatic. However, this could create problems if you are already taking insulin or oral drugs to lower blood glucose. That's why it's important to keep your doctor in the loop.

The Program in a Nutshell

Here is an overview of my program for reversing diabetes. We will discuss each aspect in detail in parts II, III, and IV.

Diet changes. The diet recommendations in this book are based on the most recent research on how your body digests and metabolizes food. Although many would label it a high-carbohydrate diet, that is a very superficial description. In the fifteen years since I wrote the first edition of this book, tremendous strides have been made in nutrition research. Even the nomenclature has changed.

No longer are "complex" carbohydrates such as grains and breads always the good guys, while "simple" carbohydrates—sugar, fruit, and the like—are always suspect. The newest research shows us that the body handles various carbohydrates within these broad classifications in different ways, depending on a food's chemical structure, fiber content, and other factors. We now know it is not appropriate to give the blessing of health to all carbohydrates.

Similarly, although this may be described as a low-fat diet, the emphasis again is on quality rather than quantity. Fats are not intrinsically bad. There are unhealthy fats (and unfortunately, these are among our favorites), but there are also fats that are essential for good health. These healthy fats are an important part of this diet. The same is true of protein. As you know, Americans have a diet that is overloaded with animal protein. Though by no means a vegetarian diet, my approach emphasizes quality of protein over quantity and contains adequate—but not excessive—amounts of healthy protein.

Exercise. Exercise enhances the body's sensitivity to insulin and significantly lowers insulin requirements. Exercise is work and requires effort, but people with diabetes should understand that the rewards are great. An exercise program should be prescribed for all diabetic patients in the same way that medication or diet is prescribed.

Nutritional supplementation. I believe that everyone should take a high-potency daily vitamin and mineral supplement. Think of it as insurance against the inadequacies of your diet and the stresses of twenty-first-century life. Although your physician may discount their value, the medical literature clearly details how and why certain vitamins, minerals, essential fatty acids, and herbs improve the diabetic condition and protect patients from the devastating consequences of elevated blood sugar and insulin. If you have diabetes, supplementation is more than important—it's vital.

The downside of drugs. Another component of this program—and one you will not likely learn about from your conventional physician—is the avoidance of drugs whenever possible. Serious long-term dangers have been associated with the aggressive use of oral diabetes drugs. Harmful side effects have also been linked to the drugs often used to treat elevated blood pressure and heart disease, which so often are part of the diabetic picture. Obviously, the more that can be accomplished with the program outlined in this book to minimize the need for medication, the better.

Everything Old Is New Again

Do not be put off by the simplicity of the program—this is powerful medicine. By following these simple steps, a majority of the thousands of patients with type 2 diabetes who have been treated at the Whitaker Wellness Institute have succeeded in managing their blood glucose without resorting to drugs. And although insulin may be a lifelong requirement for the type 1 diabetic, adherence to this program can result in better blood glucose control and a reduction in complications.

This program is backed by much more than my own clinical experience. Thousands upon thousands of scientific studies have proven the effectiveness of diet, exercise, and nutritional supplementation in the treatment of diabetes. And although advances continue to be made in the field, much of the basic research was done years ago.

James W. Anderson, M.D., professor of medicine at the University of Kentucky, has published scores of studies on the treatment of diabetes with diet, some dating back decades. He has repeatedly demonstrated that a high-fiber, low-fat diet similar to the diet regimen recommended in this book can reduce blood sugar levels and eliminate the need for insulin or oral drugs in close to 70 percent of type 2 diabetics. Yet this advice continues to be ignored, as many physicians seem to find it easier to prescribe drugs rather than take the time to truly educate their patients on the power of diet.

John Davidson, M.D., Ph.D., emeritus professor of medicine at Emory University, has been advocating a low-fat diet and weight loss as primary treatment for diabetes for most of his illustrious career. He is also a vocal critic of oral diabetic drugs and, as director of the Diabetes Unit at Grady Memorial Hospital in Atlanta from 1971 to 1991, stopped the use of these medications. Dr. Davidson's popular medical textbook, *Clinical Diabetes Mellitus, A Problem-Oriented Approach*,[1] now in its third printing, emphasizes the appropriate use of low-fat nutrition and weight loss as powerful tools for eliminating the need for medication in diabetics.

Dr. Eliott Joslin, founder of the Joslin Diabetes Center in Boston, began preaching the importance of exercise for diabetic patients in the 1920s. Yet despite his remarkable results, exercise was disregarded for decades, and few efforts were made to determine its role in the treatment of diabetes. In recent years attention has turned to the benefits of exercise in improving insulin sensitivity. However, it continues to be viewed as a lowly adjunct, rather than the powerful therapy that it is, particularly for the middle-aged, overweight type 2 diabetic patients who could benefit the most from a prescribed exercise regimen. Rarely does a diabetic patient enter the Whitaker Wellness Institute with a previously prescribed exercise program. Indeed, few of our incoming patients are aware that exercise is necessary for optimum blood glucose control.

Research dating back decades suggests that diabetics could benefit from nutritional supplementation, not only for improved blood glucose control, but also for the prevention of diabetic complications. Numerous studies have shown that diabetics are prone to having low cellular levels of several essential water-soluble nutrients. These include magnesium, deficiencies of which are associated with diabetic retinopathy, and vitamin C, a potent antioxidant that protects against free-radical damage. Research also underscores the importance of the B-complex vitamins. Vitamin B_6 protects against diabetic nerve damage, and nicotinamide or niacinamide, a form of vitamin B_3, has in some cases restored beta-cell function in newly diagnosed type 1 diabetics. Groundbreaking biochemist Roger Williams, Ph.D., who discovered pantothenic acid (vitamin B_5), has argued since the 1930s that even healthy people should take vitamin and mineral supplements as "insurance" against potential deficiencies. Yet most physicians neglect to instruct their diabetic patients, who lose untold amounts of water-soluble nutrients, to take this simplest of steps.

If this research on diet, exercise, and nutritional supplementation has been around for so long, why has it been ignored? This question is asked by almost every patient who uses the principles in this book to reduce their reliance on medication and improve blood glucose control. Why aren't all physicians enthusiastically educating and motivating their patients to make the lifestyle changes necessary to eliminate or reduce the need for medications?

Why Are These Simple, Effective Therapies Ignored?

This is a difficult question to answer, but there seem to be three prevailing trends in modern medicine that work together to discourage the use of diet, exercise, and nutritional supplementation as *primary* tools for the treatment of diabetes.

First, physicians are trained to prescribe. Doctors learn in medical school that prescription drugs are the most powerful tools we have for treating disease. Since dietary changes, exercise, and targeted nutritional supplements are almost never presented as therapeutic tools (only one-quarter of this country's medical schools require any nutrition education at all), drugs are usually viewed as the only significant therapeutic options available. If rigorous diet and exercise and the use of specific nutrients fail to solve the problem, then medications may indeed be helpful. However, the accepted way of doing things today is to prescribe first and recommend diet and exercise as an afterthought— and nutritional supplements are rarely mentioned at all.

Second, we are infatuated with new technology. In addition to the research mentioned earlier on the genetic origins of diabetes and how to manipulate genes to prevent or treat diabetes, other high-tech discoveries are generating excitement in the field. Insulin pumps continue to be improved. Scientists are working to develop an "artificial pancreas" to be implanted inside the body that would determine insulin needs and release it automatically. Pancreatic tissue transplants are being refined, as are more efficient systems for monitoring blood glucose. The FDA recently approved a device that utilizes a laser, rather than a lancet, to painlessly prick the skin. And of course, millions of research dollars are being spent for the development of new drugs, such as insulin inhalers and pills that could replace the need for frequent injections.

The mere fact that a drug, gizmo, or procedure is new and high-tech gives it enormous appeal. What many physicians and patients fail to recognize, however, is that many of these new therapies have never been shown to be better than the older, more conservative, tried-and-true methods of treatment. Controlled clinical trials to prove the superiority of some of the newer therapies used today are pending or not even on the drawing board! Yet the technology is used as if it had already been proven.

Third, there is widespread conformity of physician thought and practice. More than perhaps any other profession, medicine breeds, even demands, conformity among its practitioners. The concept of "accepted practices" carries considerable weight in the medical profession, and most doctors are predictably uniform in their treatment approaches. Conforming to today's norms guarantees a degree of safety. Regardless of the outcome of a therapy, good or bad, physicians are above censure if they have complied with the currently accepted approaches. They can take comfort knowing that they did "what was considered best." It is not hard to see how something as simple as looking to nutrition and exercise as first-line therapy for the treatment of diabetes could be discouraged, even reviled. Given the present enthusiasm for drugs and technology that is engendered by medical training and perpetuated by the forces of professional conformity, it should be expected.

My Approach

How did I come to appreciate the power of diet, exercise, and nutritional supplements as a treatment tool for diabetes? It was a fairly tortuous path, and I would like to share it with you.

All of my early medical training was geared toward a surgical specialty. I graduated from Emory University Medical School in 1970, underwent a medical/surgical internship at the Emory University Hospitals in Atlanta, and then entered a surgical residency program in San Francisco at the University of California. Two and a half years into this program, I took some time off to reevaluate my long-term goals. I wanted a year or two to think about the direction in which I was heading. I fully intended at that time to continue in my surgical training.

Until then, I had absolutely no interest in nutrition. In medical school we only had about two credit hours of nutrition, consisting of a few lectures on the properties of proteins, fats, and carbohydrates. I was convinced that the afflictions of man were either acts of God, bad luck, or both, and could be handled with appropriate drugs or surgery.

I signed on as an emergency room physician in Southern California. One day a thirty-four-year-old woman who had sprained her ankle came in for an evaluation. Except for the minor injury to her ankle, she glowed with good health. Suddenly, it dawned on me: Healthy people don't see doctors.

Like most physicians, the major portion of my training was directed toward the treatment of patients in crisis. I was curious about this healthy patient and asked her about her habits. She explained her program of diet, exercise, and vitamin and mineral supplementation. This woman believed that the way she lived determined her physical well-being. I had been studying medicine for six and a half years, but this patient was the first practitioner of *preventive* medicine I had encountered.

I read materials that she gave me and subsequently went to work with Dr. Wilbur Currier in Pasadena, California. Dr. Currier was a former ear, nose, and throat surgeon who had abandoned surgery to specialize in preventive medicine. Low-fat nutrition was his primary tool. While working with Dr. Currier, I read some monographs of a then little-known inventor, Nathan Pritikin. Mr. Pritikin, as many of you know, was a passionate crusader for the benefits of a low-fat diet and exercise.

I'll never forget my surprise when I read sections of a monograph he had written dealing with diabetes. It contained research published in the 1920s and 1930s that clearly demonstrated how excessive fat in the diet could bring on diabetes. This astounded me, for in medical school it was never taught that the *type* of food someone ate had anything to do with the onset of diabetes.

To learn more about nutrition in treating diabetes and other degenerative diseases, I worked on the medical staff of the Longevity Center directed by Mr. Pritikin from 1975 to 1976. I was amazed at the restorative power of lifestyle changes!

I left the Longevity Center to return to my own practice, and in 1979 opened the Whitaker Wellness Institute, offering patients with diabetes, heart disease, and high blood pressure a two-week residential program that taught them how to improve their health by changing their lifestyle. Over the years this has evolved into a one-week program, and the Institute now has six physicians. More than 30,000 patients have come through the Institute, and I have observed firsthand the therapeutic power of this approach. I have also learned what works, what doesn't work, and what changes patients are really willing to make. It is my experience with these patients that has provided the meat of this book: a livable, easily implemented program that can dramatically improve the diabetic condition.

What You Can Gain from This Program

This is a program designed to make your body more *sensitive* to insulin, whether it is injected or produced in your pancreas. Most type 2 diabetic patients can reasonably expect to be able to maintain near-normal blood sugar levels while lowering their doses of insulin or oral diabetic medications—and many will be able to stop these drugs altogether. Of course, a type 1 diabetic of long-standing duration should not expect to become insulin free, but lifestyle measures can certainly help keep blood sugar measurements in the normal range, most likely with lower insulin requirements.

In the past, the question of keeping glucose levels in the near-normal range was a controversial one. Some studies suggested that tight control protected patients from diabetic complications, while others hinted at the opposite. And anyway, since maintaining near-normal blood glucose levels requires considerable attention on the part of the patient—frequent monitoring and personalized adjustments in drugs—it was viewed by physicians as a lost cause.

A ten-year study conducted by the National

Institutes of Health and published in the *New England Journal of Medicine* in 1993 pretty much put this controversy to rest. The Diabetes Control and Complications Trial (DCCT) reached this conclusion: "Intensive therapy of patients with IDDM [insulin-dependent diabetes mellitus] delays the onset and slows the progression of clinically important retinopathy, including vision-threatening lesions, nephropathy [kidney complications], and neuropathy, by a range of 35 to more than 70 percent."[2]

Though this was a highly significant study, it involved only patients with type 1 diabetes. To determine if tight control would benefit patients with type 2 diabetes as well, the United Kingdom Prospective Diabetes Study was initiated in 1977. More than 3,800 patients with newly diagnosed type 2 diabetes were enrolled at twenty-three medical centers in the UK and followed over an eleven-year period. The results of this study, which were published in 1998, demonstrated that keeping blood sugars in the normal range benefited type 2 diabetics as well. Tight glucose control cut the risk of serious eye disease by one-quarter and kidney disease by one-third—although there was no significant difference in rates of heart disease.[3] However, when treatment for hypertension was added (as you recall from the previous chapter, many patients with insulin resistance and Syndrome X also suffer from hypertension), risk of heart attack and stroke also declined dramatically.[4]

Other studies have confirmed these findings and clarified the importance of keeping blood glucose levels within the normal range. A 1999 Danish study found that intensive therapy, including counseling on diet and exercise, lowered rates of kidney, eye, and nerve disease by 73 percent, 55 percent, and 68 percent respectively.[5] And researchers at several Veterans Affairs medical centers found improvements in markers of heart disease, such as normalization of blood lipids, with tight control.[6] Although most of these studies relied on the use of insulin and oral drugs to maintain close control of blood sugar levels, I know from my experience with thousands of patients that good control can also be accomplished through vigorous adherence to the lifestyle measures that are the essence of this program.

Diabetes aside, by following this program you should also see improvements in other aspects of your health. Although this is not a weight-loss regimen per se, the majority of patients who make these lifestyle changes do lose weight. This alone, as you know, will have a significant impact on many aspects of overall health. Furthermore, because of the ameliorating effects this approach has on your cells' response to insulin, you should also see improvements in other conditions related to insulin resistance. You may see substantial improvements in your blood cholesterol levels, including lower levels of artery-clogging LDL cholesterol and higher levels of protective HDL cholesterol. Your triglycerides also will likely plummet. In addition, you may see a lowering of blood pressure. More energy, increased vitality, improved memory and mental focus—these are some of the many side benefits you may experience after implementing the recommendations in this book.

Tracking Your Progress

If you have diabetes, you should be working with your doctor, as well as measuring and recording your blood glucose levels regularly on your own. If you are using insulin, it is imperative that you take readings several times a day, using one of the many home glucose monitors currently available. However, a blood glucose test has its limits. It provides a snapshot of your glucose level at any given moment, but it doesn't reflect the big picture. The most reliable indicator of longer-term glucose control is glycosylated hemoglobin (HbA1c).

Glycosylated hemoglobin (also called glycohemoglobin or glycated hemoglobin) is a measure of the degree to which glucose binds to hemoglobin in the blood. This provides an overview of blood sugar control over a period of about 120 days. Although there are variations among labs, a rule of thumb for interpreting HbA1c is as follows:

HbA1c (%)	Average blood glucose (mg/dl)
4	60
5	90
6	120
7	150
8	180
9	210
10	240
11	270
12	300
13	330

From the Diabetes Control and Complications Trial (DCCT)[7]

The target for HbA1c in diabetics is less than 7 percent. (The average in nondiabetics is less than 6 percent.) HbA1c is highly predictive of the development of diabetic complications of the blood vessels and nerves. It is estimated that for every 1 percent reduction in HbA1c, the risk of long-term diabetic complications falls by as much as 25 percent. If you have diabetes, I suggest you undergo this test twice a year.

Your Responsibility

The success of this program requires a shift in attitude. *You* own your health. It is your responsibility, not your doctor's. Patients as well as physicians are so enamored of the technological innovations of modern medicine that they often assume that whatever the problem, some new procedure or magic bullet can bail them out. While that may be true for traumatic injuries and infectious illnesses, this approach doesn't fare so well in the treatment of the major killers of this century, degenerative diseases such as heart disease, cancer, hypertension, and diabetes.

We must face up to the fact that most of the diseases and disabilities we suffer today are related more to what we do each day—the food we eat, the amount of exercise we get, and the way we handle the stress in our lives—than to almost any other factor. Take control of your health. Make a commitment to take whatever measures are necessary to get a handle on your diabetes. I will do my part in the remainder of this book by providing a road map to make the necessary lifestyle changes as easy for you as I possibly can. However, only you can take that first step on the path to optimal health.

Before we get into the nuts and bolts of the diet, exercise, and nutritional supplement program for reversing diabetes, I first want to take a hard look at the popular drug therapies used in the treatment of diabetes. While drugs are sometimes necessary (as is insulin for type 1 diabetics), they are often prescribed before safe, effective lifestyle changes have been given a proper trial. I believe that once you understand the limitations of drug therapy for the treatment of diabetes, you will be more motivated than ever to get started on the program for reversing diabetes outlined in parts III and IV.

One final note: This program is intended to be used *while under the care of your doctor.* **Please use it that way.**

PART II

Problems of Drug Therapy

CHAPTER 4

The Ins and Outs of Insulin

On December 2, 1921, twelve-year-old Leonard Thompson was admitted to the Toronto General Hospital. He had had type 1 diabetes for two and a half years, and in spite of adhering to a starvation diet, which was the only treatment available at the time, he was in the terminal stages of the disease. Knowing how bleak his situation was, Leonard and his father agreed to try an experimental new therapy developed by Frederick Banting and Charles Best. These two young Canadian physicians had been conducting experiments with diabetic dogs, utilizing pancreatic extracts to bring down blood sugar levels, with some success. Although they had not yet had a chance to conduct clinical trials, they felt they were ready to try the therapy on their first human subject.

They made a batch of extract from beef pancreas, tested it on one of their experimental dogs, and even gave each other injections. On January 11, 1922, they administered their discovery to the boy. Not much happened. They and some of their colleagues worked furiously over the next two weeks on various preparations of pancreatic extracts and came up with a more potent version. After Leonard received an injection of this newer extract, his blood sugar level fell from 520 mg/dl to 120 mg/dl, and his overall condition began to improve dramatically. He left the hospital and lived another fifteen years, dying at age twenty-seven of pneumonia.[1]

In a book about diabetes, it would be remiss not to pay homage to insulin and what it has meant to hundreds of millions of diabetics worldwide. Before the discovery of insulin, type 1 diabetes was a death sentence: Patients were destined to waste away. Insulin has made it possible for them to live long and healthy lives. The discovery of insulin, its isolation, administration, and ultimate synthesis are among the most significant achievements in medical history.

That said, it is important to remember that insulin is essential for, at most, 10 percent of all diabetics. The vast majority of the remaining 90-plus percent, those with type 2 diabetes caused by insulin resistance rather than insulin deficiency, can and should be treated with the principles outlined in this book: diet, exercise, weight control, and targeted nutritional supplements. Insulin should be the treatment of last resort for these patients.

However, insulin therapy is often started in patients with type 2 diabetes long before safer lifestyle options are exhausted. Over the past twenty-five years I have seen hundreds of patients walk into the Whitaker

Wellness Institute with a bag full of syringes and vials of insulin and walk out with a diet and lifestyle plan. Insulin simply wasn't necessary.

Like most medical therapeutics, insulin is a double-edged sword. For those who need it, it is a godsend. Yet inappropriate use can cause more problems than benefits.

Types of Insulin

Insulin is derived from a number of sources. Some preparations are made from bovine (cow) or porcine (pig) pancreas and then enzymatically modified to be exactly like human insulin. Others, called recombinant human insulin, are clones of human insulin made through recombinant DNA technology utilizing *E. coli* bacteria. A newer form of insulin, biosynthetic insulin, is an analog of human insulin, meaning that its biochemical structure has been modified.

Insulin cannot be taken orally, as it is destroyed in the gastrointestinal tract. It is administered primarily through injections with a very small needle into the layer of fat under the skin. There have been a number of advances in types of syringes over the years, and the insulin pump, which continuously injects insulin under the skin, has become increasingly popular. Clinical trials are in progress on insulin preparations that can be inhaled in aerosol form, but they are not yet available. So although refinements have been made, the general insulin delivery system remains the same as it was in the days of Banting and Best.

Rapid-, Intermediate-, and Long-Acting Preparations

Insulin is further classified by how quickly it acts. Some types go to work rapidly but are short-lived, others have a slower onset but a longer duration of activity, while still others fall somewhere in between. *Regular insulin* (Humulin R or Novolin R) is considered to be a rapid-acting insulin. Once injected, it begins to lower the blood sugar in about 30 minutes. It reaches its peak action in about two hours and will have an effect for five to six hours. It is generally injected 30 to 60 minutes before meals. A newer type of biosynthetic insulin called *insulin lispro* (Humalog) is even more rapid-acting. Taken 15 minutes before meals, insulin lispro peaks in 30 to 90 minutes. It is eliminated more quickly as well.

To slow its rate of absorption, insulin may be modified by combining it with other agents. The most commonly used preparations are *NPH* and *lente* (Humulin L and Novolin L), which are known as intermediate-acting insulin. These preparations start to work after two to three hours, have a peak action between eight and ten hours, and continue to work for about twenty-four hours. Intermediate-acting insulin is most often used to keep blood sugar in the normal range while fasting (such as during sleep), rather than to control the rises that accompany meals. The longest acting of the insulin preparations is *ultralente* (Humulin U). The effects of ultralente begin slowly over about four hours, peaking at ten to fifteen hours after injection and working for thirty-six hours.

Regular and NPH insulin are the most commonly used types of insulin. Mixtures of regular (rapid-acting) insulin and slower NPH insulin are also available. These include numbers like 70/30 or 50/50, with their names alluding to their proportions of NPH and regular. It is not uncommon for patients to use different combinations of insulin at different times of the day.

Dosage Schedules

Both the amount and the schedule of injections must be individually prescribed for each patient, and you must work with your doctor to determine what is best for you. It is important for you to be aware of the time the insulin you use reaches its peak activity, as this is the time you are most likely to have a hypoglycemic reaction. For instance, when lente or NPH is used in the morning around 8:00 A.M., its peak action occurs at 4:00 P.M., which is the most likely time for the blood sugar to fall below normal. If regular insulin is used at 8:00 A.M., its peak action occurs in mid-morning.

Many patients use combinations of NPH and regular in the morning. Some take a second dose in the late afternoon. Common protocols include a single injection of NPH and regular in the morning, or an injection of NPH and regular in the morning followed by another in the late afternoon, at around 4:30 or 5:00 before the evening meal. Generally the evening dose of insulin is much lower than the morning dose to avoid the possibility of hypoglycemic reactions in the early morning while sleeping. If hypoglycemia goes unnoticed, it can be very dangerous.

You should monitor your blood sugar levels at home regularly: when you first get up, right before lunch, and at four in the afternoon. These blood sugar levels should be recorded in a diary so that you and your physician can get an idea of the degree of control you are achieving. In addition, close monitoring will allow you to alter your insulin dosage according to recorded blood sugar levels. Your records may show fluctuations, with blood sugar levels that are too high or too low at certain times of the day. For instance, if your records show that for several days in a row you have had high blood sugar levels around noon, your doctor may suggest that you increase your regular insulin dose by about 2 units a day until your blood sugar is brought under better control. If your blood sugar level is consistently high in the afternoon around 4:00 P.M., you may be instructed to increase the NPH insulin in the morning by 1 or 2 units. Again, these adjustments vary for different patients and should be made under a physician's supervision.

Hypoglycemia

One of the most common problems of insulin therapy is hypoglycemia, particularly in type 1 diabetics. Hypoglycemia, or too-low blood sugar, most often results from taking too large a dose of insulin. People who take insulin are warned that hypoglycemia may occur and are advised to keep some type of rapidly absorbed carbohydrate, such as glucose tablets, fruit juice, or sugar, available at all times to raise blood sugar at the first signs of hypoglycemia.

Warning signs of hypoglycemia include a slowdown of reaction time, irritability, and confusion as the brain is deprived of its source of energy. Prolonged hypoglycemia is especially damaging to the brain, as starving brain cells eventually die. Severe hypoglycemia may result in loss of consciousness, convulsions, and even death. In a celebrated attempted-murder trial in Massachusetts, Claus von Bulow was accused of trying to kill his wife with insulin injections. Although he was acquitted, she never came out of her hypoglycemia-induced coma.

Hypoglycemia is clearly the most dangerous complication of insulin therapy. And it is also among the most common. In several studies documenting the frequency of this condition, it was found that more than 90 percent of diabetics on insulin reported having hypoglycemic episodes. Up to 60 percent reported having an attack at least once a month. Each year about a quarter of all insulin users will have a reaction severe enough to require assistance from another person or hospitalization. This complication of insulin therapy accounts for 3 to 7 percent of deaths in insulin-treated diabetics, and it surely has led to some degree of brain damage in a much higher percentage. Hypoglycemia is the rule, not the exception, in insulin-treated diabetics, and it represents a serious threat.[2]

For some reason, many physicians are less worried about the dangers of hypoglycemic episodes than about the consequences of elevated blood sugar levels. Often patients are "expected" to have hypoglycemic attacks as an indication of good control. I find this attitude hard to understand and certainly do not agree with it. As we shall see, hypoglycemia brought on by too much insulin is not only a clear and present danger for the diabetic but is also a major cause of poor control, as it later causes *elevations* in blood sugar levels (rebound hyperglycemia).

If you are taking insulin and are about to start the program outlined in this book, I suggest that you consult your physician regarding reducing your insulin dosage by about 25 to 30 percent. This is done routinely for all insulin-dependent patients who enter the Whitaker Wellness Institute. By making the patient more sensitive to insulin, this program lowers the insulin requirement. Therefore, it sets the stage for hypoglycemia unless the insulin dosage is reduced. If blood sugar levels rise, more insulin can be added back to the regimen. It is always safer to reestablish control of blood sugars that are moderately high than to try to raise levels that are too low.

Other Complications of Insulin Therapy

Insulin therapy also stimulates weight gain. With glucose being ushered into cells, more calories are utilized by the body rather than being lost in the urine. In addition, insulin promotes the storage of fat. This is particularly problematic in patients with type 2 diabetes who are already overweight—and the vast majority of folks with this form of diabetes do have weight problems. I have seen many patients placed prematurely on insulin gain excessive amounts of weight. As their weight goes up, so do their insulin requirements, until even with extremely high doses of insulin they remain unable to control their blood sugars. At the same time, their risk of cardiovascular disease and other diabetic complications soars.

Finally, some people may develop allergies to insulin. When insulin is injected into the body and exposed to the immune system, the body sometimes makes antibodies to this "foreign" protein, and the individual becomes allergic. This means that with each exposure, an allergic reaction may result. It may take the form of a rash or, very rarely, a severe anaphylactic reaction, in which the airways close up. Allergies to added agents may also develop. Zinc or an animal protein called protamine is added to some preparations to slow down the action of insulin. Protamine is problematic for some individuals, as it can cause the immune system to synthesize antibodies that may inactivate the insulin or cause it to be released at unexpected times.

The Somogyi Effect

Michael Somogyi, Ph.D., was a clear-thinking, sound researcher from the Jewish Hospital of St. Louis who made significant contributions in the field of diabetes from the mid-1930s to the early 1960s. He is best known for describing how large doses of insulin can be a major factor in poor diabetes control, a phenomenon that bears his name.

As we discussed at the beginning of this chapter, too much insulin causes hypoglycemia, or too-low blood sugar. Because this is a potentially life-threatening situation, the body responds by releasing insulin antagonists—cortisol and epinephrine (adrenaline) from the adrenal glands, growth hormone from the pituitary gland, and glucagon from the pancreas—to negate the effects of insulin.

Glucagon is the most powerful hormone for elevating blood glucose levels. It is made in the alpha cells of the pancreas, which are located in the islets of Langerhans, right next to the beta cells that produce insulin. Glucagon causes glycogen stored in the liver to be broken down into glucose and released into the bloodstream, raising blood sugar levels. Cortisol promotes glucose release and mobilizes fatty acids to be used as energy, while epinephrine not only elevates the blood sugar but also is responsible for the racing heart and the "cold, clammy" reaction of hypoglycemia.

These hormones are rapid and extremely powerful elevators of blood sugar and will often overshoot, causing the blood sugar level to go too high. These high levels must then be treated with *more* insulin, which may cause an even deeper plunge of the blood sugar, a higher compensatory response, and possibly even larger doses of insulin. This vicious cycle is known as the *Somogyi effect*.

To prevent this phenomenon, it is crucial to begin insulin therapy with the lowest dose possible and to increase the dosage only in very small increments. Dr. Somogyi felt that most diabetics can and should be controlled on very low doses of insulin. He stated:

> *No diabetic patient is adequately "regulated" with insulin until his daily requirement is 20 units or less, or, in exceptional cases, between 20 and*

30 units. The large doses generally used in insulin
therapy result from unawareness of the diabeto-
genic effect of hypoglycemia. Excess insulin, which
causes hypoglycemia, aggravates diabetes, and the
damage done by too much insulin is then combated
with still more insulin. This leads to a vicious cir-
cle, with an unmanageable diabetes as its product.[3]

Working on his own, Dr. Somogyi spent a good deal of his time rehabilitating diabetics who came to the Jewish Hospital of St. Louis with their blood sugar levels out of control due to excessive use of insulin. His experience with these patients led him to this conclusion:

Insulin therapy in its present way of applica-
tion serves not so much the treatment of the com-
mon, spontaneous diabetes of the patient, but the
greater part of the insulin doses administered
are consumed in arduous attempts to check and
control the new adreno-pituitary diabetes which
has been superimposed by the effects of insulin
doses that caused hypoglycemia in the course of the
treatment.[4]

The Dawn Phenomenon

Many people with diabetes have high blood sugar levels upon awakening, even though they've been fasting and had an insulin injection the night before. This has been termed the *dawn phenomenon*, and it describes a characteristic rise in blood sugar that occurs in many diabetics six to ten hours after bedtime. Its exact cause is uncertain. We do know that insulin action wanes and there appears to be a rapid clearing of insulin by the liver around this time. Dr. Peter Campbell and his associates from the Mayo Clinic in Rochester, Minnesota, have documented that most insulin-dependent diabetics have early-morning surges of growth hormone, an insulin antagonist that regularly causes elevated blood sugar readings in the morning.[5]

Whatever its precise cause, this phenomenon may create problems. The early-morning blood sugar level is the one most commonly used to establish the insulin dose for the day. If this level is high, there is a tendency to try to bring it down aggressively with larger insulin dosages in the afternoon or evening. This approach only worsens the problem by creating hypoglycemia that could elevate the early-morning blood sugar readings even more.

The bottom line is that you should be less concerned with blood sugars that are elevated (150 to 250 mg/dl) in the morning unless there is consistent elevation throughout the day.

The Insulin Pump: Is It Really an Improvement?

The last twenty years have witnessed a new era in the nuts and bolts of diabetes management. The invention of small electronic meters now allows patients to easily, reliably, and relatively inexpensively monitor their blood glucose levels several times a day. This is a powerful tool for self-management: The individual patient can determine how specific foods, supplements, exercise regimens, and drugs affect his or her blood sugar levels and can fine-tune insulin dosages in the home on a daily, even hourly basis.

Another breakthrough is the development of the various types of insulin described above. It is now feasible for diabetic patients using fast-acting insulin to keep their blood sugar levels close to those of nondiabetics. However, the innovation in diabetes care that has received the most attention is the insulin pump. This small unit, which is about the size of a pocket calculator, is connected to a plastic tube that inserts into a large needle permanently implanted in the skin, usually around the waist. The pump continuously infuses a small amount of insulin under the skin, with the patient self-administering additional boluses of insulin before meals or whenever needed.

In one sense, the insulin pump would seem to solve all the problems experienced by diabetic patients. But does it?

There is a mistaken assumption that the insulin pump measures blood sugar levels and automatically administers the required dose of insulin. It does not. Patients still have to monitor blood sugar levels frequently. Furthermore, because it is a mechanical device, it is subject to failure, blockages in the tubing, and coagulation of the insulin. One of the most frequent complications is infection at the infusion site. In addition, severe hypoglycemia caused by too much insulin occurs more frequently in users of the pump.

Although some may prefer this mode of insulin delivery, the insulin pump does not seem to improve upon the blood sugar levels achieved with close monitoring and frequent injections. Donald R. Coustan, M.D., of Brown University in Providence, Rhode Island, divided a group of twenty-two pregnant diabetic patients into two groups. Eleven used an insulin pump, while the remainder used conventional but frequent injections. Dr. Coustan found no difference in blood sugar levels or other measurements of diabetic control.[6]

In short, the insulin pump seems to have few significant advantages over regular insulin injections with close monitoring of the blood glucose level. But it certainly has some disadvantages, both physical and psychological. I want to tell you about one of my patients, G.M., who had been on an insulin pump for about two years when she arrived at the Institute for treatment. Though not a type 1 diabetic, G.M. had been started on the pump because it was hoped that it would help prevent complications down the line. However, by following our diet and exercise program, she was able to discontinue the pump altogether and use only small doses of insulin to cover occasional peak elevations of her blood sugar.

G.M. was more than happy to give up the pump. As she explained to me, it had been a constant reminder of her disease. She could never get away from her problem. So often in medicine, we vigorously treat the disease and forget what the treatment does to the patient. That the pump was to G.M. a perpetual and unpleasant reminder of her illness surely never entered the mind of the physician who prescribed it. Nor had this occurred to me until she had mentioned it, but I now consider it to be a strong argument against the use of the insulin pump.

The big advance in diabetes management is, in my opinion, not the insulin pump but the techniques that permit measurement of blood sugar levels by the patient at home. With this capability, insulin therapy can be instituted with dramatic reductions in the blood sugar level using *conventional* methods of insulin injections.

Insulin in the Non-Insulin-Dependent Diabetic

The overwhelming majority of diabetic patients (around 90 percent) have non-insulin-dependent, or type 2, diabetes. As pointed out in part I of this book, this more common form of diabetes is generally not related to a lack of insulin but to poor diet, obesity, inactivity, and other factors that render the tissues insensitive to insulin. What type 2 diabetics need is not insulin, but a program to increase insulin sensitivity, which is the essence of this book.

The primary concern in the treatment of type 2 diabetics is preventing the long-term complications associated with the condition. The most serious of these is accelerated atherosclerosis that leads to heart attacks and circulatory disorders. So when considering the potential value of insulin in type 2 diabetics, the crucial question is this: Will the use of insulin reduce the complication rate?

The University Group Diabetes Program (UGDP) was a long-term, randomized, prospective study carried out in twelve diabetic centers across the country, beginning in the early 1960s, in order to answer this question. Funded by the National Institutes of Health, the study actually had two arms. One arm examined the effectiveness of oral hypoglycemic agents in reducing the rate of diabetic complications. As you will see in the following chapter, that was its most controversial aspect.

The second arm examined whether insulin, in dosages that would significantly lower blood sugar in type 2 diabetics, would slow down the rate of complications as it was believed to do. To find out, 619 non-insulin-dependent diabetics were put in one of three groups.

◉ Group 1—insulin variable (204 patients): In this group, the dosage of insulin used was altered to achieve blood sugar levels as near normal as possible.

◉ Group 2—insulin fixed (210 patients): A fixed dose of insulin was used, calculated on the basis of body weight and height, and this was not altered for the entire length of the study, even if the blood sugar went up.

◉ Group 3—placebo (205 patients): Only dietary restrictions were used.

All the patients were followed for a minimum of nine years, and 460 of them (74 percent) were followed for fourteen years. I cannot overestimate the importance of this study, for it gives a long-term picture of what happens to type 2 diabetics when insulin is used to lower the blood sugar level.[7]

This Study Showed Little Protection from Insulin

Over the course of the study, the subjects in the insulin-fixed group (group 2) and the placebo group (group 3) had gradual increases in the blood sugar level with time, while those taking insulin in a variable dose (group 1) had very significant reductions in their blood sugar. (See figure 4.)

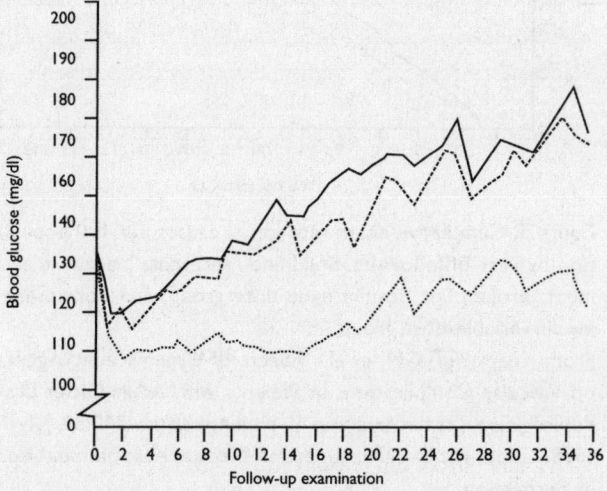

Figure 4. Average fasting blood glucose levels at the start of the experiment and at each follow-up examination from 1961 to 1974. Solid line represents placebo (group 3); broken line, insulin in a fixed dose (group 2); and dotted line, insulin in a variable dose (group 1).

From Knatterud, GM, et al. "Effects of Hypoglycemic Agents on Vascular Complications in Patients with Adult-Onset Diabetes," *Journal of the American Medical Association* 240:39, July 7, 1978. Copyright © 1978, American Medical Association. Used by permission.

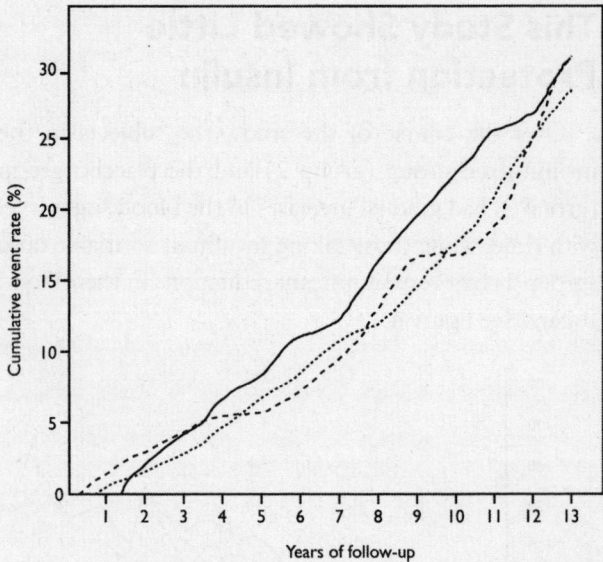

Figure 5. Cumulative death rate for all causes per 100 population by year of follow-up. Solid line represents placebo treatment; broken line, insulin fixed-dose group; and dotted line, insulin variable-dose group.

From Knatterud, GM, et al. "Effects of Hypoglycemic Agents on Vascular Complications in Patients with Adult-Onset Diabetes," *Journal of the American Medical Association* 240:39, July 7, 1978. Copyright © 1978, American Medical Association. Used by permission.

One of the most surprising findings of this study was that despite the marked difference in the average blood sugar levels, there were no significant differences in the death rates among the three treatment protocols. There also was little difference in the nonfatal complications of diabetes among the three groups. Except for slight elevations in creatinine levels in the placebo group, indicating the possibility of very slightly increased kidney damage, the researchers found no significant area where insulin in either a fixed dose or a variable dose had any beneficial result on the non-insulin-dependent diabetic when compared to placebo.

However, when the study subjects were later regrouped based on individual blood glucose control—regardless of what method they used to achieve control—the patients who had achieved good control had a reduced incidence of fatal and nonfatal events, compared to those whose control was fair or poor. Of the fatalities attributed to cardiovascular disease, almost twice as many deaths occurred in patients with fair to poor control as in those with good control. The incidence of diabetic retinopathy and elevated serum creatinine, a marker of kidney damage, was greater in the patients with poorer control. Almost 25 percent more patients with poor versus good control developed hypertension.[8]

I want to emphasize that the differences in death and disability documented in this study were related to degree of blood glucose control, not method of control. The researchers concluded:

Thus, over the time period studied with an average follow-up of 12 years, insulin used in a fixed dosage or used in a variable dosage to normalize glucose levels was no better than diet alone in prolonging life or in preventing the vascular complications considered in this report in the adult-onset, non-ketosis-prone diabetic.

The UGDP findings provide no evidence that
insulin or any other drug lowering blood glucose
levels will alter the course of vascular complica-
tions in the type of diabetes that is most common,
adult-onset diabetes. Weight reduction has been
shown to be feasible and effective in lowering blood
glucose, thus dietary management deserves greater
emphasis in this type of diabetes than it has received
to date, as others have suggested. In any case, the
UGDP results suggest that the use of any other
additional therapeutic agent must be justified on
grounds other than the prevention of macrovascu-
lar complications.

Maintaining Good Glucose Control Is Protective

The only other major large clinical trial to address insulin therapy in type 2 diabetes, the United Kingdom Prospective Diabetes Study, was begun in 1977. The goal was to determine if improving glucose control in recently diagnosed type 2 diabetics, via diet therapy, insulin, or oral drug therapy, would reduce the incidence of death and diabetic complications. The conclusion of this study, which lasted eleven years and involved more than 3,800 patients and twenty-three medical centers in the United Kingdom, demonstrated that keeping blood sugars in the normal range reduced the risk of serious eye disease by one-quarter and kidney disease by one-third.[9] However, no significant difference in rates of heart disease were observed until treatment for hypertension, which is common in type 2 diabetes, was added in a later arm of the study. With the addition of blood-pressure-lowering therapy, the risk of heart attack and stroke also declined significantly.[10]

Other than the fact that intensive insulin (and oral drug) therapy was associated with weight gain, this study did not draw any definitive conclusions about the pros and cons of insulin therapy in type 2 diabetes. (It did, however, uncover more adverse effects of oral drugs, which we will discuss in the next chapter.) Rather, it underscored the importance of obtaining near-normal blood sugar readings for the prevention of diabetes-related death and complications.

Is There Ever a Place for Insulin in Type 2 Diabetes?

Most patients with type 2 diabetes are initially told to make changes in their diet and to begin an exercise program. If that fails to lower their blood sugar levels, they are then started on one of the oral hypoglycemic agents. These usually do work and blood glucose normalizes for a time, but the natural course of these drugs is a gradual loss of effectiveness. Once this happens, the only option left, or so it is believed, is to begin the patient on insulin. Up to 50 percent of all type 2 diabetics eventually end up on insulin.

Dr. John Davidson (who as I mentioned earlier is the editor of one of the most popular medical textbooks on diabetes) and a number of other experts feel that most cases of type 2 diabetes can and should be controlled with safe, effective lifestyle measures. In a chapter in Dr. Davidson's textbook contributed by Michael Berger and Bernd Richter, the conclusion is:

> *Diet therapy, weight reduction, and increased exercise remain the rational therapeutic modalities available for the treatment of NIDDM [type 2 diabetes]. In case individual therapeutic goals cannot be achieved, appropriate insulin therapy is the treatment of choice for efficacy and safety reasons. It is estimated that, at a maximum, 20–30% of patients with NIDDM may benefit from the adjunctive use of oral antidiabetic agents.[11]*

In other words, should a patient be unable to lower blood sugars on a lifestyle regimen, the introduction of small doses of insulin is a far superior treatment to the use of oral hypoglycemic agents, which, as I will detail in the next chapter, have a number of adverse side effects.

New research also suggests that if a patient with type 2 diabetes is placed on a short course of insulin therapy during the earlier stages of the disease, improvements may be noted in insulin secretion and glucose control long after the insulin is discontinued. If patients take the opportunity to modify their diet and lifestyle while undergoing a short course of insulin therapy, they may be able to achieve normal blood sugar control thereafter, much like the newly diagnosed type 1 diabetics I told you about in the first chapter. In a study published in *Diabetes Care*, patients with recent-onset type 2 diabetes that had not responded to dietary changes were placed on intensive insulin therapy for two weeks. Following this brief period of therapy, nine of the thirteen study subjects were able to maintain adequate glucose control that lasted for an average of twenty-six months.[12]

I believe, like Dr. Davidson, that we need to change the way we think about insulin and the type 2 diabetic. Insulin is currently pulled out as a therapy of last resort after the oral drugs have lost their effectiveness. By this time the patient is likely overweight and in very poor control. I know from years of clinical experience that most type 2 diabetics can reverse their condition if they are seriously willing to embrace a dietary and exercise program and lose weight. However, if this fails, a short trial of insulin therapy, along with lifestyle changes, is warranted.

Let me make it clear that I do not view this as a substitute for a lifestyle program; it is an adjunct. I would be reluctant to put an overweight diabetic on an insulin regimen, because as I explained above, insulin promotes weight gain, which only exacerbates the diabetic condition. In any case, these are the patients whose condition most readily responds to weight loss via the diet, exercise, and supplement program described in this book.

The most popular therapy for type 2 diabetes, however, is not insulin but oral drugs, which we will discuss in the next chapter.

CHAPTER 5

The Oral Drugs

In 1978, Rebecca Warner, Sidney M. Wolfe, M.D., and Rebecca Rich, working for the Public Citizen Health Research Group of Washington, D.C., published a 121-page book provocatively titled *Off Diabetes Pills: A Diabetic's Guide to Longer Life*. The book began:

> *Warning: Antidiabetic Pills Are*
> *Dangerous to Your Health*
> *Are you taking tolbutamide (Orinase), tolaza-*
> *mide (Tolinase), chlorpropamide (Diabinese), or*
> *acetohexamide (Dymelor)? These pills could cost*
> *you your life. This booklet is written for you, to*
> *explain why you must do three things:*
>
> - *Stop taking antidiabetic pills as soon as you*
>   *can;*
> - *Go on a diet and lose weight;*
> - *Stop seeing your present doctor unless he or*
>   *she genuinely tries to help you lose weight and*
>   *agrees to switch you to insulin if you still have*

> *diabetic symptoms at or below your ideal body weight.*
>
> *These steps could mean the difference between life and death.*[1]

As you might imagine, this book, which unfortunately is out of print, stimulated considerable controversy and made a huge impact on me as a fledgling physician just beginning my medical practice. More than twenty years have passed since *Off Diabetes Pills* was published, and a lot of things have changed. The number of Americans afflicted with the disease has increased fivefold, and the incidence of diabetes-related amputations, blindness, heart attacks, kidney failure, and other complications has likewise exploded. We've also seen the advent of a multitude of new diabetes drugs, screening tools, and insulin delivery systems. Yet I believe the premise of this little booklet remains as true today as it was more than two decades ago: Antidiabetic pills can be dangerous to your health.

Types of Oral Diabetes Drugs

When the first of the oral diabetes drugs appeared on the scene some fifty years ago, they were enthusiastically embraced, no questions asked. It is not difficult to understand why these drugs were so rapidly accepted before any long-term studies had been done to prove their efficacy. First, insulin injections are never a joyful experience for either physician or patient. A pill that could be used instead of a needle to lower blood sugar was eagerly welcomed. Second, the pills represented for the non-insulin-dependent patient an alternative that would replace the need for diet, exercise, and weight loss. It became the magic bullet that relieved the responsibility of both doctor and patient to alter diet or exercise patterns.

Let's take a close look at the various types of oral drugs used to treat diabetes. My goal in this chapter is to help you understand why I rarely prescribe them for my diabetic patients.

The Sulfonylureas

The oldest and most commonly prescribed class of oral drugs for diabetes was discovered by chance in the 1940s, when physicians noted that a patient being treated for pneumonia with a sulfonamide drug had low blood sugar levels. Research began on this and related compounds for the treatment of diabetes, and in the 1950s the first of the class of oral hypoglycemic agents known as sulfonylureas was introduced. Also called insulin secretagogues, sulfonylureas act by increasing the sensitivity of beta cells in the pancreas to glucose and stimulating them to increase secretion of insulin. To a lesser extent, they also slightly enhance cellular sensitivity to insulin, and they may modestly inhibit the production of glucose in the liver.

Drugs in this class include glyburide (DiaBeta, Micronase, and Glynase), chlorpropamide (Diabinese), acetohexamide (Dymelor), tolazamide (Tolinase), glipizide (Glucotrol), tolbutamide (Orinase), and glimepiride (Amaryl). They are taken once or twice a day, usually 30 minutes before meals. Although they do lower fasting blood glucose and HbA$_{IC}$ in some patients, these drugs are ineffective in 25 percent of type 2 diabetics, and effectiveness often falls off over time.

Like all prescription drugs, the sulfonylureas have side effects, some of them quite serious. In some patients they cause significant and sometimes prolonged hypoglycemia. As we discussed in the previous chapter, hypoglycemic reactions can cause irreversible brain damage and may even be fatal. A study published in the *Journal of the American Geriatrics Society* in 1996 demonstrated that hypoglycemic reactions are particularly common in patients over the age of sixty-five who are taking these drugs. The worst offenders, according to this study, were glyburide (DiaBeta, Micronase, and Glynase), chlorpropamide (Diabinese), and acetohexamide (Dymelor) because they stay in the blood much longer. However, the other sulfonylureas were also culpable. Fears of this side effect led the Public Citizen Health Research Group, which was founded by Ralph Nader and Sidney Wolfe, M.D., as a watchdog of the drug industry, to gave a flat-out "Do Not Use" to these three types of sulfonylureas, and a "Limited Use" warning to the others.[2]

What makes this complication particularly dangerous is lack of physician awareness. All physicians know that hypoglycemic reactions can occur with insulin, but the oral drugs are not perceived to be powerful enough to have this side effect. Often when an elderly person suffers from drug-induced hypoglycemia, he or she is thought to have suffered a stroke or to be senile. That these drugs have a hypoglycemic effect in some patients and not in others probably reflects differences in rates of excretion of the drug. Furthermore, the sulfonylureas interact poorly with a long list of popular drugs. Several drugs commonly used to treat high blood pressure, heart disease, and infections (concurrent conditions with diabetes) may enhance the action of the antidiabetic drugs, making them more likely to cause severe hypoglycemia.

Another extremely common adverse effect is weight gain, which further exacerbates the diabetic condition. Other side effects include gastrointestinal upset, as well as headaches, dizziness, and other symptoms of hypoglycemia. These drugs have been known to cause hypothyroidism, skin rashes, severe allergic reactions, opacities in the cornea of the eye, water retention, elevated blood pressure, and increased stomach acid secretion. They may be inappropriate for use in elderly patients, and they are also contraindicated for patients with congestive heart failure.

However, the primary reason I am opposed to the unchecked use of the sulfonylurea drugs is because they can also have damaging effects on the cardiovascular system. The drugs most often prescribed to patients with diabetes, who are at dramatically increased risk of heart disease to begin with (three-quarters of all diabetics die of heart disease), have been shown to actually increase the risk of heart and circulatory problems. I know you're likely to balk at this idea. Your physician has probably assured you of the safety and efficacy of the sulfonylurea drugs. He or she would scoff at the very idea that these drugs used to treat type 2 diabetes may be more dangerous than the disease itself.

This is why I am going to devote several pages to the research on the suolfonylurea drugs, some of it dating back more than thirty years. For despite solid evidence that these drugs may be causing mayhem on a world-wide scale, their dangers have yet to be appreciated by most physicians.

A Landmark Study

Years after the sulfonylurea drugs were widely accepted as the first-line therapy for type 2 diabetes, the medical community finally got around to studying their benefits. The University Group Diabetes Program (UGDP) was funded with fourteen separate grants from the Public Health Service of the U.S. government. Its purpose was clear from the outset: to determine whether control of blood sugar levels with either the oral drugs or insulin in the adult-onset, type 2, non-insulin-dependent diabetic reduced the incidence of heart disease or other major vascular complications associated with diabetes. (In the previous chapter we discussed the results of the arm of the study that examined insulin.)

In 1961, 1,027 type 2 diabetic patients were enrolled in the study and were followed in twelve clinics in the United States and Puerto Rico. The study was double blinded, meaning that except for those on insulin, neither the patients nor the physicians were aware of who was taking what therapy. Each patient was put on the accepted diabetic diet of that time, which consisted of 35 to 40 percent fat calories, and was randomly assigned to one of the five treatment groups:

- Group 1: Placebo. Each patient took an inactive pill that looked like the active agents.

- Group 2: Orinase. This is a sulfonylurea drug (generic name tolbutamide).*

- Group 3: DBI (phenformin). This is another type of oral hypoglycemic drug that has since been taken off the market.

- Group 4: Insulin in a fixed dose. This means that a single dosage of insulin was calculated on the basis of body size and then given unchanged for the duration of the study.

- Group 5: Insulin in a variable dose. The dosage of insulin was varied in order to maintain as near normal blood sugar as possible.

The study on Orinase was intended to run until 1971, but the researchers stopped it in 1969 because the rate of death from heart disease among the patients taking these drugs was so high that they considered it unethical to continue the study further. Over the eight-year period of the study there were *250 percent more deaths* from heart disease in the group taking the sulfonylurea drug than in the placebo group. The group taking DBI (phenformin) fared even worse. The death rates for all causes of death were 62 percent higher than

*Note: Similar drugs include, as mentioned above, chlorpropamide (Diabinese), acetohexamide (Dymelor), and tolazamide (Tolinase). The newer and more powerful sulfonylureas are glyburide (DiaBeta, Micronase, and Glynase), glipizide (Glucotrol), and glimepiride (Amaryl). Since they all have similar actions, the studies on Orinase implicate all of them, and they all carry a strongly worded, mandatory warning about their dangers.

in the placebo group, and the deaths from cardiovascular disease increased by 300 percent!

Statistical analysis showed that these differences could not have occurred just by chance. Therefore, unless there was some other explanation, the increased death rate had to be related to the drugs themselves. Very careful analysis of all other factors was carried out to see if something had been overlooked in assigning the patients to the various groups, yet nothing could be found that would explain why those taking the drugs had a *higher* death rate from heart disease than those on placebo.

The UGDP published the results and summarized their findings as follows:

> *All UGDP investigators are agreed that the findings of this study indicate that the combination of diet and tolbutamide (Orinase) therapy is no more effective than diet alone or than diet and insulin in prolonging life. Moreover, the findings suggest that tolbutamide and diet may be less effective than diet alone or than diet and insulin at least insofar as cardiovascular mortality is concerned. For this reason, use of tolbutamide has been discontinued in the UGDR. Patients originally assigned to the tolbutamide treatment group ... are no longer being treated with tolbutamide.*[3]

In an additional publication the researchers further stated:

> *Until it is possible to find a cause or combination of causes or to discern a subgroup predisposed to this*

risk, this drug (Orinase) must be considered haz-
ardous for long-term use.[4]

Then the rebuttals started. What seemed clear suddenly became muddy. It is not difficult to understand
why. Drug interests and physician assumptions and
pride are often major obstacles to the acceptance of scientific evidence if that evidence runs counter to vested
interests or strongly held assumptions and beliefs.

The Rebuttals Begin

When the UGDP results became public, tens of millions of dollars were being spent on oral diabetic medications. If primary care physicians across the country
were to immediately stop prescribing the oral drugs
and intensify efforts in the areas of diet and exercise
instead, the drug companies profiting from the rev-
enues generated by the oral diabetic drugs would be
severely crippled. It is not surprising that the drug companies went to work immediately to cast as much doubt
as they could on the conclusions of the UGDP study.

They were unbelievably successful. Physicians have
never stopped using these drugs. Even today, more
than thirty years later, physicians are still prescribing
drugs that may be associated with several thousand
unnecessary deaths a year. Today, most physicians hon-
estly believe that the UGDP results were inaccurate.
No fault in the design or conduct of the study can be
found to support these beliefs. It is not unreasonable to
credit them to the campaign waged against the study

by the drug companies and by physicians who simply would not accept the results.

The Attack

Physician attitudes and beliefs are strongly influenced by the drug companies, more so than most physicians care to admit. One powerful tool of influence used by drug interests is the "medical tabloid," or "throwaway," which is sent to every physician without charge. I receive ten to fifteen of these weekly medical journals or newspapers. They contain little if any original scientific material. Instead they serve almost exclusively as a vehicle for the opinions of some of the experts in the field. The drug companies advertise heavily in these publications, and, more importantly, exert considerable influence on what is written.

Dr. Roger Palmer, former head of the Department of Pharmacology at the University of Miami School of Medicine, points out that many prominent physicians become unwitting spokesmen for drug interests. They are approached by the editor of a "throwaway" and asked to write, for a fee, about a drug that they favor. This opinion is then published alongside numerous advertisements for the drug. Since most physicians are too busy to read the original research, their opinions are often shaped by this obviously biased material. They are left with the assumption that a specific drug is the only reasonable treatment for a given condition. This is great for the drug interests, but not so good for patients who might possibly do just as well or even better on some less-advertised drug—or on no drug at all.

Immediately following the publication of the UGDP results, and before their implications had been discussed in legitimate scientific literature, the drug interests utilized the throwaways to discredit the study and challenge its validity. Since the drugs were already trusted, it was not difficult to discredit a study purporting to shatter that trust. By calling on physicians who were deeply critical of the study and publishing only their opinions, even when their appraisals were grossly inaccurate, these publications created the belief that the design of the study was so flawed the results could not be accepted.

Thaddeus E. Prout, M.D., F.A.C.P., associate professor emeritus, Department of Medicine at Johns Hopkins Hospital in Baltimore, and one of the primary researchers and spokesmen for the UGDP, said in a phone interview that the drug companies "got there first." Using their sophisticated avenues of communication with the medical community, they biased the nation's physicians against the results of the study before the researchers had time to clarify the importance of their findings.

Physician Pride

A second reason for the resistance to the UGDP findings and conclusions was that physicians had been using the drugs with confidence for years. In the university centers where young physicians are trained in the treatment of diabetic patients, these oral drugs were an integral part of treatment protocols. The results of the UGDP called upon the heads of departments to seriously rethink the role that the drugs had been given for so long at their medical centers. Most of them just could not do this. It was too uncomfortable. The drugs were too popular and the original assumptions about their benefit had become entrenched beliefs.

In private practice, where most diabetics are treated by their own physicians, the drugs were even more popular. They could be given to the diabetic patient with the feeling that something positive was being done. The drugs were easy to take, while the alternatives— vigorous diet and lifestyle changes, with or without insulin—required work.

The study and its conclusions just had to go, and in the minds of most physicians, that is exactly what has happened.

Just How Dangerous Are the Drugs?

The results of the UGDP study showed that the oral hypoglycemic agents increase the death rate from heart disease in diabetics by 1 percent per year. This means that each year one additional death would be expected in a group of one hundred diabetics taking the oral drugs, compared with a group of a hundred patients treated with diet alone. Over a ten-year period one could expect about ten more deaths to occur in the hundred patients taking the pill compared to those treated with diet alone.

One percent per year may seem like a small figure, and in one sense it is. But in another, more important sense, this figure is enormous.

A 1 Percent Annual Increase in Death Is Small

An increase of 1 percent annually is too small for any physician or clinic to notice in their day-to-day practice. After all, *some* diabetic patients in a physician's practice are likely to die of heart disease in any given year, especially if the practice includes many diabetic patients. One additional death is unlikely to make the physician suspect that something is wrong. It is still less likely to make him or her think that the prescribed therapy is related to that death.

Physicians characteristically feel certain that they are providing the best for their patients' well-being. Ironically, if a diabetic patient dies while taking oral drugs, the physician may come to the erroneous conclusion that the death occurred because blood sugar levels were not controlled rigidly enough. This in turn could prompt the physician to become even more aggressive in his use of drugs with other patients.

It is virtually impossible for even the most expert of physicians to "see" the toxicity of a popular remedy without the benefit of a long-term controlled study designed to uncover that toxicity objectively. Therefore, relying on "personal expertise and clinical experience" alone is foolish and extremely dangerous. However, that is exactly what many of the critics of the UGDP did. Dr. Joseph Goodman, in a letter to the *Cleveland Plain Dealer*, stated:

> *Oral antidiabetic drugs have been extensively used by the medical profession for approximately*

20 years. Doctors have considered these drugs to be effective in the treatment of diabetic patients without any fear of harmful effects and with few or no side effects.... The UGDP report of a higher rate of cardiovascular disease in persons taking antidiabetic drugs is purely statistical in a small segment of patients as opposed to the greater and longer experience of the medical profession at large.[5]

Dr. Goodman's assessment is, in my opinion, irrational. To state that the findings of an eight-year study were "purely statistical" doesn't make any sense. We physicians would love to have the opportunity to use pure statistics, not unscientific "personal experience," to guide our judgment in the treatment of any condition.

Second, that "small segment" of patients was carefully selected and randomized to accurately represent the greater number of patients who were being treated and would be treated by doctors who believed the drugs to be safe and beneficial. Given that there are literally millions of patients with type 2 diabetes who are candidates for these drugs, it is clear from this representative sample that thousands of lives could be lost each year directly as a consequence of the use of oral antidiabetic medication.

A 1 Percent Increase in Death Is Enormous

Countering Dr. Goodman's assessment of the UGDP, Dr. J. R. Carter and four other diabetic specialists replied in the same publication:

For every 100 middle-aged patients treated with tolbutamide, there would be per year about 2 deaths from cardiovascular disease as compared to about one death in 100 patients treated with insulin or diet alone. We find it impossible to believe a physician in the midst of a busy practice would be aware of one extra death per year in 100 patients whom he never originally isolated in his mind or in his records for study.[6]

The refusal of Dr. Goodman and others of his ilk to reexamine deeply held beliefs is all too common among physicians. Let's look at that 1 percent increase in another light. Take a reasonable sample of 3 million diabetic patients on a given drug. If the death rate increases by one additional death per 100 patients because of the drug, that would add up to 30,000 additional deaths per year and 300,000 more deaths in ten years! This magnitude of increased death can be determined only by a study the size and length of the UGDP in which a therapy is compared to a placebo and both groups are followed long enough to establish a difference in outcome. It could never be recognized without the aid of such a placebo-controlled study.

How Do Sulfonylureas Harm the Heart?

At the time the increase in death rate caused by the sulfonylureas was initially observed, no one was able to explain the drugs' adverse effects. There was simply no clear physiological cause. This was likely another reason why so many physicians refused to accept the findings of the UGDP. Only in the past few years has research been published that offers an explanation for the increased death rate from heart disease associated with the oral drugs.

It is now known that these drugs interfere with oxygen delivery to the coronary arteries. Under normal circumstances, when oxygen levels fall, the arteries supplying blood to the heart dilate in an effort to deliver more blood and consequently more oxygen. This is caused at least in part by the activity of potassium-sensitive channels in the arteries that prompt vasodilation. The sulfonylurea drugs block the dilation of the coronary vessels by closing these potassium channels, resulting in reduced oxygen delivery to the heart. This effect lasts for quite some time, and it has been documented with the use of both first-generation and second-generation (newer and presumably safer) sulfonylureas.[7]

Was the Study Valid?

The findings from the UGDP caught everyone by surprise. Everyone—the researchers, the drug companies, and the nation's physicians—fully expected the study to show that the drugs *reduced* deaths from heart disease. Only those who trusted the scientific method and were able to put statistical realities above empirical beliefs could adjust accordingly.

The physicians who registered the harshest criticisms about the study did so from an extremely biased position. Since they could not or would not believe the results, they reasoned that something had to be wrong with the study! As I pointed out earlier, it was these critics who, with the aid of the drug companies, received the widest exposure in the ensuing controversy.

Most of the critics felt that the excess cardiovascular deaths found in the patients taking Orinase occurred because the study was not truly randomized, that those taking the drug had more heart disease at the beginning of the study and would be expected to have more heart attacks anyway. This implies that the drug group had "bad luck at the draw." Stanley Schor, M.D., of the Department of Biometrics, Temple University Medical School in Philadelphia, summarized these and other criticisms of the study in the *Journal of the American Medical Association*.[8] In the same issue, Jerome Cornfield of the Department of Biostatistics, Graduate School of Public Health, University of Pittsburgh, answered the criticisms leveled by Dr. Schor and, using the data from the study, discounted, for the most part, each one.[9]

For instance, Dr. Schor pointed out that it was not known what percentage of each group were smokers. If the group taking the drug contained more smokers than the placebo group, they would have more deaths from heart disease as a result. Since it was not known what percentage of each group were smokers, the results were questionable.

However, the purpose of randomization, as Dr. Cornfield countered, is to distribute all factors, both known and unknown, equally into the various groups. In the case of smokers versus nonsmokers, there would be only one chance in 50,000 that a significantly higher percentage of smokers would wind up in the group taking the drug. Even if this did occur, it would result in only a 16 percent increase in cardiovascular deaths—not the 250 percent that was seen!

Dr. Schor felt uneasy with the fact that some of the patients did not take the drugs as they were supposed to or were transferred out of that group because of side effects. He suggested that this could alter the results. This happens in every study of this kind, but Dr. Schor criticized the investigators and questioned the results: "The investigators stated that the transfer problem took place in too few patients to have an effect on the mortality. This is simply not true. There seem to be many more transfers than there are deaths."

However, Dr. Cornfield pointed out that the investigators *did* record the results for the patients that adhered strictly to the drug regimen. It was found that those who took Orinase exactly as they were supposed to had an *even higher* death rate. At five years, the study subjects who strictly adhered to the Orinase regimen had a 400 percent increase in death rate compared to the recorded 250 percent increase of the group as a whole. At eight years the strict adherers had a 600 percent increase in death. On this issue, Dr. Cornfield concluded, "The analysis suggested by Dr. Schor, difficult to interpret though it is, does nothing to weaken the UGDP finding and in fact tends to strengthen it."

Dr. Schor thought it was "deplorable" that the researchers stopped the study when it became obvious that Orinase was causing a large increase in heart deaths. He felt that if the study had been continued and the increased death rate continued, no one would have argued with the results.

However, the study was not done to see whether Orinase killed people, but to determine whether it helped them! At the time the study was stopped, there was no possibility that Orinase would turn out to be beneficial. As Dr. Cornfield justifiably asked, why would anyone want to sacrifice more lives just to see how deadly the drug was?

In looking at the summaries of these two critics appearing side by side in the same journal, I was struck by the fact that Dr. Schor rarely referred to the published data in an effort to substantiate his criticisms in a factual manner. On the other hand, Dr. Cornfield extensively drew on the published material to rebut Dr. Schor's criticisms, citing page numbers and tabular information. In several instances, it appeared as if Dr. Schor's reading of the data was sketchy, if not inaccurate. Dr. Cornfield concluded:

> *None of the possible errors suggested so far do in fact account for the UGDP findings. Although further investigation, particularly if undertaken in a nonadversary framework, may still be useful, it seems likely that a point of diminishing returns may not be far off, and that continued analysis of the UGDP, in the hope of finding errors which alter the conclusions, will become increasingly unrewarding.*

An Independent Review

Both of these summaries appeared in 1971, yet the controversy continued to brew. The study was attacked from every angle, and the use of the oral drugs for the treatment of diabetes actually increased!

As a result of the ongoing controversy, Dr. Robert Marston, then director of the National Institutes of Health, contracted an independent committee from the Biometric Society, an international group of experts, to evaluate all the data generated by the study. In Feburary 1975 they reported:

> *On the question of cardiovascular mortality due to tolbutamide and phenformin, we consider that the UGDP trial has raised suspicions that cannot be dismissed on the basis of other evidence presently available.... [We] consider that in the light of the UGDP findings, it remains with the proponents of the oral hypoglycemics to conduct scientifically adequate studies to justify the continued use of such agents.[10]*

In an editorial published along with this report, Thomas C. Chalmers, M.D., of Mount Sinai Medical Center in New York, stated:

> *The probability that oral hypoglycemic agents cause premature deaths from cardiovascular disease remains valid.*
>
> *There are even more important questions to be asked as a result of the controversy over the UGDP study than how a particular diabetic patient should be managed. Assuming that the hypoglycemic drugs are actually dangerous, why have their sales continued to expand steadily in the past*

*15 years, with only a slight dip for one year after
the UGDP report?*

*One explanation is the strong desire of both phy-
sicians and patients for a way to treat diabetes that
does not involve injections, and this has resulted in
a natural reluctance to accept any possibility that
the drugs might be harmful. This has been fostered
by one-sided presentations of the controversy by one
or more of the so-called throw-away medical journals so widely read by physicians. . . .*

*Undoubtedly, the situation will improve now
that not only has the UGDP study been found to
be valid by the Biometric Society group, but also
there has been parallel confirmation in well-done
retrospective studies, analyses of deaths in coronary
care units, disturbing increases in worldwide death
rates among older diabetics, and a pharmacologic
explanation for the potential lethality of cardiovascular events.[11]*

More Bad News from the Study

A year after the publication of the results on Orinase,
the results on DBI (phenformin) were published. They
were even worse. This drug was associated with a 300
percent increase in heart-related deaths. It was found to
increase blood pressure, which probably contributed to
the increase in heart-related deaths, and had the unique
characteristic of causing lactic acid to increase to fatal
levels in the blood in some diabetics.

Interestingly, the toxicity of this agent as revealed by
the UGDP was not challenged nearly as vehemently as

that of Orinase. Because the tendency of DBI to cause fatal lactic acidosis was difficult to argue, the FDA began to move rapidly to ban the drug. Although a group of doctors called the Committee for the Care of Diabetics, formed with the support of the drug companies, attempted to block the FDA's intentions of taking DBI off the market, they failed. In 1977, in an unprecedented move, the FDA removed DBI from the market on the grounds that it was deemed "an imminent hazard." At that time, 336,000 diabetics were taking the drug.

Strong Labels Finally Appear

The Committee for the Care of Diabetics also lobbied long and hard against putting warning labels on Orinase and similar diabetic drugs. However, in March 1984, the FDA finally succeeded in its attempts to put strong warning labels on oral hypoglycemic drugs. The warning for the drug Diabinese and other sulfonylureas reads:

Warnings: SPECIAL WARNING ON INCREASED RISK OF CARDIOVASCULAR MORTALITY

The administration of oral hypoglycemic drugs has been reported to be associated with increased cardiovascular mortality as compared to treatment with diet alone or diet plus insulin. This warning is based on the study conducted by the University Group Diabetes Program (UGDP), a long-term prospective clinical trial designed to evaluate the effectiveness of glucose-lowering drugs in preventing or delaying vascular complications in patients with non-insulin-dependent diabetes. The study involved 823 patients who were randomly assigned to one of four treatment groups (Diabetes 19 [suppl. 2]: 747–830, 1970).

UGDP reported that patients treated for 5 to 8 years with diet plus a fixed dose of Orinase (1.5 grams per day) had a rate of cardiovascular mortality approximately 2½ times that of patients treated with diet alone. A significant increase in total mortality was not observed, but the use of Orinase was discontinued based on the increase in cardiovascular mortality, thus limiting the opportunity for the study to show an increase in overall mortality. Despite controversy regarding the interpretation of these results, the findings of the UGDP study provide an adequate basis for this warning. The patient should be informed of the potential risks and advantages of DIABINESE and of alternative modes of therapy.

Although only one drug in the sulfonylurea class (tolbutamide) was included in this study, it is prudent from a safety standpoint to consider that this warning may also apply to other oral hypoglycemic drugs in this class, in view of their close similarities in mode of action and chemical structure.[12]

This warning remains on the labels of this and other sulfonylureas to this day. Although the basis for this labeling was the UGDP studies, and plans for the labeling were made soon after the results were published, the Committee for the Care of Diabetics was successful in delaying this action by the FDA for almost thirteen years! At present, many physicians still feel comfortable prescribing these drugs, in spite of the fact that they are clearly labeled as being associated with an increased risk of death from cardiovascular disease—the very fate that both diabetic patients and their physicians fear most.

If ever there were an example of entrenched belief winning over rigorous scientific research in the practice of medicine, it is the continued use of these oral hypoglycemic drugs.

The New Generation of Sulfonylurea Drugs

In addition to tolbutamide (Orinase), the first-generation sulfonylurea drugs, as noted earlier, include chlorpropamide (Diabinese), tolazamide (Tolinase), and acetohexamide (Dymelor). These drugs are very similar to Orinase and thus are incriminated by association with the negative findings on Orinase.

There are also several newer sulfonylurea drugs that became available in the late 1970s or thereafter, long after the UGDP studies were completed. These second-generation drugs include glyburide (DiaBeta, Micronase, and Glynase), glipizide (Glucotrol), and glimepiride (Amaryl). The newer sulfonylurea drugs have the same mechanism of action as the older ones. Therefore, although they have not been studied in the long-term controlled manner that was afforded Orinase, these drugs should also be suspected of causing an increase in heart attack rates. Indeed, they carry the same warning label that is required of Orinase and Diabinese about the potential increased risk of heart attack. Some briefer studies indicate that with respect to increased heart attack rate, the newer drugs may be safer than the older drugs if used in patients who have already obtained optimal weight and are following a good diet and exercise program. But the truth is that their safety regarding the cardiovascular system with long-term use has not been proven.

Also of concern, as I mentioned above, is that because these second-generation drugs have a long duration of action, they have an increased potential to create severe and prolonged hypoglycemic reactions. Because symptoms of hypoglycemia could be misdiagnosed as senility or a stroke, these drugs are particularly dangerous for patients over sixty-five. However, other known complications of the older sulfonylureas seem to be less of a problem with these newer drugs.

In addition to the sulfonylureas, three other classes of oral drugs are currently used to treat diabetes: two varieties of insulin-sensitizing drugs, and a drug that affects carbohydrate metabolism.

Metformin Improves Insulin Sensitivity

Insulin sensitizers, or insulin enhancers, work on a completely different principle than the sulfonylureas, which stimulate insulin secretion. As their name implies, these drugs come at the problem from the opposite direction: They increase the cells' ability to utilize insulin. In other words, they reduce insulin resistance.

The most popular of these drugs, metformin (Glucophage), belongs to a class of drugs known as biguanides. Their formulation was inspired by the use in medieval Europe of a medicinal herb called *Galega officinalis* and known as goat's-rue or French lilac. The active ingredient in this herb, guanidine, was used in preparations to treat diabetes in the 1920s.

Two biguanides, metformin and phenformin, were introduced in the late 1950s. Phenformin (DBI), as you will recall, was the other oral diabetes drug used in the UGDP study. Like Orinase, phenformin proved to be associated with an increase in deaths attributed to heart disease—by 300 percent compared to placebo! It was also found to raise blood pressure. Even more alarming, in some patients, particularly those with impaired kidney function, phenformin caused a condition known as lactic acidosis. Lactic acidosis is a life-threatening condition; in fact, it is fatal in half of all cases. In 1977, when the toxicity of this drug became evident, the FDA removed it and other drugs of its class, including metformin, from the market.

Metformin never really went away, however. Because it was considered to be much safer than phenformin, it remained available in Europe, where it is currently the second most commonly prescribed oral diabetes drug, and was reintroduced in Canada within a few years. However, the FDA ban remained in place until 1994, when it again became available in this country.

Metformin increases insulin sensitivity by enhancing the uptake of glucose by the cells, particularly in the muscles. It also inhibits the production of glucose in the liver. It increases the binding of insulin to insulin receptors and boosts the activity of GLUT-4 transporters. In addition, it slows the absorption of glucose from the gastrointestinal tract. Although some studies have suggested that metformin is superior to other oral drugs in controlling diabetes over the long term, other research efforts do not support this claim. Because this drug improves insulin sensitivity, it also ameliorates other conditions caused by insulin resistance. It improves cholesterol levels and ratios, triglyceride levels, and to a very slight degree, blood pressure. Furthermore, unlike many of the diabetes drugs, it promotes modest weight loss in some patients.

Fairly common side effects of metformin, especially with higher doses, are gastrointestinal symptoms, including diarrhea, nausea, and abdominal upset. Some patients experience a metallic taste in the mouth. The drug may also interfere with the absorption of folic acid and vitamin B_{12}. As I mentioned above, however, the most significant adverse effect of metformin is the risk of lactic acidosis. According to its manufacturer, Bristol-Myers Squibb, the risk of this potentially fatal condition in patients treated with metformin is one-tenth to one-twentieth that of phenformin. However, patients with kidney or liver disease, cardiac or respiratory problems, severe infections, or alcoholic abuse are at increased risk and should avoid the drug.

Metformin and Sulfonylurea Drugs Do Not Mix

In the previous chapter I told you about the United Kingdom Prospective Diabetes Study. This was one of the few large-scale studies that have been conducted to examine the effects of long-term drug use on outcomes in type 2 diabetics. One of its findings, which unfortunately has not received enough attention, is that there was an increase in mortality in the study subects taking both metformin and a sulfonylurea drug. Patients taking the two drugs in tandem had a 96 percent increase in diabetes-related deaths and a 60 percent increase in death from all causes, compared to those taking a sulfonylurea alone or using diet therapy exclusively. Follow-up studies were unable to come up with any satisfactory explanations of these findings, so they have more or less been ignored. The American Diabetes Association continues to include in its recommendations concurrent use of the two types of drugs.[13]

Thiazolidinediones: Dangerous Drugs?

A newer class of insulin-sensitizing drugs are the thiazolidinediones, which attempt to correct insulin resistance at the cellular level. The drugs in this class, which are also called "glitazones," are rosiglitazone (Avandia) and pioglitazone (Actos). A third, troglitazone (Rezulin), was removed from the market by the FDA in 2000 because of extreme liver toxicity. These drugs improve insulin sensitivity and utilization in muscle and fat tissues by binding to a receptor site in the nucleus of cells called peroxisomal proliferation activated receptor gamma (PPAR-gamma). This in turn regulates genes that are involved in insulin-stimulated glucose transport and uptake. The result is an increase in activity of the GLUT-4 transporters that usher glucose across the cell membrane. In addition, these drugs enhance the liver's sensitivity to insulin, prompting a reduction in release of glucose from the liver.

Because these drugs address the basic issue of insulin resistance, they have proved to be quite popular in the treatment of type 2 diabetes. The thiazolidinedione drugs lower both insulin and fasting glucose levels; however, they aren't that effective at lowering HbA$_{1C}$, a measure of long-term glucose control. Several studies have demonstrated that when patients switch from other oral drugs, such as sulfonylureas, to a glitazone, this indicator of diabetes control actually deteriorates.

In addition, the thiazolidinediones have numerous adverse side effects. They raise LDL cholesterol by 7 to 10 percent and may cause mild anemia and fluid retention. Weight gain is also common in patients taking these drugs. In the clinical trials carried out prior to FDA approval, diabetics taking Rezulin gained from 1.1 to 7.7 pounds.[14] Although the precise explanation for this is unclear, it is likely caused by a conversion of glucose to fat. As you know from our earlier discussions in this book, extra weight is a decided negative for the type 2 diabetic. It increases insulin resistance and is a significant contributor to the development of the condition.

Most alarming, these drugs are associated with serious liver damage. Rezulin (troglitazone) was launched to great fanfare in March 1997, only to be implicated in thirty-five cases of liver damage and one death within its first seven months on the market. By December 1997 the number of adverse events had climbed to 150, including three deaths, prompting the United Kingdom to pull the drug from the British market. The response of federal watchdogs in the FDA? Stating that the drug's benefits outweighed its risk, they issued a recommendation for new warnings on drug labels and new prescribing guidelines for physicians to warn of potentially fatal liver damage occurring even after short-term use.

In February 2000, FDA medical officer Robert I. Misbin, a veteran diabetes specialist who is employed by the agency to evaluate the safety and effectiveness of proposed and existing drugs, publicly chastised his superiors at the FDA for turning a blind eye to the dangers of this drug. He urged the withdrawal of the drug from the U.S. market. He was joined in short order by other experts, including Dr. Janet B. McGill, a St. Louis physician who had been involved in the early clinical testing of the drug. Dr. McGill stated that the drug's manufacturer, Warner-Lambert, "clearly places profits before the lives of patients with diabetes."[15] Only then—after more than eighty-nine cases of liver failure and sixty-one deaths were attributed to this drug—did the FDA take action and follow the lead of UK regulators by banning the sale of Rezulin.

The newest of the thiazolidinediones, which were approved by the FDA in 1999, are rosiglitazone

(Avandia) and pioglitazone (Actos). They also appear to have some liver toxicity, although it may be less than that of Rezulin. Regardless of degree of toxicity, there are enough red flags and clanging bells associated with these drugs that the regulators who approve new drugs for the European Community have refused to allow Avandia on the market. This governing board is not convinced of the drug's safety, nor is there enough evidence to prove to them that Avandia is effective on its own in treating diabetes.[16] I strongly suggest that you avoid this class of drugs.

Drugs That Affect Carbohydrate Metabolism: Acarbose

Among the most recently approved oral diabetes drugs is acarbose (Precose). It works by slowing the absorption of glucose into the bloodstream. Known as an alpha-glucosidase inhibitor, it blocks the pancreatic enzyme (alpha-glucosidase) in the gastrointestinal tract that breaks down carbohydrates into small glucose molecules that can easily pass through the intestinal walls. Taken just before meals, it targets the spikes in blood sugar experienced by diabetics after eating.

Acarbose causes numerous gastrointestinal problems. When carbohydrates linger in the intestines, they are partially fermented by the bacteria that reside in the gut. This commonly results in diarrhea, abdominal pain, bloating, and flatulence. In fact, in one placebo-controlled study, one-third of the patients taking this drug had diarrhea, and three-fourths experienced excess gas.[17] But there's more. The Japanese Ministry of

Health reported in 1998 that fifty-seven patients taking acarbose had reported liver dysfunction, and two had died. And close examination of the package insert reveals that 15 percent of the patients involving in the premarketing clinical trials of this drug had changes in liver function tests.[18]

Acarbose is at best an expensive and superfluous drug. You can get the same effects by altering your diet, as described in chapters 6 and 7. At worst, it spells liver toxicity for untold numbers of diabetics. Stay away from this drug.

You Do Have Options

The current reliance on the oral drugs, in my opinion, reflects to some extent laziness and a failure to understand (or a refusal to acknowledge) the underlying factors in type 2 diabetes. While there is a small population of type 2 diabetics who could derive benefits from oral drugs, the vast majority can achieve healthy blood glucose levels through a combination of diet, exercise, and targeted nutritional supplementation. Dr. Michael Berger, M.S., professor of medicine in the Department of Medicine, Dusseldorf University in Germany, has this to say about the overreliance on oral diabetes drugs. Although he is addressing the sulfonylureas in particular, I believe his comments encompass all classes of oral diabetes drugs:

> *Unfortunately the use of sulfonylurea drugs has become entrenched as the "treatment of laziness," both on the part of the physician and the patient.*

How much easier it is to prescribe or swallow a pill than to explain or observe a weight-reducing diet in combination with increase in caloric expenditure [exercise]. The central problem of the syndrome for which Sims had coined the term "diabesity" (representing more than 90 percent of the patients with NIDDM in the industrialized world) is insulin resistance due to hyperinsulinemia [excessive insulin secretion by the pancreas] associated with obesity/hyperphagia [overeating] and immobilization. Any rational attempt to treat this disorder should be based upon attempts to decrease, rather than increase, insulinemia in order to improve sensitivity to endogenous insulin. Thus, hypocaloric [low-calorie] dieting and increased physical activity must remain the basis for therapy for overweight patients with non-insulin-dependent diabetes mellitus. Only if patients are still hyperglycemic despite significant weight loss of several weeks or if they are already of normal weight and reasonably physically active, is the use of sulfonylurea drugs justified, and in a high percentage of patients, will prove successful.[19]

One physician who has steadfastly refused to buy into the "treatment of laziness" is Dr. John K. Davidson, whom I have referred to several times in this book. He has been a leader in the campaign to minimize the use of the oral drugs and implement lifestyle programs that encourage weight reduction and other measures to naturally increase insulin sensitivity. Following the publication of the UGDP studies and his careful reading of them, Dr. Davidson, then head of the Diabetes Unit at Grady Memorial Hospital, Emory University Medical School in Atlanta, took 1,500 diabetic patients being seen at the hospital off oral medications. He instituted a policy that staff physicians put greater emphasis on diet and weight control. In addition, he suspended the use of insulin in all patients who were above ideal body weight, using diet and weight control only as therapies for diabetes. Eighteen months later, he found that 60 percent of his patients had experienced no increase in blood sugar levels when the drugs were stopped and diet therapy alone was used.[20]

The Drug Merry-Go-Round

As I reflect on the current recommendations for the treatment of type 2 diabetes, I am struck by the cavalier manner in which physicians approach drug therapy. General recommendations are to begin the patient on sulfonylureas. These drugs usually keep blood sugar levels down for two or three years, then they are *expected* to fail. So the patient is then moved on to metformin, which may work for a while before it too loses its effectiveness. If metformin fails, then the patient might be started on a thiazolidinedione, before being prescribed a two- or three-drug combination. This is not conjecture, folks. According to a long-term, large-scale British study, after three years only half of the study subjects were able to maintain adequate glucose control on one drug. After nine years, three-quarters of them required multiple drugs.[21]

Then there is the plethora of drugs that many patients with type 2 diabetes are prescribed for hypertension, high cholesterol, heart disease, and other manifestations of insulin resistance—and the drugs some patients require to clear up problems caused by their drugs! Drug dependency is a merry-go-round that spins faster and faster as the years go by. The solution? Don't get on it in the first place.

Now that you know the real risks of the drugs used to treat diabetes, I hope you will be motivated to implement the effective natural therapies for reversing diabetes detailed in part III of this book. My wish for you is that you achieve optimal health via the safest route possible.

The Whitaker Wellness Institute Program for Reversing Diabetes

CHAPTER 6

A Diet to Improve Insulin Sensitivity

It is generally accepted by medical professionals that diet is an important therapy for diabetes. However, passively accepting a concept and actively embracing it and stressing its importance to patients are two different things. Virtually all of the diabetic patients who have come to the Whitaker Wellness Institute over the past twenty-two years have been given vague admonitions by their doctors to "eat right." Most have been told to avoid eating too much sugar, and some have been given leaflets from the American Diabetes Association with lists of "exchanges." Few, however, have had a doctor sit down with them and help them understand how powerful dietary changes can be in improving their insulin sensitivity and controlling their diabetes. And virtually none were educated in how to make these changes. At most, they were handed a meal plan and a few recipes and told that if this didn't bring their blood sugar down in a few weeks, they would be started on medication.

Why don't physicians stress the importance of diet in the treatment of diabetes? As we discussed earlier, I believe that there is an inherent bias in the medical profession against nutrition and in favor of using drugs to treat patients. Equally important, I am convinced that most physicians underestimate the determination and willpower of their patients. It is the responsibility of the doctor to stress the urgency of dietary changes and to provide instruction and guidance in how to do so. But it is the responsibility of the patient to actually implement a dietary program. And most doctors seem to have little faith in their patients' ability to do this. "Patients are not compliant with diet recommendations," they claim. "They aren't willing to make the changes required."

This is nonsense. My experience has shown me that if patients are educated about the tremendous impact eating right will have on their diabetes as well as their overall health, they sit up and take notice. If they are truly made aware of the downside of conventional treatment modalities (i.e., drugs and more drugs, which we covered in detail in part II), motivation increases. And if they are given the proper instruction in how to get started and the encouragement to stay on track, they are willing and able to do what it takes.

Is There an Ideal Diet for All Diabetics?

What should you eat if you have diabetes? Well, it depends on whom you ask. Some experts promote a low-carbohydrate diet for diabetics, claiming that all carbohydrates are bad because they increase glucose and insulin levels—and these authorities have the research to back up their claims. Others insist on lots of carbohydrates and very little fat, contending that fat decreases insulin sensitivity. They too are able to cite research that supports their position. Still others call for extra protein, declaring it to have ameliorating effects on diabetes. They also can prove it. The presence of so much contradictory advice about the ideal diet makes things terribly confusing for patients who are serious about utilizing diet as a therapeutic tool for diabetes.

For almost thirty years now I have closely followed the medical literature on how diet affects diabetes, and I'm familiar with the research quoted by all sides. I've also seen fad diets come and go—and some come back for a second round—and I've followed numbers of patients who have jumped from one bandwagon to another. I have observed people who have lived a long, illness-free life eating food that no one on earth could possibly label healthy, and I've also watched patients who rigorously followed an excellent diet and still got sick. If I had to say one thing for certain, it would be that there is no one absolutely perfect diet that fits each and every person. We are all unique, as different in our biochemical makeup as we are in physical appearance and personality.

Although there is no one perfect diet that will affect everyone in exactly the same way, there are some basic principles regarding food and health that are indisputable. In the next two chapters I'm going to tell you about a diet that, in my experience, comes pretty close to being perfect. It takes into consideration the totality of the medical research on diet, diabetes, and insulin resistance, some of it hot off the press, some dating back eighty years. And it works for the majority of patients with diabetes for several reasons.

First, it takes into account how the food we eat affects glucose and insulin levels, and it helps normalize them over the short term and the long term. Second, it isn't too complicated. One of the major complaints of my patients is that they are forever counting calories or figuring out combinations or exchanges or what have you. This food plan is pretty straightforward: selections within broad categories and portion control, yes; obsessing over grams and percentages, no. While there are guidelines for overall dietary composition, and even recommended percentages of fat, protein, and carbohydrate, the focus is on *quality* of food. Third, the food selections are varied and tasty. I don't care how healthy a diet is—if it is too restrictive or doesn't taste good, few people are going to stick with it. And finally, the dietary recommendations I make in these next two chapters don't address only diabetes: They will improve every aspect of your health.

In this chapter, I want to explain the rationale behind my diet for diabetes and why I believe that the *right kinds* of carbohydrates are an excellent therapeutic tool for improving insulin resistance. In the next chapter, we will discuss how protein and fat fit into this picture. Then in part IV we'll get into the "meat" of it, and I'll tell you how you can easily and inexpensively make this health-enhancing diet a part of your life.

What Is the Human Body Designed to Eat?

Most of the degenerative diseases that afflict our population can be traced at least in part to the high-calorie, fatty, processed foods that make up the bulk of the American diet, and diabetes is no different. We have witnessed over the past half century a growing trend in the food industry toward packaged, prepared convenience foods. Few people buy flour and yeast—they purchase packaged bread and other baked goods. They buy fewer fresh foodstuffs and more canned goods and frozen items. Couple that with the enormous popularity of calorie-dense but nutrient-poor fast food, and we've got a nutritional crisis on our hands. Is it any wonder that rates of diabetes and other "lifestyle" diseases are soaring?

Granted, it is human nature to eat what tastes good. Fat tastes good, and animal fat tastes really good. This taste for fat is advantageous when it comes to evolutionary survival, as we discussed in our example of the Pima Indians in chapter 2. Eat up during times of feast, for famine may be just around the corner. Furthermore, our food choices are strongly affected by our culture. Animals for the most part follow strict dietary patterns regardless of where they live and what choices they have. They have instinctual barriers that ordinarily prevent them from eating foods that are not good for them. Humans, on the other hand, have no instinctual controls on their food intake. We learn what is "good" from our culture. Often we develop preferences for foods that are alien to our physiological makeup and decidedly unhealthy.

Since the diet of humans is so diverse and is not instinctively controlled, we can best estimate which food groups best suit human physiology by comparing humans with other mammals whose food patterns are instinctively controlled. In terms of dietary habits, there are three general categories of mammals. Carnivores, such as lions, dogs, and cats, eat meat exclusively. Leaf, grain, and grass eaters include herding animals like cows, horses, and antelopes. Members of the third group, which includes monkeys, gorillas, baboons, and chimpanzees, eat mostly fruit. Figure 6 presents

Meat Eater	Has claws	No pores on skin; perspires through tongue to cool body	Sharp, pointed front teeth to tear flesh	
Grass and Leaf Eater	No claws	Perspires through millions of pores on skin	No sharp, pointed front teeth	
Fruit Eater	No claws	Perspires through millions of pores on skin	No sharp, pointed front teeth	
Human Being	No claws	Perspires through millions of pores on skin	No sharp, pointed front teeth	

Figure 6. Comparison of humans with three types of mammals in terms of diet.
From Parham, B. "What's Wrong with Eating Meat?" Denver: Ananda Marga Publications, 1981. Used by permission.

the basic physiological differences among humans and these three groups of mammals.

This table makes it clear that the human physiology is similar, if not identical, to that of fruit eaters. Our bodies are not designed to handle a lot of meat. While the first humans, without tools or weapons, would have had trouble acquiring much meat, carnivores are ideally suited for such. They have exceptionally strong jaws with sharp, pointed fangs to kill other animals and tear their flesh into chunks that can be swallowed, as these animals do not chew their food, but swallow it whole.

Small salivary glands in the mouth (not needed to predigest grains and fruits)	Acid saliva; no enzyme ptyalin to predigest grains	No flat, back molar teeth to grind food	Much strong hydrochloric acid in stomach to digest tough animal muscle, bone, etc.	Intestinal tract only 3 times body length so rapidly decaying meat can pass out of body quickly
Well-developed salivary glands, needed to predigest grains and fruits	Alkaline saliva; much ptyalin to predigest grains	Flat, back molar teeth to grind food	Stomach acid 20 times less strong than meat eaters	Intestinal tract 10 times body length, leaf and grains do not decay as quickly so can pass more slowly through the body
Well-developed salivary glands, needed to predigest grains and fruits	Alkaline saliva; much ptyalin to predigest grains	Flat, back molar teeth to grind food	Stomach acid 20 times less strong than meat eaters	Intestinal tract 12 times body length, fruits do not decay as rapidly so can pass more slowly through the body
Well-developed salivary glands, needed to predigest grains and fruits	Alkaline saliva; much ptyalin to predigest grains	Flat, back molar teeth to grind food	Stomach acid 20 times less strong than meat eaters	Intestinal tract 12 times body length

The carnivore's mouth and teeth structure are ideally suited for hunting and for defense. A man in the wild without tools is more likely to *be* an animal's dinner than to eat one for dinner. He is more adept at food gathering, and the structure of his mouth and teeth is designed for plant foods that must be chewed well and mixed with the digestive enzymes in his saliva.

There are other significant differences in the digestive systems among these groups. The meat eaters have twenty times the amount of hydrochloric acid in their stomachs as fruit eaters. Protein requires copious amounts of concentrated acid for digestion; plant matter does not. In addition, the intestinal tract of the meat eater is much shorter than that of the fruit eater—about four times the length of his body trunk as measured from the hips to the shoulders. For a meat eater the size of man, with a distance from hips to shoulders measuring about four feet, the intestinal tract would be about sixteen feet long. This relatively short intestinal tract is best suited for meat, which putrefies rapidly. Plant matter, which unlike meat contains fiber, requires significantly more time in the intestines for adequate assimilation. Therefore, the intestinal tract of the fruit eaters is proportionately longer, measuring about twelve times the body trunk length. The human intestinal tract, which measures forty-eight feet in length, fits the proportions of the fruit eaters much more closely than it does those of the meat eaters.

Since lions are not partial to salad, why do we flood our system with meat? It is like putting diesel in the gasoline tank of your car. No one would do that. It is against the design specifications of the machine.

However, that is exactly what we do when we regularly load each meal with meat and other animal proteins.

We will take a closer look at protein and fat in the next chapter, but now let's examine the role of dietary carbohydrates—the foods our body was designed to eat—as a therapy for diabetes and insulin resistance. Keep in mind as you read these two chapters that the prevailing theme is not so much *quantity* of a single dietary component but overall *quality* of the bulk of the foods eaten.

Carbohydrates in the Treatment of Diabetes

No component in the diabetic diet is the subject of as much controversy and confusion as carbohydrates. The pendulum has swung from one side to the other, from blessing this essential dietary constituent to damning it and back again. This stems, I believe, from an erroneous and enduring oversimplification of what carbohydrates really are.

The Evolution of Understanding

Before insulin was discovered in 1921 by two young Canadian physicians, Frederick Banting and Charles Best, there was simply no effective treatment for the type 1 diabetic, whose body does not produce insulin. The patient was usually put on a starvation diet with no carbohydrates at all. The reasoning behind carbohydrate restriction went like this: The basic problem in diabetes is elevated blood glucose; since carbohydrates are broken down into glucose and enter the blood as such, they obviously should be restricted, even eliminated from the diet. However, in the absence of insulin, the result of this restricted diet was invariably rapid weight loss and early death.

After insulin was discovered, patients with severe type 1 diabetes no longer followed the traditional path to emaciation and death, and insulin was rightly heralded as one of this century's greatest breakthroughs. Soon after, astute scientists began to challenge the dogma of carbohydrate restriction. One of the first to report better results with diabetic patients using a higher-carbohydrate, lower-fat diet was Dr. W. D. Samsum, of Santa Barbara, California. In the *Journal of the American Medical Association* on January 16, 1926, he reported how he simply stumbled onto this in the process of treating a patient:

> *Ever since the discovery of insulin by Banting and Best, we have hoped to be able to use better diets.... Our first experiment was instigated, however, to satisfy a discontented patient:*
>
> *A man, aged 51, who, in the past, had been able to do big things in the business world, was admitted to the clinic from Denver, March 9, 1924, with the usual symptoms of a mild diabetes. His weight was normal at 140 pounds (63.5 kg.) net. There were no complications except for a very mild chronic interstitial nephritis, as evidenced by an occasional hyaline cast in the urine. The highly intelligent cooperation of both him and his wife enabled them to learn the diabetic routine rapidly. At the end of*

three weeks, he was discharged from the hospital on a diet containing 120 gm. of carbohydrate, 80 gm. of protein and 195 gm. of fat, totaling 2,555 calories. [The caloric composition of this diet regimen was 19 percent carbohydrate, 13 percent protein, and 68 percent fat.] He was sugar-free, had a normal blood sugar and did not take insulin, nor did we advise its use.

He returned to the clinic October 20, to be carefully checked up, stating frankly that he had gained nothing by the six months of treatment, and that there must be something wrong either with him or with our diet. He had adhered faithfully to the weighed diet prescribed. He had remained constantly sugar-free, and his blood sugar had been normal whenever it had been taken. His weight had remained constant. We felt that he had managed his case as well as it could have been done. For theoretical reasons, we advised the use of a diet with a slightly higher proportion of carbohydrate to fat and small doses of insulin, although his diet then did not contain as much fat as was usually given. He refused, however, to be annoyed with insulin injections and returned home after a stay of seven days.

The patient returned to the clinic November 16, with the intention of staying many months in a warmer climate at a lower altitude, in the hope that a long rest would bring about the desired improvement. In the meantime, although sugar-free, his blood sugar had risen slightly above normal, and on our advice he had reduced the carbohydrate and raised the fat so that his diet contained 80 gm. of carbohydrate, 88 gm. of protein and 207 gm. of fat, totaling 2,535 calories. [13 percent carbohydrate, 14 percent protein, 73 percent fat] This diet brought about no improvement in his blood sugar, and he felt even worse than he did before. On this admission, we again advised the slightly higher carbohydrate diet with small doses of insulin. This he willingly agreed to. We gave him a diet consisting of 119 gm. of carbohydrate, 78 gm. of protein and 200 gm. of fat [18 percent carbohydrate, 12 percent protein, 70 percent fat], totaling 2,588 calories, with 30 units of insulin daily. He reported that on this diet he felt better, and with his approval we planned a radical experiment with a high carbohydrate diet. December 26, we gave him a diet containing 278 gm. of carbohydrate, 85 gm. of protein and 117 gm. of fat [44 percent carbohydrate, 14 percent protein, 42 percent fat], totaling 2,505 calories. Within twenty-four hours, he noticed a change, and eight days later he felt so much better that he left the hospital and returned to work. We found that on this diet, 112 units of insulin was required to keep him sugar-free and with a normal blood sugar. He has written us a letter each month, and again and again has asserted that the diet with insulin has fully restored him to his former pre-diabetic state of mental and physical activity. He has been able to reduce his insulin dosage gradually, and August 16, 1925, still using the same diet, he was taking only 34 units a day.

Dr. Samsum went on to use higher-carbohydrate diets in 150 diabetic patients and found significant improvement in almost all his cases:

> *In many instances, both with insulin and non-insulin patients, we have frequently substituted carbohydrate for fat without the appearance of sugar in the urine in the non-insulin cases or without raising the insulin dosage in the insulin cases... From the patients' standpoint, the most striking advantage gained by the use of these high-carbohydrate diets has been the improvement in physical and mental activity.[1]*

The typical diabetic diet used by many physicians in Dr. Samsum's day was the "Woodyatt formula," which had a caloric composition of 14 percent carbohydrate calories, 7 percent protein calories, and 79 percent fat calories. According to almost all of the experts at that time, the best diet for diabetics consisted of large quantities of animal lard, fatty meats, and high-cholesterol foods, including copious amounts of mayonnaise and egg yolks, while such foods as fruits and vegetables were forbidden. Considering the time when Dr. Samsum was making these changes and observations, his departure from the dogma of the day was remarkable.

Others picked up on this line of research. One was H. P. Himsworth, M.D., an astute clinician from University College Hospital in London, who, as I will describe in the next chapter, conducted studies in which he showed that a high-fat diet could actually *cause* insulin-resistant diabetes. Another was I. M. Rabinowitch, M.D., of Canada's McGill University, who put the high-carbohydrate diet to work in his patients and published numerous articles on its benefits. In 1930, he outlined his departure from the generally accepted methods of the day, stating that "fat-protein diets from which carbohydrates are excluded find no logical place in the present day management of the diabetic."[2]

In 1935, Dr. Rabinowitch summarized his results with fifty diabetic patients who had been followed closely on a high-carbohydrate, low-calorie diet for five years. Twenty-four percent of these patients were successfully withdrawn from insulin, and insulin requirements were reduced in almost all patients who still required it. The patients felt better, had more energy, and noted improvements in quality of life. Dr. Rabinowitch concluded, "I believe that in the data presented here there is incontestable evidence that the high carbohydrate–low calorie diet is more effective in controlling diabetes than all other methods of treatment reported hitherto."[3]

All Carbohydrates Are Not Created Equal

When you read about these studies dating back seventy to eighty years supporting the therapeutic value of carbohydrates in the treatment of diabetes, what do you imagine these diabetics were eating? Bagels, rice cakes, fat-free chips and cookies, and other popular carbohydrate foods we eat today? Don't count on it. There were very few processed and packaged items back then.

Food was pretty much in its natural state in those days. Sure, people ate bread and other things made with flour, and they also included a little sugar in their diet. But other than that, foods that fell into the category of carbohydrates were fiber-rich and nutrient-dense whole grains, vegetables, and fruits.

Jump to the early twenty-first century and what do we eat? White bread, french fries, and all kinds of fat-free products that are loaded with sugar and white flour. The point is that all carbohydrates are not created equal. Candy bars and sodas are primarily carbohydrates. So are apples and beans. Some carbohydrates you shouldn't touch with a ten-foot pole, while others should be the foundation of your diet. To say that carbohydrates shouldn't be eaten, or that a certain percentage of your diet should be carbohydrates, ignores the tremendous differences among carbohydrate foods. What we need, rather than lists or edicts that lump all carbohydrates together, is a realistic look at the quality of the carbohydrates we eat.

Healthy Carbohydrates Contain Fiber

Carbohydrates are found in plants. Meat and eggs contain only protein and fat, and while dairy products do have some carbohydrate, the primary source of this nutrient is plants. One of the unique features of carbohydrate-rich plant foods is dietary fiber, which is the undigestible components of plant cell walls. There are two general types of fiber. Insoluble fiber is the "roughage" found in vegetables and the skins and outer coatings of grains, fruits, and legumes. Soluble fiber, so called because it dissolves or forms a gel-like substance when mixed in water, is abundant in beans, oats, and fruits.

It is hard to believe that the importance of fiber was all but ignored until the early 1970s. Today most people are aware that fiber plays a significant role in health maintenance. (Not that they do anything about it. The average American gets only one-third to one-half of the recommended 30-plus grams of fiber per day!) It is widely recognized not only for its protective role in disorders of the gastrointestinal tract, from constipation to hemorrhoids to colon cancer, but also as an excellent therapy for lowering cholesterol. Adding just 5 to 10 grams of fiber to your daily diet can result in a five-point drop in cholesterol—which translates into a 10 percent reduction in risk of heart disease.

Less well known, however, are fiber's tremendous benefits for diabetics. A high-fiber diet is highly protective against the development of insulin resistance and diabetes. In a 2000 study involving almost 36,000 women living in Iowa, a high intake of whole grains and dietary fiber had a dramatic effect on the risk of developing diabetes. Women consuming the most fiber had a 22 percent decrease in the incidence of diabetes, compared to women with the lowest intake.[4] A study conducted in Great Britain in 1999 was even more impressive. It showed that men and women who year-round frequently ate salad and raw vegetables had an 80 percent lower risk of type 2 diabetes than people who ate vegetables less often.[5]

Fiber is also an excellent therapy for people who

already have diabetes, for this humble dietary component helps maintain glucose control. It delays gastric emptying, or the pace at which food passes through the stomach. This allows a slower rate of absorption of glucose into the bloodstream, which reduces the ups and downs of blood sugar levels. It also improves the body's sensitivity to insulin, combating insulin resistance and helping insulin do its job of ushering glucose into the cells.

One of the earlier studies demonstrating the power of dietary fiber in the treatment of diabetes was conducted by Perla M. Miranda, R.D., M.S., and David L. Horwitz, M.D., Ph.D., F.A.C.P, and published in the *Annals of Internal Medicine* in 1978. Each of eight subjects who had insulin-dependent diabetes consumed either 20 grams of dietary fiber per day in the

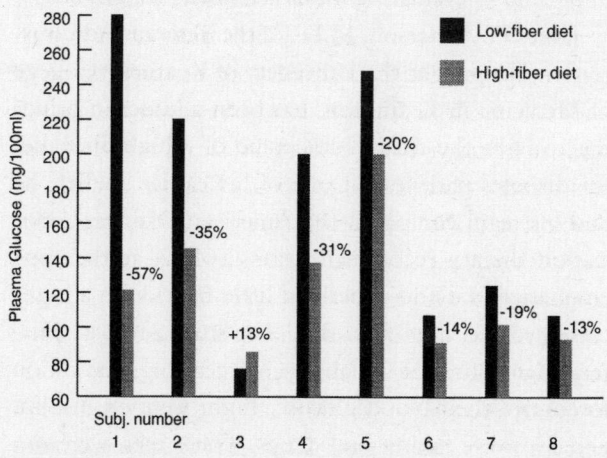

Figure 7. Effects of fiber in type I diabetics.
Used by permission.

form of high-fiber bread or a mere 3 grams of fiber. All other factors of the diet were kept constant, as was the patients' insulin dosage. On the low-fiber intake, the average blood glucose level of the patients was 169.4 mg/dl. During the period of higher fiber intake, the mean blood sugar level was 120.8 mg/dl.

The authors of this study pointed out that several of the subjects had such dramatic declines in their glucose levels when placed on the high-fiber diet that they had to lower their insulin dose. They concluded, "It may no longer be adequate to think in terms of the traditional diabetic 'exchange' lists, where foods may be freely substituted if equal in calories, carbohydrate, fat, and protein. We must also now think of the fiber content of the individual foods. For instance, apple juice contains 0.1 g of fiber per serving; an apple contains close to 10 g of fiber."[6] In a nutshell: Once again, what's most important in evaluating foods is *quality*, not *quantity*.

James W. Anderson, M.D., of the Veterans Administration Hospital at the University of Kentucky College of Medicine in Lexington, has been a leader in bringing to light the therapeutic value of a high-fiber diet for diabetes patients. In one of his earlier studies, he and his team compared the American Diabetes Association dietary recommendations (which at the time emphasized fat and contained little fiber) with a high-carbohydrate, high-fiber diet. The study involved thirteen men with type 2 diabetes, all receiving medication to control their blood glucose. Eight were on insulin, and five were taking oral drugs. These men were not newcomers to diabetes; they had had the condition for an average of eight years.

During the first week these patients were fed an ADA diet that contained 43 percent carbohydrate calories and only 4.7 grams of fiber. They were then shifted to a diet containing 75 percent carbohydrate calories, only 9 percent fat calories, and 14.2 grams of fiber. The results were almost unbelievable. Of the eight who had required insulin injections, four were able to come off insulin, and one reduced his insulin requirement from 28 units to 15. Of the five who had required the oral diabetic medications, all were rendered drug free. And all this occurred with a meager 14 grams of fiber—and in just two weeks![7]

One of the more recent studies examining the impact of a high-fiber diet on type 2 diabetes was published in 2000 in the *New England Journal of Medicine*. Study subjects were divided into a high-fiber group and a low-fiber group, and their fasting blood sugars were periodically tested. The researchers found that blood sugar levels were reduced by about 10 percent in the diabetics consuming the high-fiber diet—an effect equal to that of oral antidiabetic drugs![8]

It is hard to overstate the significance of these studies. In these diabetic patients, simply adding fiber (and in some cases, reducing fat) allowed many of them to discontinue their drugs. This suggests that of the millions of diabetics in the country who are taking some kind of diabetic medication, given the proper diet, a significant percentage of them could become drug free.

Whole Plant Foods Are Nutrient-Rich

In chapter 9 we will focus on specific nutrients that are beneficial for individuals with diabetes. Guess where most of these essential nutrients are found? In plant foods! This abundance of vitamins, minerals, essential fatty acids, and phytochemicals is yet another reason why carbohydrate-rich plant foods should form the foundation of a healthy diet. Certain fruits, vegetables, and grains contain large amounts of antioxidants, nature's antidote to harmful free radicals. Low blood levels of antioxidants are associated with an increased risk of virtually every degenerative disease, including diabetes and especially its complications. Protective B-complex vitamins are also abundant in plant foods, particularly in nuts, beans, and whole grains, as are minerals important for the diabetic, such as magnesium, chromium, and vanadium. Essential fatty acids, which improve insulin sensitivity and protect against the complications of diabetes, are also found in plant foods. In the chart below, you can see the most concentrated food sources of these important nutrients.

Nutrient-Dense Foods for Diabetes

Beans and legumes	Magnesium, zinc, B-complex vitamins
Whole grains	Magnesium, chromium, vitamin E, B-complex vitamins
Leafy greens	Magnesium, calcium, vitamin A, B-complex vitamins, carotenoids
Orange/yellow fruits and vegetables	Vitamin C, vitamin A, beta-carotene
Citrus fruits	Vitamin C

Peppers	Vitamin C, vitamin A
Broccoli and other cruciferous vegetables	Vitamin C, vitamin A
Raw nuts and seeds	Calcium, magnesium, zinc, B-complex vitamins, vitamin E

Simple Versus Complex, or High Versus Low?

The primary dietary guideline I formerly gave my patients was to eat complex carbohydrates and avoid simple sugars. Back in the good old days, it was generally accepted that there are two basic types of carbohydrates, simple and complex. Simple carbohydrates are one- or two-molecule sugars that are quickly broken down into glucose, enter the bloodstream rapidly, and cause a fast rise in blood glucose, accompanied by a rise in insulin. Foods in this group include not only sugars of every kind but also grain-based products that have been processed and stripped of their fiber, such as white flour, white rice, and many cereals.

Complex carbohydrates, which include whole grains, beans and legumes, vegetables, and fruits, are made up of many sugar molecules bonded or chained together. Their sugars are released more slowly into the bloodstream, a process made slower still by the fiber in these foods, and they cause a gradual, more sustained rise in blood sugar.

However, research carried out over the past twenty years by David Jenkins, M.D., and colleagues at the

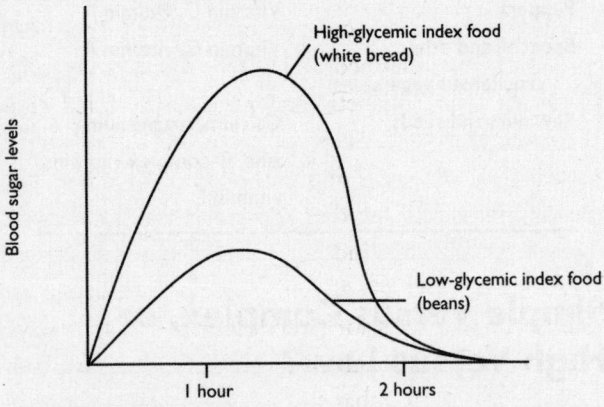

Figure 8. Comparison of glucose levels after eating high- and low-glycemic-index foods.

University of Toronto has added a twist to the simple/complex carbohydrates concept: the glycemic index. It is a way of evaluating foods according to how quickly they are metabolized into glucose. The glycemic index is based on the blood glucose elevation caused by eating a specific quantity of either glucose or white bread. (Many of the more recent indexes use white bread, since it is a commonly eaten food.) Foods with a high glycemic index enter the bloodstream rapidly, causing a spike in glucose followed by a similarly abrupt rise in insulin, while low-glycemic foods promote a more gradual release of glucose and insulin. This obviously has particular significance for patients with diabetes and insulin resistance.

The therapeutic effects of a low-glycemic-index diet for people with type 1 and type 2 diabetes have been demonstrated in a number of studies. Blood sugar levels are easier to control when patients adhere to such a diet, and improvements in markers of both short-term and long-term control have been reported. A low-glycemic diet improves diabetic complications as well. In a 1999 Swedish study published in *Diabetes Care*, two groups of twenty type 2 diabetic patients each were fed diets that were identical in proportions of carbohydrate, protein, and fat, and amount of fiber, but had one major difference: One diet contained foods that were low on the glycemic index, while the other was based on foods with a high glycemic index. Each group ate one of the two diets for twenty-four consecutive days, then switched to the other diet. At the end of the study period, it was found that those diabetic individuals eating a low-glycemic-index diet had lower LDL cholesterol levels and a decrease in PAI-1 activity (a measure of blood clotting discussed in chapter 2), resulting in a decreased risk of heart disease. This study suggests that eating foods with a low glycemic index may be an excellent therapy for insulin resistance and diabetes.[9]

Figuring out where foods fall on the glycemic index is to some extent intuitive. Generally speaking, it is easy to figure out, because most of the carbohydrates we think of as complex have a low glycemic index value, and most simple sugars have quite high values. Products that contain a lot of sugar and white flour obviously have a high glycemic index and should thus be avoided. The majority of vegetables and fruits have a low glycemic index and are excellent choices. However, there are a few surprises. Some complex carbohydrates behave more like simple sugars, with a quick release of glucose, and vice versa. For example, most of the foods we think of as starchy, such as potatoes, have a moderate to high glycemic index—even though they are complex carbohydrates. I will provide detailed lists of recommended foods with low to moderate glycemic indexes in part IV, but for now, let me give you an overview of where some common foods fall on the glycemic index.

The Glycemic Index of Common Foods

Low	Moderate	High
(recommended in abundance)	(recommended in moderation)	(not recommended for diabetes or insulin resistance)
Green vegetables	Stone-ground whole wheat bread	Bagels
Tomatoes		White bread
Beans and peas		Rice cakes
Pasta	Rye crackers	Pretzels
Apples	Brown rice	Most cold cereals
Berries	Sweet potatoes	White rice
Citrus fruit	Grapes	White potatoes
Oatmeal	New potatoes	Pineapple
100% bran cereal	Whole wheat tortillas	Dates
Sprouted grain bread	Kiwi	Ripe bananas

Refined Sugar and Flour: Dietary Disasters

As I have made clear in this chapter, I am a big fan of carbohydrate-dense plant foods. But what happens when you take these vital, life-sustaining foods and process them? You strip them of their beneficial fiber and rob them of vitamins and minerals. This is what occurs when white flour is milled from whole wheat, when high-fructose corn sweeteners are made from corn, and when sugar is refined from sugar beets.

One of the most unhealthy components of the American diet is white flour, yet we eat it like there is no tomorrow. The average American may eat toast, pancakes, or bagels for breakfast, a sandwich or hamburger for lunch, and rolls with dinner. That adds up to a whole lot of refined, processed, fiberless white flour with a very high glycemic index that shoots up glucose levels. Furthermore, many of the flour-based foods we eat, such as cookies, cakes, and pastries, also contain sugar.

Sugar is another dietary disaster, and one that we eat way too much of. When George Washington was alive, Americans consumed about 20 pounds of sugar a year. Today we are approaching 150 pounds, which is what I would call one large sweet tooth. In addition to causing dental caries (cavities), depressing the immune system, and providing a lot of empty calories that contribute to weight gain, sugar has other detrimental effects, especially for diabetics.

Excessive consumption of sugar has recently been identified by some researchers as the single most important dietary risk factor for heart disease in women. According to a study published in the *Journal of Orthomolecular Medicine*, sugar also poses a similar risk in men, albeit less significant than animal fat. Researcher William Grant, author of this study, estimates that sugar intake may account for more than 150,000 premature deaths from heart disease in the U.S. each year.[10] Given the close association between diabetes and heart disease, diabetics should sit up and take note.

Consuming large quantities of readily absorbed carbohydrates such as sugar also stresses your body's blood sugar control mechanisms, causing sharp rises in glucose and insulin, followed by precipitous drops. Furthermore, some studies show a link between high sugar intake and chromium loss, which may also contribute to insulin resistance and diabetes. That's a steep price to pay for a food that is devoid of everything but calories—particularly when you eat sugary, processed foods at the expense of whole natural foods.

Many of my patients tell me that they eat no sugar, that their sugar bowl is a relic of the past. But even if you don't add sugar to your food, you are likely eating more than you think, for most of the sugar we eat is hidden in processed and prepared foods. This isn't always readily evident by reading food labels. Manufacturers add sugar in different forms to make their products appear to have less sugar than they actually do, so you have to read between the lines to discover what is really in the foods you're eating. Common names of added sweeteners include sucrose; dextrose; fructose; lactose; high-fructose corn syrup; corn, rice, and barley malt syrups; maple syrup or solids; fruit juice concentrates; mannitol; and sorbitol.

You might think that replacing white sugar with honey, molasses, and other "healthy" sweeteners is the way to go. Unfortunately, just like refined white sugar, almost all natural sweeteners have a high glycemic index and provoke a sharp glucose release. The one "natural" sweetener that is low on the glycemic index is fructose. However, fructose poses problems of its own, especially for diabetics. It is a primary culprit in glycosylation, the chemical binding of sugars to proteins, which, as I explained in the first chapter, is one of the mechanisms behind the cascade of complications in diabetes.

Fructose is a highly reactive molecule that readily attaches to proteins, changing their structure and interfering with their normal activity. Studies show that fructose accelerates glycosylation, damaging proteins to a significantly greater degree than sucrose or glucose.[11] Yet we consume this harmful sweetener like it is going out of style. In a highly processed form (high-fructose corn syrup), it is the primary ingredient in soft drinks, sales of which have gone through the roof in recent years. More than 25 percent of the beverages Americans consume are sodas. In 1997 Americans purchased 14 billion gallons of "liquid candy"—more than 576 12-ounce servings per person per year![12] Fructose is one sweetener that I recommend diabetics stay away from.

What about artificial sweeteners, such as aspartame (NutraSweet and Equal)? While it is true that aspartame does not alter blood glucose levels, I recommend that you avoid this chemical additive like the plague. It is broken down in the body into harmful components, including formaldehyde (a known toxin and carcinogen), formic acid (the poison in ant stings), and methanol (a nervous system toxin also known as free methyl alcohol or wood alcohol). In addition, the two amino acids that comprise aspartame, phenyl-alanine and aspartic acid, can bypass the blood-brain barrier and enter the brain, upsetting the balance of neurotransmitters and brain chemistry. High intake of aspartame has been linked with a number of adverse effects, including headache, vision loss, seizures, mood disorders, and other nervous system problems.

I recommend approaching other artificial sweeteners with caution as well. Saccharin, the oldest of the noncaloric sweeteners, has been linked to tumors of the bladder—although in 2000 the FDA removed saccharin from its official list of substances that may cause cancer. Acesulfame K (Sunette or Sweet One), the sweetener in Pepsi One, has been sold as a sugar substitute since 1988 and is growing in popularity. According to the Washington, D.C.–based Center for Science in the Public Interest, however, the FDA approval process for acesulfame K was inadequate. Questions remain regarding the potential of this additive to cause cancer, as it has been shown to be carcinogenic in animals.[13] Sucralose (Splenda), which is derived from sucrose, is growing in popularity because it doesn't have the aftertaste that many artificial sweeteners have. Yet it is not without problems. The most significant one for diabetics is that, although it does not affect blood sugar levels, in one small study it raised levels of HbA_{1c}. This suggests that it may worsen the diabetic condition. Until all safety questions are cleared up, stay away from sucralose.

Skip the sugar *and* the artificial sweeteners and try the sweeteners we use at the Whitaker Wellness Institute: stevia and xylitol. Stevia is extracted from an herb native to South America, where it is known as "honey leaf." Intensely sweet, a few drops of a liquid extract or a dusting of stevia powder provide adequate sweetening for a cup of tea or a bowl of cereal. Xylitol is a unique sweetener obtained from birch trees that essentially looks and tastes like white granulated sugar. Unlike stevia, xylitol is not calorie free. However, it has been demonstrated in repeated clinical studies to be very slowly metabolized. Therefore, it causes none of the abrupt rises and falls you get with other sweeteners. In addition, this unique sweetener has been studied for its ability to prevent dental caries: Over time, chewing xylitol-sweetened gum can change the bacterial makeup in the mouth and eliminate cavity-causing pathogens. Xylitol is also being studied for its ability to prevent ear infections in children. (Sorbitol and mannitol, which are in some ways similar to xylitol, are often found in many sugar-free or dietetic candies and food. The primary problem with these sweeteners is that they can cause diarrhea when consumed in large amounts. In some people, children in particular, even small amounts of sorbitol and mannitol may cause loose stools.) We'll discuss healthy sweeteners in greater detail in part IV.

Can Diabetics Drink Alcohol?

For more than twenty years we've known that people who drink moderate amounts of wine, beer, and spirits have increased levels of protective HDL cholesterol and a reduced risk of heart attack.[14] However, because alcoholic drinks contain a fair amount of calories derived from sugars, it used to be recommended that diabetics avoid alcohol. We now know that rather than worsening the diabetic condition, judicious use of alcohol actually improves insulin sensitivity. In one study published in *Diabetes Care*,

Dr. Gerald Reaven and colleagues at Stanford University enlisted twenty men and women who drank light to moderate amounts of alcohol and twenty others who did not drink at all. Measurements were taken of their glucose and insulin levels, as well as their HDL cholesterol. The "social" drinkers scored better in all areas.[15]

Alcohol is a double-edged sword. The majority of people who drink do so in moderation and clearly derive benefits from it. While I would never recommend that anyone start drinking alcohol for their health, if you are currently drinking modest amounts of alcohol, there is no harm in continuing as long as you don't exceed moderate intake: one drink for women and two drinks for men per day. (One drink equals a 12-ounce beer, a 5-ounce glass of wine, or a shot—1½ ounces—of hard liquor.) Be aware, however, that habitual abuse of alcohol affects roughly 10 percent of the drinking population and requires treatment.

This has been a rather exhaustive review of the pros and cons of carbohydrates in the diabetic diet. The bottom line is that the bulk of vegetables, fruits, grains, beans, legumes, nuts, and seeds in their natural and unprocessed state are an excellent foundation for a therapeutic diet aimed at improving insulin sensitivity and treating diabetes. Refined sugars, white flour, and other processed foods, as well as the few natural plant foods that have a high glycemic index rating, should be avoided.

In the next chapter we will look at the other two major dietary components, protein and fat, and see how they fit into the picture.

CHAPTER 7

The Diabetic Diet: Where Do Protein and Fat Fit In?

The high-protein, high-fat animal foods that make up a significant portion of the typical diet eaten in this country are not keeping us healthy. More than half of all Americans are overweight, and we are suffering in record numbers from degenerative diseases such as diabetes, heart disease, and hypertension that are caused in part by what we eat.

As I made clear in the previous chapter, the human body is engineered to eat plant foods: clean-burning, fiber-rich carbohydrates. Moderate amounts of lean protein and healthy fats are fine, but the degree to which we indulge in high-fat animal protein is just plain wrong for our systems. Let's continue our discussion of the therapeutic diet for diabetes and see precisely where and how protein and fat fit in.

Protein: A Little Dab'll Do You

Protein is one of the most important nutrients required by your body. It is necessary for the construction of muscles, hair and nails, nerves, skin, and internal organs. Protein and its component amino acids provide the building blocks for enzymes, hormones, neurotransmitters, blood plasma, sperm, and saliva. They are essential for growth and tissue repair and act as a carrier of important components in the blood. Adequate dietary protein is essential. However, too much can be harmful, especially for patients with diabetes. Let's take a close look at some of the protein propaganda—specifically, the unfounded claims made by the proponents of a high-protein diet.

How Much Protein Do We Really Need?

The idea that we need huge amounts of protein goes back to the mid-1800s. Carl Voit, a prominent German scientist, observed the dietary habits of German workers who were eating a meat-based diet and calculated that they took in an average of 120 grams of protein per day. Because he considered these men to be in good health, Dr. Voit concluded that the optimum protein intake for humans was 120 grams per day.

Justus von Leibig, another well-known German researcher, made what seems even today to be a reasonable assumption: Muscle strength depends on the amount of protein ingested. Drs. Voit and von Leibig were highly respected in their time, but we now know that their assumptions about the protein needs for humans were just plain wrong. Nevertheless, their ideas have held sway ever since. The mistakes of the great are far more damaging than the mutterings of the multitudes.

True scientific evaluation of protein requirements has been carried out in the intervening years, with many of the studies looking at what is known as *nitrogen balance*. In a healthy individual eating an appropriate amount of protein, the amount of nitrogen ingested (protein is about 16 percent nitrogen) equals the amount that is excreted in the urine and feces. When protein breakdown and excretion exceed intake—an unhealthy state associated with stress, injury, illness, or inadequate protein consumption—the body is in negative nitrogen balance. On the other hand, when a person is in positive nitrogen balance, he or she is taking in more protein than is excreted. This would be expected during pregnancy and the growth spurts of childhood or following an illness. Nitrogen balance can also be used to accurately assess protein requirements.

Such measurements have become more and more sophisticated over the years, and we now know that the amount of protein needed for optimum health is quite small. The consensus among international experts, including those representing the World Health Organization, is that the human body requires 0.5–0.8 grams of high-quality protein per kilogram (g/kg) of body weight. For a 150-pound person this equals 35–55 grams of protein per day. Some experts recommend even less. Dr. W. C. Rose of the University of Illinois found that 20 grams of high-quality protein would sustain an adult in good nitrogen balance if all other aspects of his diet were adequate.[1]

However, in this land of plenty, we eat considerably more protein than we need—an average of 70–120 grams per day. And the folks promoting protein power seem to suggest that the sky's the limit. This is a mistake, for excess protein intake may lead to several problems.

Excessive Protein Is Hard on the Kidneys

When we eat too much carbohydrate or fat, the body stores this extra energy as fat. While this may be unsightly and unhealthy, it is not as damaging to the body as excessive protein. The body cannot store excessive protein. It must be broken down, and its waste products must be excreted by the kidneys. When we consistently eat 300 to 400 percent more protein than we need, tremendous stress is placed upon the body, and particularly the kidneys. As John M. Hindhede, a Danish physiologist of the late nineteenth century, pointed out, there is a fundamental incompatibility between the design of the human kidney and the amount of protein it is called upon to process from the typical Western diet.

For patients with diabetes, this incompatibility is of particular concern because the diabetic condition itself stresses the kidneys, making them even more vulnerable to disease and degeneration. Excess glucose in the bloodstream damages the small blood vessels in the kidneys, which impairs the filtering process and may ultimately lead to complete kidney failure. Diabetics rarely die from elevated blood sugar levels. Instead, they have to contend with long-term complications of their condition, and one of the most serious is kidney failure. *Diabetes is the number one cause of kidney failure.* It accounts for the majority of patients receiving dialysis as well as most recipients of kidney transplants.

Kidney function can be accurately assessed by measuring the amount of protein breakdown products found in the blood and urine. Blood levels of urea nitrogen (BUN) and creatinine rise when the kidneys are failing. Another, more accurate test for kidney damage is the creatinine clearance test, in which the amount of creatinine excreted in the urine over 24 hours is measured. The BUN blood test can be confounded by several factors: If you are dehydrated or have been eating a lot of protein, the BUN level can rise; if you've been drinking a lot of water, it can fall. Creatinine, on the other hand, is not affected by these variables and is thus a more accurate measure of kidney function. When the level of creatinine in the urine goes up, you know that kidney damage is under way.

Diabetic patients with slightly elevated creatinine levels are usually told that sometime down the line they will need dialysis, and sure enough, a few years later they do. At that time, they are put on a very low-protein diet. When you are on dialysis, the more protein you eat, the more frequently you require the machine. A steak dinner can land such a patient in the hospital.

However, diabetic patients are rarely told to reduce their protein intake *before* kidney failure becomes a reality. Kidney damage does not happen overnight. Red flags appear early on, in plenty of time to change its course by restricting protein intake. One of the very first signs of kidney damage is the presence of a protein called albumin in the urine, and the best time to take action to protect the kidneys is when it first appears. By the time creatinine levels climb, kidney damage has already begun. By failing to jump on a low-protein diet at the first sign of kidney damage, the patient misses the opportunity to slow it down or, in some cases, to stop it altogether.

The therapeutic value of a low-protein diet in the treatment of kidney disease is undisputed. William E. Mitch, M.D., of Harvard Medical Center, and Mackenzie Walser, M.D., of Johns Hopkins University, examined the effects of a very low-protein diet on the progression of kidney failure in seventeen patients. These patients had kidney problems arising from a variety of causes (four from diabetes), and all were progressing toward complete kidney failure. They were placed on a very low-protein, primarily vegetarian diet with supplements of some amino acids. This regimen slowed the rate of kidney destruction in ten patients and stopped it altogether in seven in whom it had not already progressed too far. The researchers concluded that early detection followed by a change in diet could result in a delay in progression for large numbers of patients and substantially reduce the need for dialysis.[2]

Some experts recommend a daily protein intake of 0.55 grams per kilogram of body weight for patients with compromised kidney function. This diet, which is labeled a "low-protein diet" for such patients, falls within the international recommendations for protein intake for all adults! In other words, the protein intake that is being recommended as a *therapy* for a serious illness is in reality what we should *all* be eating.

The recipes and meals in part IV of this book will help you develop a low-protein diet that would be well suited for you if you have any evidence of kidney dysfunction. But the mere fact that you have diabetes is reason enough to reduce your protein intake to protect your kidneys and lessen the likelihood of problems down the road.

A High-Protein Diet Is a Primary Cause of Osteoporosis

Your kidneys are not the only organs threatened by excess protein consumption. Excessive intake of protein-rich foods—including dairy products—also contributes to osteoporosis, or thinning of the bones. I know this goes against everything you've ever been told, but bear with me as I explain.

As I mentioned above, our bodies have no way of storing the extra protein we take in. Instead it is broken down to urea, creatinine, and uric acid, which are eliminated through the kidneys. These breakdown products create an acidic condition in the blood. The body tolerates only very narrow changes in pH (acid-alkaline balance), so to return the blood to its optimal pH, it calls on an alkalinizing agent. The most readily available of these agents is calcium, which is stored in the bones. When you eat excess protein, calcium is literally leached from your bones. Unfortunately, once the body brings blood pH back into balance, calcium is not returned to the bones. Instead it is excreted in the urine, along with the protein breakdown products. So you can see how a high-protein diet can gnaw away at your bones over the course of a lifetime.

Nancy E. Johnson, of the Department of Nutritional Sciences at the University of Wisconsin in Madison, explored the effects of a high-protein diet on calcium loss by measuring calcium balance. This is determined by comparing the amount of calcium taken in to the amount lost either by lack of absorption or by urinary excretion. She found that a high-protein diet would put healthy young men in negative calcium balance even if they were taking in more calcium than the Recommended Dietary Allowance (RDA). She gave her study subjects 1400 milligrams of calcium daily, while placing them on either a low-protein diet (48 grams) or a high-protein diet (141 grams).

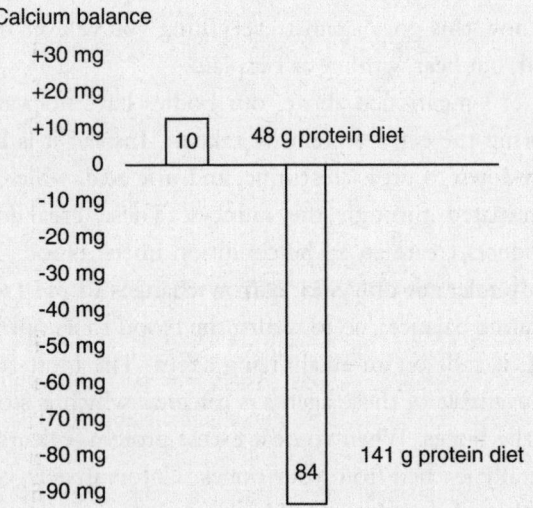

Figure 9. A high-protein diet promotes calcium loss.

On the low-protein diet, the young men were in positive calcium balance. They retained 10 milligrams of calcium per day to be deposited into their bones, increasing their strength. On the high-protein diet, all the subjects were in negative calcium balance, losing on the average 84 milligrams per day. This means not only that all of the calcium they ingested was lost (1400 milligrams), but also that an additional 84 milligrams of calcium was taken from their bones and lost as well![3]

What is interesting about this study is that increasing calcium intake did not diminish the negative effects of protein on calcium balance. On the high-protein diet, a negative calcium balance of minus 84 milligrams per day occurred, despite the high calcium consumption of 1400 milligrams. Osteoporosis is epidemic in this country, and there are constant warnings that we should consume lots of calcium. However, what is important is not how much calcium we consume daily but how much we are able to deposit into our bones. This study and others like it suggest that in the presence of our high-protein diet, such deposits are not being made.

The Lowdown on Protein

In summary, our ingrained belief that more is better when it comes to protein just isn't true. The amount of protein I recommend to my patients is about 20 percent of total calories, again emphasizing quality over quantity. Lean animal protein, particularly poultry, fish, egg whites, and reduced-fat dairy products, is a useful addition to a therapeutic diet for treating diabetes. Beans, whole grains, and "meat substitutes" made primarily from soybeans are excellent plant sources of protein. Although most plant proteins, unlike animal proteins, do not contain all of the essential amino acids (those your body cannot produce on its own), as long as you eat a varied diet that includes both legumes and grains, it doesn't matter whether or not specific foods are "complete" proteins. With a little awareness, even strict vegetarians are perfectly able to obtain adequate and balanced protein.

The Skinny on Fat

Fat is an essential nutrient with multiple roles in the body. It cushions and insulates our organs, is an integral component of cellular membranes, and serves as the precursor to important messenger molecules called prostaglandins. Fat is a primary fuel for many of our body's cells, and it provides us with a source of stored energy. But it is also what pads our hips, dimples our thighs, and protrudes from our bellies.

In addition, fat is intimately related to diabetes. As we discussed in part I, around 90 percent of all type 2 diabetics are overweight, and diabetes is rare in cultures that consume little fat in their diets. Excess fat—in the tissues, in the bloodstream, and in the diet—is an underlying cause of insulin resistance and type 2 diabetes. It elevates levels of free fatty acids in the blood, and this continual exposure to excessive fat takes its toll on the organs involved in blood sugar regulation.

Fat can hurt the body in numerous ways. First, it interferes with the proper functioning of the beta cells of the pancreas. Under its influence, they don't seem to get the message to increase insulin production after a meal, when glucose levels rise and insulin is needed most. Second, it contributes to insulin resistance of the muscle cells, reducing the ability of insulin to move glucose into the cells. Third, it prompts the liver to spew out excessive amounts of stored glucose, raising glucose levels yet higher. Furthermore, many diabetics share another common problem. Whereas under normal circumstances fatty acids are released from the fat cells only in the absence of glucose and insulin, the fat cells of type 2 diabetics tend to release large amounts of free fatty acids into the blood at inappropriate times. After a meal, free fatty acid levels should come right down; in diabetics they do not. These consistently high levels of free fatty acids result in further interference with blood sugar metabolism—and pose a significant risk for heart disease and other conditions as well.

This is why I believe a low-fat diet is crucial for the prevention and treatment of diabetes. However, as with carbohydrates, quality is the issue: Some fats are good, some are not so good, and some are simply terrible. Let's take a close look at the different types of fat and see where and how they fit into a diet aimed at increasing insulin sensitivity and reducing the risk of diabetic complications.

Fat and Insulin Sensitivity

For many years the prevailing belief in medicine was that fats were the preferred foods for diabetics, and carbohydrates were off limits. This belief actually makes sense on one level. Carbohydrates are broken down into glucose and cause a rise in blood sugar. And while both protein and carbohydrates stimulate the release of insulin, dietary fat does not.

One of the first clinicians to challenge this belief was H. P. Himsworth, M.D., of the University College Hospital in London. He published several articles in the early 1930s demonstrating that rather than improving glucose control, a high-fat diet could actually bring on marked glucose intolerance (pre-diabetes), even in a normal individual. Furthermore, the condition could be reversed by switching the patient to a carbohydrate-rich diet.

Dr. Himsworth gave volunteers in this experiment one of seven different diets. (Figure 10 shows the diets and figure 11 shows the blood sugar fluctuations.) Diet No. 1 was a very high-fat, low-carbohydrate diet with 240 grams of fat (2160 calories, 80 percent of total), 80 grams of protein (320 calories, 12 percent), and only 50 grams of carbohydrates (200 calories, or 8 percent of total calories). This diet was almost identical in composition to the diet used in treating diabetic patients during Dr. Himsworth's time. He found that individuals who consumed this diet for a week before taking the glucose tolerance test would have positive results on the test, indicating the presence of impaired glucose tolerance. He then began replacing the fat with carbohydrate and found that with each increase in carbohydrate at the expense of fat, the diabetic condition as shown by the glucose tolerance test improved.[4]

Dr. Himsworth's work should be required reading for all physicians who treat patients with diabetes,

Diet No.	Carbohydrate calories	Protein calories	Fat calories	Total
1	200	320	2160	2680
2	500	320	1860	2680
3	800	320	1560	2680
4	1100	320	1260	2680
5	1400	320	960	2680
6	1700	320	660	2680
7	2000	320	360	2680

Figure 10. Caloric composition of diets used in Himsworth's experiment.
Himsworth, HR. "The Dietetic Factor Determining the Glucose Tolerance and Sensitivity to Insulin of Healthy Men." *Clinical Science* 2: 67–94, 1935.

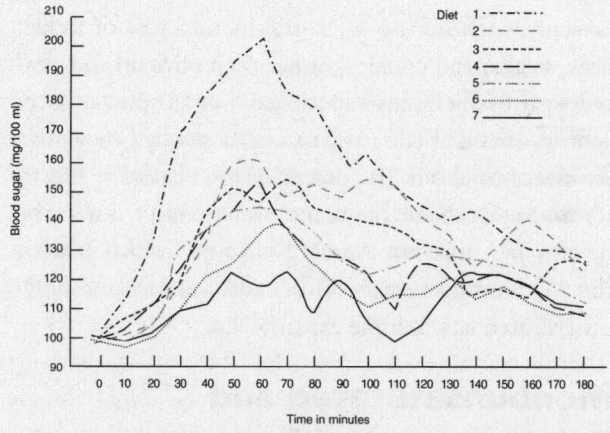

Figure 11. The seven glucose curves produced in one subject as a result of seven diets with differing proportions of carbohydrate and fat.
Himsworth, HR. "The Dietetic Factor Determining the Glucose Tolerance and Sensitivity to Insulin of Healthy Men." *Clinical Science* 2: 67–94, 1935.

for, seventy years later, some of the popular diet gurus continue to urge a high-fat diet to control diabetes and insulin resistance. I simply cannot endorse these best-selling diets that severely restrict carbohydrates and allow unlimited fat. There is just too much research on the harmful effects of certain fats to condone a no-holds-barred high-fat diet for the treatment of diabetes—or any medical condition, for that matter.

This is not to say that you should avoid fat—you just need to eat the right types of fat. Mediterranean populations, which have among the lowest rates of heart disease and the longest life spans of any in the world, thrive on a diet that contains up to 40 percent fat. If you carefully control the types of fats you eat, then consumption of this much fat might be acceptable. Unfortunately, such license often results in a diet of french fries, steaks, and cookies, rather than olive oil and avocados. It has been my experience over the past quarter century that diabetic patients fare best when they limit fat intake to about 20 percent of total calories. But to return to our theme of quality over quantity, it must be healthy fat: monounsaturated olive oil (which is what the Mediterranean people eat) and unprocessed polyunsaturated fats. Let me explain why.

Monounsaturated and Polyunsaturated Fats: A Boon for Good Health

The most important of all dietary fats are the polyunsaturated fats, for among their ranks are the essential fatty acids (EFAs), which are crucial for optimal health.

From these vital fats, which cannot be produced in the body and must be obtained through food or supplements, the body is able to synthesize every other type of fat it needs. EFAs have a number of important functions that are particularly valuable to diabetics. They facilitate the burning of free fatty acids in the liver, which enhances weight loss. In addition, they are a key component of the structure of healthy cellular membranes. As you know, insulin resistance is largely an issue of disruptions in cellular communication. Insulin binds to receptor sites on the surface of the cell, but the message to open up and let glucose in isn't getting through. It is easy to see how keeping cellular membranes as healthy and fluid as possible by making sure you get adequate EFAs may improve the diabetic condition.

We will explore EFAs in greater detail in the chapter on nutritional supplements, chapter 9. For the purposes of this discussion on dietary fats, the important thing for you to understand is that there are two types of EFAs, omega-3 fatty acids and omega-6 fatty acids, and that optimal health requires a balance between the two. Unfortunately, achieving this balance isn't so easy. Omega-3 EFAs are found in few foods that Americans eat regularly—the best sources are fatty fish like salmon, mackerel, and sardines, and flaxseed. Omega-6 EFAs, on the other hand, are easily obtained, as they are present in commonly eaten vegetable oils, nuts, and seeds. You can see how the balance between these two types of fat might tilt toward the omega-6s. And for most Americans, tilt it does. While many experts consider the ideal ratio between omega-6 and omega-3 fatty acids to be 1:1 or 2:1, the current ratio for the average American is 20:1 or 30:1!

Make a concerted effort to increase your consumption of omega-3 EFAs by eating salmon, mackerel, sardines, and other cold-water fish several times a week. Use flax-seed oil in salad dressings and other recipes that do not require heating of the oil. (EFAs are quite fragile and are easily damaged by heat.) Another way to add omega-3s to your diet is to grind whole flaxseed, which is available in most health food stores, in a coffee grinder. Then sprinkle these nutty-tasting seeds on your cereal or salad, or mix them in a drink. This is one of my favorite ways of ensuring adequate omega-3 consumption, because in addition to EFAs, flaxseed contains an abundance of healthful fiber. To get the benefits of the omega-6 fatty acids, make sure the vegetable oils, nuts, and seeds you eat are in their natural state. Select unrefined, expeller-pressed oils you'll find in your health food store, and eat your nuts and seeds raw rather than roasted. Exposure to heat, light, and even oxygen damages these fragile oils and reduces their beneficial properties.

Another type of fat that merits a place in a diet for reversing diabetes is monounsaturated fat. Though this type of fat, which is abundant in olive, canola, peanut, and almond oils, does not contain the essential fatty acids found in polyunsaturated oils, it is still among the healthiest fats you can eat. Monounsaturated fats are particularly protective against heart disease, which is a real concern for people with diabetes. They keep arteries flexible and have been demonstrated to help lower blood pressure.

One of the best properties of monounsaturated fats

is their stability. Unlike polyunsaturated fats, they can withstand heat without breaking down into harmful substances, so they are a superior choice for cooking. The king of the monos is olive oil, for its extraction and processing do not call for the harsh methods that hard seeds and nuts require. I highly recommend olive oil for cooking, but it should not be used exclusively in place of EFA-rich polyunsaturated fats.

Saturated, Hydrogenated, and Trans Fatty Acids

Unlike polyunsaturated and monounsaturated oils, saturated fat is solid at room temperature. It is the fat that marbles prime rib and the hard white grease that's left in the pan after you cook hamburgers. Red meat is the most abundant source of saturated fat in the American diet, although it is also found in egg yolks, butter, cheese, and other whole-fat dairy products, as well as in tropical oils such as palm and coconut. Saturated fat raises levels of LDL cholesterol and increases heart disease risk. It is also associated with cancers of the lung, colon, rectum, breast, prostate, and endometrium.

Although saturated fat should not be a mainstay of your diet, an occasional egg yolk, a small serving of lean meat, or a little cheese is perfectly acceptable. People have been eating these sources of saturated fats for thousands of years. I'm more concerned about trans fatty acids, for they are like nothing Mother Nature has ever seen before. These chemically altered fats are cropping up everywhere: in margarine, hydrogenated oils, peanut butter, baked goods, and fried foods. Recent research suggests that trans fatty acids are even more harmful than saturated fats. They increase the risk of heart disease to a greater degree than saturated fats, for in addition to raising total cholesterol, they lower protective HDL cholesterol. They also have been implicated in cancer of the breast and prostate, diabetes, immune dysfunction, and infertility. Drs. Walter Willett and Alberto Ascherio of the Harvard School of Public Health have estimated that 30,000 premature deaths every year are attributable to our consumption of trans fats.[5] The good news about these harmful fats is that they are very easy to avoid. Select whole and natural foods over prepared, fried, and processed and you will escape these highly damaging fats.

What About the ADA Diet?

Most diabetics at one time or another have followed the diet recommendations offered by the American Diabetes Association (ADA). Just the mention of "exchanges" or an "exchange list" conjures up a familiar picture: six exchanges—milk, fruits, vegetables, breads, meat, and fat—with instructions to eat from each exchange in a balanced way to provide a specified amount of calories each day. Up until 1979, the balance of calories obtained from carbohydrate, protein, and fat in the ADA diet did not differ significantly from the balance of calories contained in the average American diet. The diet served only to control the number of calories consumed; it did not alter their composition. In short, it simply ignored all the research, some of it dating back to the 1920s and 1930s, showing that the balance, or composition, of calories is one of the most important therapeutic aspects of a diet for diabetics.

Beginning in 1979, the ADA finally started paying attention to the medical research and began changing its recommendations. Modifications have been made over the years in caloric composition, and the current ADA recommendations call for reasonable amounts of carbohydrate, protein, and fat. In addition, the value of dietary fiber has also been figured in. These improvements are definitely a step in the right direction, but in my opinion they fall short. Too much emphasis is placed on broad categories and not enough on the quality of various foods within those categories. As I hope I've made clear in these past two chapters, there may be a world of difference between one food that is primarily carbohydrate—or protein or fat—and another. It's the difference between a cookie and a stalk of broccoli, between cured ham and salmon, between lard and flaxseed oil.

Quality Is Paramount

Let's review these past two chapters. I believe that the foundation of the optimal diet for diabetics should be unprocessed plant foods, primarily those that are low on the glycemic index. More than half of your caloric intake (60 percent) should be obtained from these types of carbohydrates. The remainder of your diet should contain approximately equal amounts of high-quality fat (20 percent) and lean protein (20 percent). We'll get into the specifics of the diet as well as how to shop, cook, and plan meals, in part IV.

I want to make a few concluding points. The recommendations in these two chapters are general guidelines. The quality of the food you eat is more important than the precise percentages of this and that. By making intelligent choices among a wide variety of healthful foods, you can improve your cells' sensitivity to insulin, lower blood sugar levels, and reduce or eliminate your need for medication. You will also likely decrease your chances of developing diabetic complications—and above all, increase your likelihood of a long and healthy life. Although there is no one diet that works equally well for everyone, I have found that this one does pretty well for the vast majority of patients with diabetes. The proof of what's working for you will be right there in your glucose tests and other measures of blood sugar control.

CHAPTER 8

Exercise: A Powerful Therapy for Diabetes

Exercise may get more lip service but less action than any other therapy for diabetes. Almost all of the textbooks and scientific journals as well as the books and articles written for the public about treating diabetes mention exercise as a powerful therapeutic tool. However, among the vast numbers of diabetic patients who have come to the Whitaker Wellness Institute from all over the country, it is exceedingly rare to find one who arrived with an exercise prescription in hand. I find this hard to comprehend. Exercise is so effective a therapy that when used appropriately it often allows diabetics to reduce or even eliminate their medication requirements.

Every diabetic, regardless of age, current state of health, or type of diabetes, should be on an exercise program. For those with insulin-resistant or type 2 diabetes, regular exercise can mean the difference between dependency on medications and drug-free blood sugar control, between having mild insulin resistance and full-blown type 2 diabetes. For those with type 1 diabetes, exercise can dramatically lower insulin requirements and help stave off the devastating complications of the condition.

Exercise Clears the Blood of Glucose

Exercise acts in a sense like an insulin shot: It reduces blood glucose levels. The cells of exercising muscles obviously have huge energy needs. In order to satisfy these needs, nature has devised a system by which muscles in motion are able to extract glucose from the blood much more efficiently than resting muscles.

The glucose-reducing action of exercise was first demonstrated more than a hundred years ago, and a number of theories have been developed to explain how it works. One theory is that by dilating (opening) the blood vessels, exercise allows even small amounts of circulating insulin to be utilized, resulting in a fall in blood glucose. Another is that the exercising muscle may release some substance that acts like insulin and allows circulating glucose to enter the cells. It has also been postulated that since exercising muscles produce lactic acid and carbon dioxide, these substances might somehow unlock receptors in the muscle cells, letting glucose enter. Or that calcium, which becomes more concentrated within muscle cells during exercise, might play a role in letting glucose in.

There is a new theory explaining how exercise provides a stimulus similar to insulin at the cellular level, and it is growing in acceptance. As you may recall from our discussion of insulin resistance in chapter 2, glucose is ushered into the cell by special proteins called GLUT-4 transporters. Insulin stimulates GLUT-4 transporters to rise to the surface of the cell and take glucose inside. Well, exercise appears to do the same thing. Like insulin, it causes GLUT-4 transporters to rise to the surface of the cellular membrane, where they can shuttle circulating glucose into the cell.[1]

Although we do not completely understand the unique effects of exercise on blood glucose metabolism, one thing is certain: Exercise is a powerful tool to clear the blood of glucose and control diabetes. D. M. Klachko and colleagues from the University of Missouri demonstrated this thirty years ago in a study in which his team took continuous measurements of blood sugar in normal and insulin-dependent diabetic subjects during exercise. The subjects took half-mile walks on a treadmill at a relatively brisk pace of four miles per hour. The treadmill was elevated at either 2.5 or 5 degrees. For the nondiabetic subjects, the less strenuous walk dropped the blood sugar level an average of 5.3 mg/dl, while the more strenuous walk produced an average drop of 11.7 mg/dl. The diabetics, however, recorded an average drop of 24.5 mg/dl for the less strenuous walk and 30.0 mg/dl for the more strenuous one. And although the blood sugar level in the diabetics rose after exercise, it remained below the level recorded before the walk. These little bursts of exercise took only seven and a half minutes, but the drop in blood sugar was substantial.[2]

It has been repeatedly demonstrated that exercising after eating, when blood glucose levels are at their highest, lowers blood sugar. Moreover, exercising after breakfast appears to make physical activity later in the day, after lunch and dinner, even more powerful in keeping the blood sugar under control. Here at the Whitaker Wellness Institute, we see to it that all of our diabetic patients get some exercise—eight to twelve minutes' worth—directly after each meal, and we instruct them to continue this practice at home. (A note of caution: If walking after meals brings on angina, or chest pain, you should not walk immediately after eating. Instead, you should wait for a few hours before exercising.)

Exercise Increases the Cells' Sensitivity to Insulin

Besides having the immediate effect of clearing the blood of glucose, exercise has far-reaching benefits for individuals with diabetes. For the 90 percent of diabetics who have type 2 diabetes, the most valuable benefit of an exercise program is likely the long-term increase in insulin sensitivity. One way in which exercise improves insulin sensitivity is by promoting weight loss, which in some cases in and of itself normalizes blood sugar levels. Another is by clearing the blood of free fatty acids, which, as we discussed in the previous chapter, decrease insulin sensitivity and raise glucose levels. Furthermore, exercise (particularly strength training) increases muscle mass. As the ratio between lean body (muscle) mass and body fat (particularly in the abdominal area) increases, insulin sensitivity improves.

But even if you don't lose weight or gain muscle through your exercise program, other mechanisms are at work to improve the diabetic condition. Regular exercise increases the number of GLUT-4 transporters, the proteins that rise to the surface and carry glucose into the cells. This is a dose-dependent relationship: The more you exercise, the more GLUT-4 transporters your body will make. So the benefits of exercise last long after you've taken off your walking shoes.

In a 2000 study carried out at Case Western Reserve University School of Medicine and published in the *Journal of Applied Physiology*, researchers studied the effects of long-term exercise on insulin sensitivity. They did this by tracking and comparing the activity of insulin and insulin-signaling molecules (which regulate GLUT-4 transport in muscle tissue) in eight athletic men and women and eight sedentary subjects. According to muscle biopsies, insulin concentrations were similar in both groups, but insulin was 30 percent more effective in moving glucose into the cells in the exercise-trained group than in the sedentary individuals. In other words, their cells were much more sensitive—and less resistant—to the action of insulin. Furthermore, the activity of the insulin-stimulated messenger molecules was almost twice as great in the athletes as in the couch potatoes. Although these chemical messengers are not yet completely understood, this study revealed a clear association between the activation of these signals and the rate at which glucose was utilized.[3]

Other measurements have been employed to ascertain the effects of exercise on long-term insulin sensitivity. Dr. Oluf Pedersen of the Department of Internal

Medicine at County Hospital in Århus, Denmark, measured the binding of insulin to various cells in the body and found that exercise increased insulin binding to certain blood cells by 30 percent. In addition, he determined that increased insulin binding, and thus increased insulin sensitivity, was dependent on the degree of exercise conditioning.[4] Researchers at Yale University School of Medicine also found that exercise dramatically increased insulin binding and insulin sensitivity. They concluded, "Physical training may have a role in the management of insulin-resistant states, such as obesity and maturity-onset diabetes, that is independent of its effects on body weight."[5]

In addition to treating diabetes, exercise can also prevent it. The Finnish Diabetes Prevention Study is an ongoing trial designed to assess the effectiveness of an intensive diet and exercise program in preventing impaired glucose tolerance or insulin resistance from progressing into type 2 diabetes. This study involves 523 people at high risk for developing diabetes. At the study's onset, they were overweight and had abnormalities on fasting glucose and glucose tolerance tests. After one year of exercising regularly (and eating a healthy diet), these people had significantly greater reductions in fasting glucose and improvements in glucose and insulin tests than the control group, which did not engage in lifestyle changes. In addition, their blood pressure and triglyceride levels were lower. Furthermore, most of these beneficial changes were sustained over two years.[6]

TV Increases Risk of Diabetes

Every hour you spend in front of the television increases your risk of type 2 diabetes, according to a study reported by the American Diabetes Association. Researchers followed 41,811 men, ages forty to seventy-five, over a ten-year period. A direct association was observed between television watching and risk of developing diabetes. The men who reported sitting in front of a TV more than 19 hours per week were over 150 percent more likely to become diabetic than those who watched less than three hours a week.[7]

No, your television set doesn't exude mysterious rays that raise your blood sugar levels. This is all about exercise, or rather lack of exercise, along with other factors such as snacking and weight gain. Watching a lot of television is simply a marker for a sedentary lifestyle. Before you shrug this off, keep a tally of the number of hours you spend in front of your TV for a couple of weeks. Forty hours a week seems like a lot, but it sneaks up on you. The average American watches more than 30 hours per week. Do yourself a favor—turn off the TV and get active. You'll lose weight, reduce your risk of a number of degenerative diseases, and, according to one study, even make more money!

Exercise Is Essential for Weight Loss

As we have discussed in previous chapters, carrying extra weight is a significant risk factor for type 2 diabetes, and in many cases weight loss alone is enough to completely reverse the condition. Here's an area in which the value of exercise is paramount, for successful and sustained weight loss is next to impossible without regular exercise. We've all been teased by fad diets that promise to melt away pounds with little effort on our part. In the past few years we've seen expensive prescription weight-loss medications gain immense popularity among dieters, only to be removed from the market for their harmful, even lethal side effects. We are inundated with books and tapes, powders and pills that guarantee a trimmer torso by following some special diet or taking some "magical" potion.

Guess what? They don't work! Even if these quick fixes do result in initial weight loss, rarely is it permanent. In almost all cases weight loss or gain is a question of calories in/calories out. If you eat more calories than you burn, you'll gain weight. Conversely, if you burn more calories than you take in, you'll lose weight. The most efficient means of burning extra calories is physical exercise.

Furthermore, as you exercise you build up more muscle tissue and decrease your stores of body fat. There is a direct association between insulin resistance, muscle, and fat. Remember, the higher your ratio of lean muscle mass to abdominal body fat, the more sensitive you tend to be to insulin. In other words, more muscle equals better blood glucose control.

Exercise Protects the Cardiovascular System and Helps Prevent Diabetic Complications

The benefits of exercise do not end with improvements in insulin sensitivity. Physical activity also has ameliorating effects on the cardiovascular system that spell significant protection for diabetics. Virtually every complication that plagues diabetic patients, from kidney and eye disease to amputations and problems with memory and erectile function, is in some way related to decreased circulation. Although exercise alone won't reverse all of these problems, it is a much more powerful tool than most recognize. Diabetic patients should never forget that the number one cause of death in people with this diagnosis is heart disease—it is what ultimately kills three-quarters of all diabetics. Anything you can do to improve your circulation and enhance the health of your heart and circulatory system is well worth the effort required.

Exercise Improves Blood Flow

Your circulatory system, that vast network of arteries, veins, and capillaries that carry nutrient- and oxygen-rich blood to every cell of your body, functions best when the blood is fluid rather than viscous, as this enables it to flow easily through the tiny capillaries that nurture your tissues. This is an important issue in diabetes, for excess glucose in the blood, along with high levels of blood lipids such as triglycerides and cholesterol so common in type 2 diabetes, causes the blood to become more viscous.

One measure of the fluidity of the blood is the "stickiness" of the platelets, small particles that are important for the normal formation of blood clots. Despite their usefulness in stopping bleeding, platelets can be a hazard if they precipitate a clot in a blood vessel. By blocking one of the large vessels going to the brain or heart, such a clot, or *thrombus*, can result in a stroke or heart attack. In addition, smaller clots can block the tiny vessels that nourish the eyes and the kidneys. This kind of blockage is thought to be one of the causes of the blindness and kidney failure so common in diabetics.

Greg Peterson, research assistant to Peter Forsham, M.D., at the University of California School of Medicine in San Francisco, measured the effect of exercise on platelet stickiness in insulin-dependent diabetic patients. He did this by passing a blood sample through a tube of glass beads and measuring the percentage of platelets that stuck. Before exercise, 74 percent of the platelets stuck to the beads; however, 30 minutes on the treadmill or bicycle reduced this to 53 percent. Such an improvement in fluidity can only help protect the eyes and kidneys from diabetes-induced damage.

Exercise Elevates HDL Cholesterol

The level of cholesterol in the blood is highly predictive of risk of heart disease. As cholesterol goes up, the chances of having a heart attack or stroke increase. This is true for low-density lipoprotein (LDL) cholesterol, very-low-density lipoprotein (VLDL) cholesterol, and total cholesterol. There is one form of cholesterol, however, that actually decreases the likelihood of heart disease: high-density lipoprotein (HDL) cholesterol.

All cholesterol molecules are carried in the blood attached to complexes of fat and protein called lipoproteins. The most dangerous form of cholesterol is called low-density lipoprotein (LDL) cholesterol because it is attached to complexes that are mostly fat and thus are very light. When a sample of blood is placed into a centrifuge and very rapidly spun, LDL complexes come to the top. These cholesterol complexes plug up the arteries and contribute to strokes and heart attacks.

HDL cholesterol is attached to carriers made up mostly of protein, which is denser than fat. HDL particles are heavier than the LDL fraction and gravitate to the bottom when blood is centrifuged. These beneficial complexes do not stick to the walls of the arteries. In fact, HDL cholesterol helps clear the body of harmful cholesterol by mobilizing cholesterol attached to the arteries and transporting it to the liver where it can be turned into bile, excreted into the intestinal tract, and eliminated from the body.

Exercise is one of the few things that has been shown to elevate the HDL cholesterol level. It seems to burn up the fatty complexes that .make up the dangerous LDL fractions, replacing them with the denser HDL variety. This has a favorable effect on the arteries and thus protects against heart attacks and strokes.

Exercise Lowers Triglycerides

Triglycerides are molecules of fat in the blood. As you may recall from our discussion in chapter 2, insulin resistance causes the liver to make more VLDL (very-low-density lipoprotein) cholesterol, which is the primary carrier of triglycerides in the blood. Therefore, many type 2 diabetics have elevated levels of both VLDL cholesterol and triglycerides. Elevated triglycerides are a decided risk factor for heart disease. A 1999 review of seventeen studies examining the link between triglyceride levels and cardiovascular disease revealed a 76 percent increased risk in women and a 31 percent increased risk in men for each 86-point rise in triglycerides.[8] (Normal triglycerides are 40–160 mg/dl; ideal is less than 140.) Regular exercise lowers triglyceride levels and helps the body burn fats more efficiently. In patients with triglyceride levels in the 250–350 mg/dl range, exercise has been shown to bring the level down to normal in less than a week.

Exercisers Have Stronger Hearts

The heart of a well-conditioned individual is so much stronger and more efficient than the unconditioned heart that it has a special name: the athletic heart. The characteristics of an athletic heart are:

- ⦿ *A slower resting pulse rate.* The normal resting heart rate is between 60 and 90 beats per minute. However, after a few weeks of conditioning exercise the resting pulse rate may fall to 45 to 60 beats per minute. Because it is stronger, the conditioned heart pumps more blood with each beat, thus needing fewer beats to pump the same amount of blood.

- *A slower exercise heart rate.* The well-conditioned heart develops the capacity to work more efficiently in response to exercise than the unconditioned heart. During exercise, when the call for more blood goes out, the athletic heart can meet this demand with fewer beats.

- *A larger stroke volume.* Stroke volume refers to the amount of blood delivered with each beat. In the well-conditioned heart each stroke is stronger, and thus the amount of blood delivered with each stroke is increased. This makes the heart much more efficient.

Exercise Strengthens the Diseased Heart

Even patients with very severe heart disease can benefit from some form of regular exercise, modified for their special needs and carried out under professional supervision. Doctors make a terrible mistake when they decide that a patient is too ill to start a mild exercise program. This may be especially true of patients with diabetes. Researchers from University Hospital in Grenoble, France, followed 158 high-risk patients with type 2 diabetes who had complicating conditions that limited their ability to exercise. Some had heart disease, others had peripheral neuropathy or pulmonary disease, and still others had chronic fatigue. The researchers found that after six years, the patients who had not exercised were seven times more likely to die from heart attack than those who had exercised.[9]

In his book *Cardiovascular Rehabilitation: A Comprehensive Approach,* Dr. Lyle Peterson, director of the Comprehensive Rehabilitation Center in Houston, reported quite remarkable results with a mild exercise program in twelve severely ill heart patients. These patients, all registered and waiting to undergo a heart transplant operation, were referred to Dr. Peterson's center for evaluation and for mild exercise conditioning in order to strengthen them for surgery. Because of the severity of their illness, they had to be closely monitored during any physical activity.

Much to the surprise of Dr. Peterson and his staff, six of the twelve improved so much that they were taken off the heart transplant list and went home to live essentially normal lives. One patient maintained his improvement during the five-plus years he was monitored, and he continued to work out regularly on an exercise bicycle. Dr. Peterson's results indicate that the power of exercise to rehabilitate damaged hearts extends even to those who have almost surely been told by their physician not to exercise. Obviously, when patients are this ill, the exercise needs to be carefully prescribed and monitored. Nevertheless, it is a powerful tool to strengthen a weakened heart.[10]

Exercise Builds "Collaterals"

When arteries to the heart muscle start to fill with fatty deposits, the body's normal defense is to build additional blood vessels around them to ensure continued blood flow. These new vessels are known as *collateral* circulation. Many times a coronary artery will close completely, but a heart attack is avoided because collateral arteries have developed around the blockage.

The dreaded condition of atherosclerosis of the coronary arteries is like a race: The major arteries are being plugged by fat and cholesterol, and the body is building collateral blood vessels to bypass the blockages. Which side will win? Don't passively wait to find out. Regular exercise will give the edge in building of collateral circulation and help reduce your risk of heart attack.

Dean Ornish, M.D., demonstrated in a 1990 clinical study published in the *Lancet*, complete with before-and-after pictures of artery blockages, that regular exercise, along with a low-fat diet and stress reduction program, can reverse the process of atherosclerosis. You can also speed up the development of collaterial circulation. But you can't do it without exercise.[11]

Additional Benefits of Exercise

Exercise is particularly therapeutic for diabetics, but the general benefits of vigorous activity are more than enough reason for anyone—with or without diabetes—to start an exercise program.

If you were looking at two men of the same body build and weight, it might be difficult to tell which one was active and well conditioned. However, the changes that could be measured on the inside are astounding. Exercise has a beneficial effect on every system in the body!

Exercise Elevates Mood

Every day, joggers, bicyclists, and walkers hit the road by the millions in this country. Ever wonder why? Are they trying to lower their blood sugar level and combat diabetes? Are they trying to prevent or treat heart disease? No. For most, exercise is a "pepper-upper." Who has not felt his mood lift with a brisk walk? Who hasn't cleared her mind and solved some problem while engaged in physical activity? Exercise simply makes you feel better.

The positive effect of exercise on our psyche results from the elevation of certain chemicals in the brain called endorphins. Exercise promotes an increase in these very potent mood elevators. In fact, it is their effect on the same systems in the brain that allows the drugs morphine and Demerol to relieve pain and create a feeling of euphoria. With exercise, endorphins go up naturally: Mood is elevated, thinking is clearer, life is just better. Numerous studies have found that exercise is an excellent therapy for depression, anxiety, and stress.

Exercise Improves Oxygen Utilization

When you exercise, you flood your system with oxygen. If the exercise is vigorous enough, your uptake of oxygen can increase 1000 percent. One of the first signs of conditioning is the body's improved utilization of oxygen, both during exercise and at rest. The well-conditioned body simply extracts oxygen from the blood more efficiently, benefiting every system in your body.

One sign of aging is decreased ability to utilize oxygen during exercise. During maximum exercise, a man of fifty will use less oxygen than a man of twenty-five under the same conditions. However, this is one mechanism of aging that you can slow down, and even reverse. The maximum uptake of oxygen can be increased in anyone at any age with regular exercise. With adequate training, a well-conditioned man or woman of fifty can match a twenty-five-year-old in this measure.

Exercise Is a Whole-Body Tune-up

Although I've touched on the most important benefits of exercise, you should be aware that physical activity rejuvenates virtually every organ in your body, adding energy to your days and years to your life. Exercise builds stronger bones, alleviates asthma, prevents migraine headaches, and strengthens the immune system. It sharpens the mind and promotes good sleep. It even reduces the risk of some forms of cancer. Some of the most common diseases of aging can actually be prevented, postponed, or reversed through physical exercise. Exercise is simply one of the healthiest habits you can incorporate into your life.

A Word of Warning

Although exercise is one of the safest, most beneficial of all therapies, there are a few caveats you should be aware of. Diabetics who are using insulin or oral diabetes medications that increase insulin output must observe a few precautions when undertaking exercise. The normal response of the pancreas to exercise is to slow down or stop insulin secretion, since exercise in and of itself lowers blood glucose. However, if additional insulin is thrown into the mix by injections or oral drugs, it is possible for exercise to drive blood glucose too low.

For type 1 (insulin-dependent) diabetics, particularly those who are thin and active, physical activity can make matters worse, as exercise may cause a severe drop in blood sugar (hypoglycemia). Insulin-dependent diabetic patients should know that *they must closely monitor their blood glucose levels and substantially reduce their insulin dose* on the days they plan vigorous activity. It is important not to start exercise with blood sugars in the low-normal range. The patient should always carry some source of carbohydrate, such as glucose tablets, to be eaten if signs of hypoglycemia occur. The reduction in insulin dosage when embarking on an exercise program should be worked out under a physician's care. For a well-controlled type 1 diabetic the reduction could be as much as 80 percent on the mornings when a long bike ride or some other form of protracted activity is planned.

If a patient with type 1 diabetes starts exercise with very high blood sugars, problems may also arise. In these patients, blood sugar levels may not fall. In fact, exercise could cause levels to rise even more. This sequence could bring on the dangerous condition known as ketoacidosis, which in some cases becomes so severe as to require hospitalization. Fortunately, the threat of ketoacidosis with physical exercise applies only to thin insulin-dependent diabetics. All type 1 diabetics should discuss their exercise plans with their doctor.

Exercise poses little danger for individuals with type 2 diabetes who are treated with lifestyle measures. Of course, they too should consult a physician before beginning an exercise program. However, there is virtually no likelihood that exercise will cause an elevation in blood sugar leading to ketoacidosis. Nor is exercise likely to cause hypoglycemia in type 2 diabetics treated with diet and exercise only.

Caution should be taken, however, by patients with type 2 diabetes who are utilizing insulin or an oral hypoglycemic drug that prompts insulin secretion (a class of drugs known as sulfonylureas, which we discussed in detail in part II). In such drug-dependent patients as in type 1 diabetics on insulin, exercise can cause dangerously low blood sugars. The drug-free body "knows" to turn off insulin secretion once blood glucose levels fall during exercise. However, you can't turn off the effects of these drugs, and the combination of exercise-induced falling blood sugars and extra insulin can be problematic. This is one reason why I am so averse to this class of oral diabetic drugs.

Another group of patients who should approach exercise with caution are those who have complications involving fragile blood vessels, such as diabetic retinopathy. This by no means rules out exercise. Rather, these individuals should be carefully not to exercise too strenuously. Intense exertion could cause rupture of the small vessels of the eyes and other organs. This is particularly dangerous in the out-of-shape diabetic who begins exercising after years of being sedentary.

These precautions should be taken seriously, and I want to stress again that professional supervision is necessary for all diabetics who engage in an exercise program, particularly those using insulin or sulfonylureas. However, for the vast majority of diabetics, exercise, if started and carried out properly, is an exceptionally powerful therapy that will significantly improve the diabetic condition.

In part IV I will give you some important tips on how to get started on—and stay on—an exercise program.

CHAPTER 9

Nutritional Supplements for Diabetes

Nutritional supplements are a must for anyone with diabetes. Vitamins, minerals, essential fatty acids, and herbs are naturally occurring compounds that, if used rationally and in a balanced manner, can have profoundly positive effects on blood glucose levels. They can also offer protection against the debilitating consequences of diabetes, from eye and kidney problems to heart disease and premature death.

This isn't conjecture—it's fact. The annals of medicine are filled with thousands upon thousands of studies examining these natural agents and their beneficial effects on all manner of health challenges. Nevertheless, there is a strong bias in medicine against using nutritional supplements unless a classic deficiency exists. In fact, this bias is so entrenched in some circles that it is considered "unprofessional" to recommend a nutritional supplement to anyone unless there is a gross nutritional deficiency.

The Roots of the Professional Bias against Nutrition

J. S. Goodwin and M. R. Tangum wrote a compelling article, published in the *Archives of Internal Medicine* in 1998, entitled "Battling Quackery: Attitudes about Micronutrient Supplements in American Academic Medicine." They observed that this bias is marked by

> *uncritical acceptance of bad news about micronutrient supplements (reports of toxic effects were rarely questioned and widely quoted); by the scornful dismissive tone of the discussions about micronutrient supplementation in textbooks of medicine, a tone avoided in most medical controversies; and by the skeptical reaction greeting any claim of efficacy of a micronutrient, relative to other therapies, indeed, most claims were simply ignored....*
>
> *There are only three important questions when evaluating a potential treatment. Does it work? What are the adverse effects? How much does it cost? Ideally, issues such as the theory underlying the treatment or the guild to which the proponents of the treatment belong should be irrelevant to the fundamental questions of efficacy, toxicity, and cost. The history of the response of academic medicine to micronutrient supplementation suggests that we have not attained that ideal.*[1]

Why is there such a negative bias among physicians against nutrition in general and nutritional supplements in particular? One reason is that physician education gives clinical nutrition scant attention and completely ignores nutritional supplements. When I was in medical school in the 1960s, nutrition was dismissed with a few lectures on the general digestion and breakdown of fats, carbohydrates, and proteins. Vitamins and minerals were covered in simplistic lectures that described only their most basic functions and the effects of gross deficiencies. And herbs? They were relegated to the kitchen. Some strides have been made over the years, yet to this day a mere one-quarter of all medical schools in this country require any education in nutrition at all!

Consequently, even today physicians graduate from intensive and grueling programs with little understanding that what people eat has a profound effects on their health. And most of them have no inkling that adding targeted nutritional supplements to a healthy diet is an extremely powerful therapeutic tool.

Nutritional Supplements: Dispelling the Myths

There are many misperceptions about nutritional supplements, not only among physicians but also among some of you reading this book. Before we get into the particulars about the specific supplements I recommend for improving diabetes, I would like to address these fallacies.

Myth #1: If You Eat Right, You Don't Need to Take Vitamins

I'm often asked, "I eat a balanced diet. Why should I take nutritional supplements?" My first response is to question these patients about their diet, for most Americans don't come close to eating a healthy diet. Fewer than 10 percent eat even the minimum daily recommended amount of plant foods: a paltry five servings. A U.S. Department of Agriculture study further showed that on an average day, 41 percent of those surveyed ate no fruit, 72 percent had no vitamin C–rich fruits, 82 percent ate no cruciferous vegetables (such as broccoli and cabbage), and 84 percent consumed no fiber-rich whole-grain foods (such as whole wheat bread).[2]

Our fast-paced lives leave little time or desire for cooking. The number of families who sit down together for a home-cooked meal most evenings has fallen dramatically in recent years. Eating out has gone from being a luxury to a necessity. And many restaurant meals are obtained from fast food outlets. Furthermore, even if you are eating well, there is no guarantee that your food contains the nutrient levels you would expect it to contain. As we discussed in chapters 6 and 7, much of the food eaten in this country has been processed and is sorely lacking in important nutrients. Cooking and storage also affects vitamin and mineral content. The potential for mineral deficiencies is particularly high, because the amount of minerals in the soil and water, and therefore in plant foods, varies greatly from region to region.

At the very least, taking a daily vitamin and mineral

supplement will help cover the nutritional "gaps" in your diet. Think of supplements, if you will, as insurance against the potential inadequacies of your diet.

Myth #2: It Is Important to Follow the RDAs

The Recommended Dietary Allowances (RDAs) were established by the Food and Nutrition Board of the National Academy of Sciences "to set levels of intake of the essential nutrients considered, in the judgement of the Food and Nutrition Board on the basis of available scientific knowledge, to be adequate to meet the known nutritional needs of practically all healthy persons." In a nutshell, this means that *healthy* individuals who are consuming food containing the RDAs of the essential nutrients should not develop any nutritional deficiency diseases related to these nutrients.

There are several fallacies in this rationale. First, who is healthy? Take a look at how many Americans are afflicted with these serious medical conditions:

Arthritis	50 million
Diabetes	16 million
Heart disease	58.8 million
Hypertension	50 million

Clearly, a significant percentage of Americans are less than healthy. Furthermore, the RDAs are "one size fits all." The obvious differences among people in such characteristics as height, hair color, temperament, athletic ability, musical talent, and intelligence are minor when compared to the tremendous variations that exist under the skin. As an example, the gastric fluids of one "normal" man may contain 400 percent more pepsin (a digestive enzyme) than his equally "normal" neighbor. There are numerous examples illustrating that the differences between normal individuals may vary by as much as 500 to 1000 percent! These variations suggest similar differences in nutrient requirements among individuals. What may be an optimal amount of a nutrient for one individual could be completely inadequate for another.

In addition, the optimal vitamin or mineral intake for any individual may vary with time and circumstances. Several studies show, for instance, that stress dramatically increases the need for vitamin C and some of the B-complex vitamins. The thinking behind the RDAs simply ignores the reality that we are all unique, with individualized requirements for certain nutrients, and that various factors likely alter our nutritional needs at any given time.

Finally, the RDAs are designed to prevent deficiencies, not promote optimal health. Many vitamins and minerals at doses higher—sometimes much higher—than the RDA have been demonstrated to have positive therapeutic effects in certain conditions, and with no toxicity. Let's at look at vitamin C. The RDA of 75 to 90 milligrams for vitamin C is the amount that will prevent scurvy, the vitamin C deficiency disease. However, several studies have shown that 2000 to 3000 milligrams of vitamin C per day can enhance the function of the body's white blood cells and elevate production of several types of immune cells that increase resistance and fight disease. Other studies have demonstrated that daily doses of vitamin C in the 300–500 milligram range are protective against heart disease.

Another example is vitamin E. The RDA for this fat-soluble vitamin, which is a potent antioxidant, is 15 milligrams (24 international units). However, a huge body of clinical and epidemiological research suggests that what might be considered "megadoses" of this vitamin are extremely beneficial for a number of conditions. Two Harvard studies, one involving 87,245 female nurses and another involving 39,910 male health care professionals, studied the effects of supplemental vitamin E on the risk of heart disease. It was discovered that women who took at least 100 international units of vitamin E daily had a 41 percent reduction in risk, compared with those study subjects who did not take vitamin E supplements.[3] For men, a daily intake of 30 international units of vitamin E conferred a 37 percent decreased risk of heart disease.[4]

But that's not all. A study published in the *New England Journal of Medicine* in 1997 showed that a daily intake of 2000 international units of vitamin E (more than 100 times the RDA!) slowed the progression of Alzheimer's disease by several months. And, in the words of the researchers involved in the study, "it's inexpensive, easily available, and safe."[5]

When we are misled into believing that the RDAs are the only yardstick for determining safe and appropriate doses of vital nutrients, we are missing the opportunity to protect ourselves from health challenges much more common than these rare deficiency diseases.

Myth #3: Supplements Do Nothing beyond Making Expensive Urine

It is true that water-soluble vitamins, which include the B-complex vitamins and vitamin C, may be excreted in the urine. Since these vitamins are not stored by the body, the purpose of supplementing them is to saturate the metabolic systems that require these nutrients. Saturation may require dosages that ultimately show up in the urine. Some physicians conclude that if the vitamin is being excreted in the urine, the dosage being taken is more than is needed for a beneficial effect. This is just not accurate. Many water-soluble vitamins continue to exert beneficial effects, even though the threshold for urinary excretion has been exceeded. This phenomenon occurs with prescription drugs as well.

Myth #4: Vitamins and Minerals Are Dangerous

There is a perception among many that vitamins and minerals, particularly when taken in amounts well above the RDAs, are dangerous. This is utter nonsense. I would be hard-pressed to count on my fingers the number of fatalities attributable to any nutritional supplement. True, fat-soluble vitamins, particularly vitamin A and vitamin D, do have the potential of toxicity. They collect in the fat cells and could conceivably build up to dangerous levels. However, that would require taking many, many times the recommended doses over a long period of time. Furthermore, symptoms of toxicity give warning signs, and they rapidly subside after the vitamin is discontinued. Rarely are there any lasting effects.

Compare this to the well-documented 106,000 deaths per year that result from prescription drugs used as directed by doctors. This makes them, according to a 1998 study published in the *Journal of the American Medical Association,* the fourth to sixth leading cause of death (depending on which database is used to calculated such statistics). Prescription drugs kill more people than automobile accidents, breast and prostate cancer, and AIDS![6]

There are other myths about nutritional supplements that we will attempt to dispel as we cover individual nutrients later in this chapter. For now, suffice it to say that targeted nutritional supplements, even if taken at therapeutic levels far higher than the RDAs, are a safe and powerful adjunct to diet and other lifestyle measures in the treatment of diabetes.

The Times They Are a-Changin'

Regardless of what the medical establishment thinks about nutritional supplements, they have been heartily embraced by the American public. More than half of all Americans take supplements, and sales of vitamins, herbs, and other supplements have grown by leaps and bounds in recent years. Americans are also flocking to health care practitioners who utilize nutritional supplements and other "alternative" therapies. In 1993, David Eisenberg, M.D., of Harvard Medical School, published a survey indicating that in 1990 more than one-third of Americans made a total of 425 million visits to practitioners of alternative medicine.[7] (Alternative care was defined as therapies that were not taught in medical schools or used in hospitals and included things such as chiropractic, acupuncture, massage, and the use of diet and nutritional supplements to treat disease.)

When Dr. Eisenberg repeated this survey in 1997, the number of visits had increased to 629 million—more than the total number of visits to conventional doctors. Alternative therapies were being used by almost half of the population. For these therapies, Americans paid an estimated $27 billion out of pocket, a figure comparable to the out of pocket expenditures (those not covered by insurance) for all conventional physician services.[8]

Among those pursuing alternative therapies are patients with diabetes. A paper presented at the 1999 Scientific Sessions of the American Diabetes Association revealed that more than one-third of 502 diabetics surveyed by researchers at the University of Alberta in Edmonton, Canada, admitted to using therapies other than the drugs prescribed by their doctors.[9]

Many doctors may be standing around scratching their heads about this "vitamin craze," but patients certainly are not. Physicians are no longer the one and only source of medical information. The public now has at its disposal instant access to medical facts and figures via the Internet and a plethora of printed materials. Rarely a day goes by that a story on some aspect of health does not make the headlines or the evening news. Regarding some aspects of medicine—for example, alternative therapies—patients are better informed than their physicians! Changes in our health care system to incorporate more of these alternative therapies, led by a proactive, well-educated populace, are gaining momentum. The medical profession is going to have to jump on the bandwagon or be left at the station.

Targeted Nutritional Supplements for Diabetes

Over the past twenty-two years, I have treated thousands of patients with diabetes at the Whitaker Wellness Institute. Many come into the clinic after fifteen to twenty years of drug therapy with serious heart disease, visual impairment, or kidney or nerve damage. Some patients with a similar history of diabetes and insulin therapy, however, have virtually no complications. What accounts for these differences?

Of course, keeping blood glucose as near to normal is a big part of it. But my impression is that most of those patients who have avoided the debilitating complications of diabetes have also been conscientious about taking vitamin and mineral supplements. Diabetes is a disease of nutritional wasting brought on by the excessive urination that is characteristic of this disorder. As I explained earlier, under normal circumstances glucose, along with other water-soluble nutrients, is reabsorbed by the body. However, when glucose rises to levels above 160 to 170, as it does frequently in diabetic patients, it acts as an *osmotic diuretic*, overwhelming the system and causing substantial losses of these nutrients that pass out in the urine. It is my opinion that nutritional deficiencies brought on by the diabetic condition are a significant contributor to diabetic complications.

Vitamin and mineral deficiencies are quite common in diabetics. In a review article of 247 studies, published in the *American Journal of Clinical Nutrition,* it was found that type 1 diabetics generally had deficiencies in zinc, calcium, magnesium, and vitamin D. Many were also low in vitamins B_6 and B_{12}. Individuals with type 2 diabetes were frequently found to be low in zinc and magnesium, and, in many cases, in vitamins B_6 and C.[10,11]

Let's take a close look at the specific supplements we utilize at the Whitaker Wellness Institute for the treatment of diabetes. Some of them we recommend simply to ensure adequate levels of nutrients important for overall health. Others, however, have specific effects on glucose metabolism and may help improve insulin sensitivity. Still others have been found useful in fending off or treating complications associated with diabetes. It may seem like quite a list to you at first, but believe me, the cost and effort it may take to implement a comprehensive nutritional supplement program will pay off in big improvements in your health.

Vanadium Acts Remarkably Like Insulin

In my opinion, the single most effective and intriguing weapon for combating diabetes is the mineral vanadium. Numerous animal studies and a small but growing body of human research show that vanadium compounds, most notably vanadyl sulfate, markedly improve fasting glucose and other measures of diabetes.

Recent research suggests that vanadium acts in a manner very similar to insulin. Insulin's primary activity in blood glucose metabolism is to stimulate GLUT-4 transporters to rise to the surface of the cell and carry glucose inside. Vanadium has been identified as one of the few compounds other than insulin that can activate GLUT-4 transporters.[12] In essense, it mimics the action of insulin. Amazingly, vanadium's benefits often extend for weeks after the supplement is discontinued. In one animal study, for example, three weeks of treatment resulted in complete resolution of diabetes, which lasted for ten weeks after the mineral was stopped.

This phenomenon has been demonstrated in humans as well. In a 1996 study, eight men and women with type 2 diabetes received 50 milligrams of vanadyl sulfate twice a day for four weeks, followed by a placebo for four weeks. A 20 percent average reduction in fasting glucose was noted, which extended into the placebo period. The only side effect was some initial gastrointestinal upset during the first week of supplementation.[13]

The compound has also been studied in patients with type 1 diabetes. Ten patients, half with type 1 diabetes and half with type 2, were administered 125 milligrams per day of sodium metavanate (another form of vanadium) for two weeks. Although the insulin-dependent patients had no significant change in blood glucose, they required significantly less insulin while taking vanadium.[14]

For some reason, there is a commonly accepted belief, even among practitioners of alternative medicine, that vanadium is toxic. According to John McNeill, Ph.D., dean of the faculty of Pharmaceutical Sciences at the University of British Columbia and one of the world's leading experts on vanadium, these rumors of toxicity are based on studies done by one—and only one—researcher. That researcher's results have never been replicated by anyone else and are in fact at odds with the toxicity studies carried out by other scientists.

Although vanadium is indeed retained in the tissues, it is safe and well tolerated by most people at dosage levels in the 100–150 milligram range. In a study presented at a worldwide symposium on vanadium in November 1997, doses as high as 400 milligrams per day were utilized. Although the patients using these higher doses reported having diarrhea, there were no serious side effects. I and other physicians have utilized vanadyl sulfate with hundreds of diabetic patients in doses up to 150 milligrams per day with remarkable success and absolutely no adverse reactions, save slight gastrointestinal distress in a few individuals.

For my diabetic patients I recommend an average of 100 milligrams a day of vanadyl sulfate, although some patients require as little as 45–50 milligrams.

Important note: You should be under the supervision of your doctor and monitor your blood sugar levels closely when you begin taking this mineral, as dramatic drops in blood glucose may result. Modifications in medication or insulin dosage may be required.

Chromium Improves the Action of Insulin

The therapeutic potential of chromium was first recognized in 1957, when researchers isolated a previously unknown compound from pork kidney. When they have this substance to laboratory rats with glucose intolerance (a pre-diabetic condition marked by impaired ability to metabolize carbohydrates), it caused such significant improvements that they named it *glucose tolerance factor* (GTF). This unique compound was shown to improve the activity of insulin and facilitate the uptake of glucose into cells. Research efforts intensified, and in 1959 the active ingredient of GTF was identified: chromium, a trace mineral with no previously defined function in the body.

Chromium now has more than forty years of research behind it, much of it involving its effects on insulin. As you know, if cells do not respond to insulin—the essence of insulin resistance and the cause of most cases of type 2 diabetes—nutrients simply cannot enter cells. Chromium doesn't cause the body to make more insulin; it just makes insulin work better.

At least fifteen well-controlled clinical trials examining the effects of chromium supplementation on patients with diabetes, insulin resistance, and other blood sugar abnormalities have shown that chromium improves glucose metabolism. This mineral is beneficial in gestational diabetes (diabetes that develops only during pregnancy) and steroid-induced diabetes, as well as the far more common adult-onset diabetes associated with insulin resistance.

Much of the early chromium research was carried out by Dr. Walter Mertz of the U.S. Department of Agriculture. In a 1975 study, he gave chromium supplements to six diabetics, and three of them demonstrated improved glucose control.[15] A more recent and much larger study was conducted by the U.S. Department of Agriculture's Human Nutrition Research Center and Beijing Medical University in China. Researchers divided 180 type 2 diabetics into three groups and assigned each group a specific protocol: supplements containing 100 micrograms chromium picolinate, supplements containing 500 micrograms chromium picolinate, or a placebo, twice a day. No other changes were made in their medications, diets, or activity levels. When their blood sugar levels were tested after four months, the patients taking chromium had reductions in blood sugar, insulin, cholesterol, and gluosylated hemoglobin (a longer-term measure of blood sugar control). Those taking 500 micrograms per day generally had greater reductions than those taking the lower dose.[16]

Another way chromium may benefit patients with diabetes is by facilitating weight loss. As you know, excess weight, particularly in the abdominal area, is part and parcel of type 2 diabetes. Although this mineral is not a miracle cure for obesity, chromium has been demonstrated to improve body composition by increasing muscle mass and decreasing body fat. As we discussed in the previous chapter, this in and of itself helps improve insulin sensitivity.

Two of the most compelling studies on chromium and weight loss were conducted by Dr. Gilbert R. Kaats. In his most recent study, published in June 1998, 122 subjects were given either 400 micrograms of chromium picolinate per day or a placebo, while their diets and exercise regimens were monitored. After ninety days, adjusting for caloric intake and expenditure, it was determined that chromium did indeed have positive effects on weight and body composition. Those taking chromium lost more weight (and average of 17.1 pounds compared to 3.9 pounds for the placebo group), fat mass (16.9 pounds versus 3.3 pounds), and percentage of body fat (6.3 percent versus 1.2 percent).[17]

Concerns have been raised in recent years about the safety of chromium. The press picked up on a couple of, in my opinion, insignificant studies on chromium picolinate and, in an astounding leap of illogic, proclaimed that chromium was not only ineffective, but also dangerous. The "evidence" they used to support this conclusion came from two test-tube studies—not human studies, not even animal studies, but test-tube studies. In one of the studies, published in 1996, hamster cells were exposed to extremely high concentrations of chromium (3,000 times higher than the amount supplement takers are exposed to), and researchers concluded that this concentration of chromium picolinate could cause chromosomal damage in hamster cells.[18] They then jumped to the well-publicized, but what I consider to be irrational, conclusion that chromium causes cancer in humans.

The most recent study was, from my viewpoint, even less relevant. Researchers merely observed a chemical reaction between chromium, vitamin C, and other antioxidants, and found that interactions between chromium picolinate and antioxidants caused free-radical damage that may lead to mutations in DNA. Now, all biochemists know that these same interactions occur with numerous minerals commonly found in food and supplements. Such alarmist reporting only causes undue panic. More important, it scares away people who would benefit from this mineral.

The truth is that numerous animal and human studies, which are more reliable (though less sensational) than the lab studies described above, have demonstrated that chromium is extremely safe. In one toxicity study, rats fed 100 milligrams per kilogram of body weight of chromium picolinate daily (equal to several thousand 200-microgram tablets for a 150-pound human) showed no signs of toxicity. Safety studies conducted by the U.S. Department of Agriculture have similarly found no toxicity or adverse effects with high doses of chromium. The Ames test, commonly used to identify potential cancer-causing substances, has given chromium the thumbs-up, as do standard medical reference books. *Modern Nutrition in Health and Disease* notes that "chromium becomes toxic only at extremely high amounts—chromium then acts as a gastric irritant rather than as a toxic element."[19]

Chromium deficiencies are common in this country, probably because high consumption of sugar and refined grains depletes chromium reserves. Dr. Mertz, who as I mentioned above was one of the pioneering researchers on this mineral, noted that chromium concentration in the tissues of Americans declines with age and that this may be one of the reasons for the significant increase in the incidence of diabetes as we get older. Government surveys suggest that most Americans fail to get even 50 micrograms of chromium per day. Although I recommend that all my patients supplement with 200 micrograms of this important mineral every day, I suggest that my diabetic patients double that dose to 400 micrograms daily. The best-absorbed forms are chromium picolinate and chromium polynicotinate.

Magnesium Guards against Diabetic Complications

Magnesium is an essential mineral involved in hundreds of biochemical functions in the body. Among its many, many actions, magnesium has a relaxing effect on the smooth muscle tissues that line the arteries. Therefore, it helps improve blood flow, lower blood pressure, and reduce the likelihood of arterial spasms that may contribute to heart attacks. Deficiencies in this mineral are strongly linked with heart disease.

The medical literature also contains many studies showing that diabetic patients have below-average blood levels of magnesium and higher urinary losses of this mineral. The diabetic condition itself, as discussed above, may cause magnesium and other essential minerals and trace elements to be lost in the urine. In addition, when insulin-dependent diabetics go into ketoacidosis (insulin coma) there is marked mineral depletion. Furthermore, many diabetics who also have hypertension are taking diuretics to control their blood pressure. Although diuretics are notorious wasters of all minerals, potassium is the only mineral that is routinely replaced. The others, including magnesium, are ignored altogether.

H. M. Mather of the Department of Medicine, St. George's Hospital in London, measured the blood magnesium level in 582 consecutive diabetic patients visiting the hospital's outpatient clinic. He also measured the magnesium levels of 140 nondiabetic subjects. He found that the diabetics had significantly lower blood magnesium levels. In fact, 25 percent of the diabetics tested had lower levels than all of the nondiabetics except one. Dr. Mather pointed out that magnesium has a fundamental role in carbohydrate metabolism in general, and a very specific role in the efficient action of insulin itself. A low level of magnesium can certainly contribute to poor control of the diabetic condition. But he also concluded "that it is at least conceivable that the hypomagne-saemia [low magnesium levels] occurring in diabetic patients may predispose to their markedly increased incidence and morbidity of ischemic heart disease."[20]

In addition to being an independent and verifiable risk factor for premature heart attack, magnesium deficiencies are also associated with diabetic retinopathy. A landmark study by Dr. P. McNair, entitled "Hypomagnesemia, a Risk Factor in Diabetic Retinopathy," revealed that diabetics with the lowest magnesium levels had the most severe retinopathy. Dr. McNair further concluded that low magnesium levels were more significantly linked to retinopathy than any other factor.[21] It only stands to reason that if a diabetic patient is put on magnesium supplementation, blood and cellular levels of magnesium will increase, and the risk of blindness and cardiovascular complications will likely decrease.

The recommended daily dose of magnesium for people with diabetes or heart disease is 1000 milligrams per day. Magnesium should be balanced with calcium so that the ration of calcium to magnesium intake is between 2:1 and 1:1. In other words, for every 1000 milligrams of calcium you take, you should also be taking 500 to 1000 milligrams of magnesium. In addition to this oral dose, almost every diabetic patient at the Whitaker Wellness Institute receives a series of three or four injections of magnesium sulfate (1 milliliter of a 50 percent solution of magnesium sulfate mixed with 1 milliliter of heparin in a 1:1000 solution and injected intramuscularly). On leaving the Institute, many of our patients carry with them a prescription for one or two of these injections per month, in addition to oral magnesium.

Antioxidants: A Must for the Diabetic

Living is risky business, and it is particularly risky for diabetics. Oxidation, the process of generating the energy in our cells that ultimately keeps us alive, has a dark side: the formation of destructive by-products called free radicals. Free radicals are unstable molecules that, in an attempt to complete themselves, grab electrons from neighboring molecules, damaging and destabilizing them and initiating a chain reaction of molecular and cellular destruction. This is known as free-radical or oxidative damage, and it is felt to be a principal cause of a number of degenerative diseases, as well as the aging process itself. High levels of glucose accelerate the production of free radicals, placing diabetics at increased risk.

Nature has devised an elegant system for counteracting

oxidative damage: antioxidants, compounds that give up electrons to stabilize and neutralize free radicals. These beneficial substances, which include a number of enzymes and vitamins produced in the body, as well as certain nutrients found in food and supplements, work in synergy to revitalize one another and keep the body in tip-top shape. The best-known of the antioxidant supplements are vitamin A, vitamin C, vitamin E, beta-carotene, selenium, and lipoic acid. A number of herbs, phytonutrients (chemical compounds found in plants), and amino acids also have antioxidant activity.

I *advise* all my patients to supplement with anti-oxidants, but I *insist* that my diabetic patients do so. First, they are likely deficient in the water-soluble anti-oxidants. Second, certain antioxidants improve insulin sensitivity. And third, these important nutrients protect the cardiovascular system. The metabolic processes that the diabetic condition unleashes on the body may, as we discussed in chapter 2, result in a constellation of medical conditions (Syndrome X) that often appear alongside type 2 diabetes. These include hypertension, blood lipid abnormalities, and an increased risk of cardiovascular disease. A plethora of research suggests that free-radical damage is at work here, and that by supplementing with antioxidants, we may be able to slow it down. Let's examine the antioxidants that are of particular benefit to the diabetic.

Vitamin C

Because insulin helps transport vitamin C into the cells, it is not surprising that diabetics are prone to having low intracellular concentrations of this vitamin—even if blood levels are normal. This may lead to several problems, for vitamin C plays multiple crucial roles in the body. It strengthens the blood vessels, especially the small capillaries, and boosts the activity of the immune system. Deficiencies in vitamin C may result in capillary fragility and delayed wound healing, conditions that are particularly problematic in diabetics.

Vitamin C also protects against cardiovascular disease, another concern in this patient population. In one of the most remarkable studies examining the effects of vitamin C on the heart and vascular system, researchers analyzed the vitamin C intake of 11,348 adults over five years. They found that men with the highest intakes of this vitamin (more than 300 milligrams per day from food and supplements) had a 45 percent lower risk of death from cardiovascular disease than men with the lowest intakes (less than 50 milligrams).[22]

Several studies have also suggested that taking high doses of vitamin C may protect against other destructive processes brought on by the diabetic condition. One of these is glycosylation, the chemical alteration of proteins, which, as we discussed in chapter 1, is one of the mechanisms that leads to diabetic complications of the eyes and nerves. Vitamin C may also reduce the accumulation of sorbitol in the cells, another probable cause of diabetic complications. In a 1994 study published in the *Journal of the American College of Nutrition*, researchers followed young adults with insulin-dependent diabetes who, according to food diaries, had been getting adequate (RDA) amounts of vitamin C. They first measured the amount of sorbitol in the patients' red blood cells, and found that it averaged twice the normal level. The patients were then given either 100 milligrams or 600 milligrams of supplemental vitamin C daily for fifty-eight days. With repeated measurement, the concentration of sorbitol within the red blood cells had normalized in these patients after just thirty days of supplementation! The researchers concluded that vitamin C supplementation was a highly effective therapy for diabetics.[23]

My recommended dose of vitamin C is 2000 milligrams per day. Some individuals report gastrointestinal upset or loose stools with doses this high. To avoid this possibility, I suggest starting with a lower dose, say 500 milligrams, and building up to the therapeutic dose by adding another 500 milligrams every few days, as tolerated. Vitamin C is otherwise well tolerated and very safe.

Vitamin E

Vitamin E is the premier antioxidant in your body's fatty tissues. Interestingly, some studies indicate that tissue and plasma levels of vitamin E may be higher than average in patients with diabetes. This is likely nature's response to the destructive nature of the condition: More vitamin E is utilized to protect against the free-radical damage that is accelerated in these patients.[24]

Vitamin E has multiple benefits for diabetics. It has been shown to confer protection against glycosylation, a destructive mechanism related to elevated glucose levels.[25] In addition, vitamin E appears to directly improve insulin sensitivity. In one study, researchers administered quite high doses of vitamin E (1350 international units per day) for four months to healthy subjects and to subjects with type 2 diabetes. Before-and-after glucose tolerance tests revealed improvements in insulin sensitivity in both groups, but improvements were most pronounced in the diabetics.[26]

Vitamin E is best known, however, for the protection it confers against cardiovascular disease. This was clearly demonstrated in the 1996 double-blind, placebo-controlled Cambridge Heart Antioxidant Study (CHAOS). The 2002 patients involved in this study were divided into two groups. One group took 400–800 international units of vitamin E, while the other received a placebo. After an average period of 510 days, the patients taking supplemental vitamin E had 75 percent fewer heart attacks than those on the placebo. This study has important ramifications for diabetics, since the vast majority of these patients concurrently suffer from heart disease.

Drs. Ishwarlal Jialal and Sridevi Devaraj of the University of Texas Southwestern Medical Center in Dallas believe that high doses of vitamin E may not only prevent cardiovascular complications in diabetics but may even serve to prevent the metabolic syndrome that leads to diabetes. In a 2000 study published in *Circulation*, these researchers studied the effects of 1200 international units of natural vitamin E on fifty subjects with type 2 diabetes, half with no vascular complications and half with cardiovascular disease. They found that even in the diabetics who had no signs or symptoms of heart disease, there was evidence of accelerated free-radical activity, as well as inflammation, another factor in vascular damage. Once they gave the study subjects high-dose vitamin E, there was, as expected, a fall in free-radical activity. However, there was also—and this was a novel finding—a marked reduction in inflammatory markers.[27] These researchers are currently planning a trial to determine if vitamin E might prevent heart disease and stroke in diabetics.

The suggested daily dose of vitamin E for diabetics is 800 international units. If you are having problems getting your blood sugar under control, consider upping your dose to 1200 international units. Make sure you purchase natural vitamin E, not synthetic. Natural vitamin E is referred to as *d-alpha-tocopherol* (or tocopheryl). *Dl-alpha tocopherol*, which is synthetic vitamin E, has been shown to be less effective than natural E.

Lipoic Acid

Lipoic acid, also known as alpha-lipoic acid or thioctic acid, is a small sulfur-containing compound that is essential for two important energy-producing reactions in the body. In addition to these vital roles, lipoic acid is an exceptionally powerful and versatile antioxidant, as it is both water-soluble and fat-soluble and can enter virtually all areas of the cells to neutralize free radicals. By comparison, vitamin C can only work in the water-based portions, and vitamin E only in the lipid-based parts.

Lipoic acid has proven to be a very useful supplement in the treatment of diabetes. In addition to its potent antioxidant effects, it has been demonstrated to improve insulin sensitivity. It is believed to do this by increasing the activity of the GLUT-4 transporters, the proteins that rise to the surface of the cells and usher in glucose.[28] In a 1999 placebo-controlled study involving seventy-two subjects with type 2 diabetes, Dr. S. Jacob and his German colleagues gave study subjects oral supplements of lipoic acid in daily doses of 600, 1200, or 1800 milligrams for four weeks. Another group received a placebo. Glucose uptake by the cells increased by an average of 63 percent in the individuals taking lipoic acid, regardless of the dose, and the supplement outperformed the placebo by 300 percent.[29]

Lipoic acid also protects against diabetic complications. It reduces the degree of glycosylation in tissues, improves circulation, and even stimulates the regeneration of nerves. More than fifteen clinical trials have examined the effects of lipoic acid on diabetic neuropathy. Although some of these studies have utilized intravenous administration of lipoic acid, many of the more recent ones demonstrate that oral supplements are also effective. One of these studies, which was published in 1999, involved type 2 diabetics who had neuropathic symptoms of pain, burning, and numbness in the feet. These patients were administered either 600 milligrams of lipoic acid or a placebo three times a day for three weeks. At the study's conclusion, significant improvements were noted in the patients taking lipoic acid.[30] In Germany, where much of the research has been carried out and the benefits of this powerful therapy are better known, lipoic acid is the preferred treatment for diabetic neuropathy.

Lipoic acid may also be helpful in protecting against diabetes-induced damage to the eyes. Lester Packer, Ph.D., a noted researcher at the University of California,

Berkeley, who has published at least sixty-five studies on lipoic acid, feels that this antioxidant may be a valuable therapy for several eye disorders. Its small molecular size allows it to enter both aqueous and fat tissues of the eyes, so it offers protection to both the lens and the retina. It has also been shown to increase the levels of vitamin C and vitamin E in eye tissues, both of which are important for healthy eye functioning.[31] Although research on diabetic retinopathy is preliminary at this stage, patients suffering with this disorder may do well to consider supplementing with lipoic acid.

Lipoic acid should be a mainstay in a nutritional supplement program for treating diabetes. The recommended dose is a minimum of 200 milligrams per day, going up as high as 600 milligrams for patients with diabetic neuropathy. Because lipoic acid may lower blood sugar levels, diabetics taking this supplement should be monitored by their doctors, as medication doses may need to be reduced.

The Benefits of the B-Complex Vitamins

The family of nutrients that make up what are commonly referred to as B-complex vitamins contains four members that are particularly important for diabetics.

Vitamin B_3

Vitamin B_3 is a player in many pivotal functions in the body, including energy production and nerve impulse transmission. It is also, along with chromium, a component of glucose tolerance factor, which we discussed above, and as such is involved in the metabolism of carbohydrates and the action of insulin.

As a nutritional supplement vitamin B_3 comes in two forms—niacin (also called nicotinic acid or nicotinate), and nicotinamide (also called niacinamide). The nicotinamide form of vitamin B_3 has been demonstrated to preserve pancreatic function and actually reverse diabetes in some type 1 patients when administered within the first few years of diagnosis. As you may recall from chapter 1, type 1 diabetes results from destruction of the insulin-producing beta cells in the pancreas. This is an autoimmune condition, like rheumatoid arthritis and multiple sclerosis, in which the body's immune system attacks and ultimately destroys its own tissues. Free-radical damage is known to be involved in this process, and one of the ways in which nicotinamide intervenes is by inhibiting free-radical generation.

In addition, nicotinamide may also help curtail other autoimmune mechanisms. One of the specific actions recently discovered to be involved in the destruction of the beta cells is overproduction of an enzyme known as poly-ADP-ribose synthetase (PARS). Excess amounts of this enzyme deplete cellular stores of ATP, the energy that runs the cells, leading to cell death. Nicotinamide is believed to inhibit the PARS enzyme.

At least ten studies have examined this phenomenon, and although some of them have demonstrated no effect, others have shown excellent results. In one such study, seven patients with recent-onset type 1 diabetes were administered daily doses of nicotinamide while nine others received a placebo. When the patients were followed up in six months, five of the seven taking nicotinamide and two of the nine on placebo had not yet had to start taking insulin. After one year, three of the patients in the nicotinamide group were considered to be in remission; none of those who had taken a placebo were.[32]

Nicotinamide may also have a useful role in patients who are at high risk of developing type 1 diabetes. As I mentioned in chapter 1, the presence of islet-cell or beta-cell antibodies in the blood is often a harbinger of autoimmune destruction of the insulin-producing cells. A five-year intervention trial was conducted in New Zealand to see if nicotinamide offered any protection to patients with this risk factor. Researchers screened 20,000 five- to seven-year-old children to determine islet-cell antibody levels and offered nicotinamide therapy to the high-risk children, those with elevated antibody levels. Over five years there was an average 50 percent reduction in the development of the disease in the at-risk children taking nicotinamide, compared to those who chose not to take the therapy or who were not involved in the initial screening.[33,34]

The amount of nicotinamide used for new-onset type 1 diabetics is based on weight: 25 milligrams per kilogram. **This protocol should be undertaken only under the supervision of a doctor.**

The recommended daily dose of niacin or nicotinamide (niacinamide) for type 2 diabetics and those with long-standing type 1 diabetes is 100 milligrams per day. Higher-dose niacin, in the range of 3000 milligrams per day, is an effective therapy for lowering cholesterol and triglyceride levels, which are often elevated in type 2 diabetics. Doses above 100 milligrams have traditionally not been recommended for diabetics, as it is widely believed that niacin impairs glucose control. New research, however, does not support this belief, suggesting that high-dose niacin is an excellent alternative to the commonly prescribed cholesterol-lowering drugs, even for diabetics.[35]

Biotin

Biotin, a B-complex vitamin produced by bacteria that reside in the intestinal tract, is required for the metabolism of fats and amino acids. It also improves insulin sensitivity and, equally important for diabetics, the activity of glucokinase, an enzyme involved in glucose utilization in the liver. Glucokinase levels are often quite low in people with diabetes. However, levels of this important enzyme may be raised by supplementing with high doses of biotin. This results in increased activity of glucokinase and improvements in glucose metabolism.

Biotin has been studied as a therapy for both type 1 and type 2 diabetes, and it has been shown to lower blood sugar in both types. In one study, type 2 diabetics were given 9 milligrams a day for one month, along with an antibiotic to ensure that the supplemental biotin would not be affected by bacteria in the gut. Compared to a similar group of patients who took a placebo, the subjects taking biotin experienced an average drop of 45 percent in their blood glucose levels.[36] Similar improvements were noted in another study of type 1 diabetics taking 16 milligrams of biotin per day.[37] As an added bonus, biotin has also been demonstrated to improve diabetic neuropathy.

I recommend 8 milligrams of biotin twice a day for patients with diabetes. Please follow your blood sugars closely when you first begin this therapy, as insulin or medication doses may need to be reduced. Biotin is very safe and no side effects have been reported.

Vitamin B_6, Vitamin B_{12}, and Folic Acid

Vitamins B_6 and B_{12} and folic acid have made headlines in recent years since it was discovered that they dramatically reduce the risk of cardiovascular disease. Because heart disease afflicts so many diabetics, maintaining adequate levels of these nutrients is crucial. However, these B-complex vitamins play other roles as well. Of all the B-complex vitamins, vitamin B_6 (pyridoxine) and vitamin B_{12} (cobalamin) may be the most important for the prevention of diabetic neuropathy. Deficiencies in these vitamins are associated with nerve damage, even in individuals who do not have diabetes. In addition, vitamin B_6 supplementation has been shown to be a safe treatment for gestational diabetes (diabetes that develops during pregnancy). In one clinical trial of this therapy, published in the *British Medical Journal*, twelve of fourteen women with gestational diabetes taking 100 milligrams of vitamin B_6 for two weeks had a complete reversal of their diabetes.[38]

I recommend a baseline dose of 75 milligrams of vitamin B_6, 100 micrograms of B_{12}, and 400 micrograms of folic acid. As we age, our absorption of vitamin B_{12} is often impaired. Therefore, if you are over sixty-five years old, consider upping your intake with monthly B_{12} injections (talk to your doctor about this) or daily 1000-microgram oral or sublingual supplements. Vitamin B_{12} is quite safe. However, very high intakes of vitamin B_6 (more than 500 milligrams per day for prolonged periods) may be toxic and cause nerve damage. Folic acid is also safe, and an increase to 800 micrograms per day is suggested if you have heart disease as well as diabetes.

Essential Fatty Acids Are Essential for Health

Americans have a love-hate relationship with fat: We hate to love it, and we love to hate it. But as I made clear in chapter 7, not all fats are created equal. There are some fats that are so important for optimal health that they are called *essential fatty acids* (EFAs). They earn their name by virtue of the fact that because they are not manufactured in the body, it is essential for you to get them from dietary of supplemental sources. The health benefits of EFAs stem from their unique chemical structure, which makes them highly biologically active. They are able to perform functions in the body that other fats cannot.

EFAs are important structural components of all cellular membranes. A lot of action takes place at the membrane, or outer surface, of the cell. This is the point of entry for substances coming into or leaving the cell, and it is where much of the intercellular communication takes place. The healthiest cellular membranes contain a variety of specialized fats, including EFAs. These essential fats help keep the membrane fluid and responsive to chemical messengers, including insulin's signals to let glucose into the cell.

In addition, EFAs are precursors to powerful chemical messengers called prostaglandins that have a multitude of effects in the body, from stimulating the inflammatory response to affecting the thickness of the blood. Optimal health requires that these prostaglandins be in balance. Unfortunately, because our dietary sources of fat are decidedly out of balance, the equilibrium between the various prostaglandins is thrown off, which sometimes causes things to get out of whack. Let's examine how the two classes of essential fatty acids, omega-3 and omega-6, affect, and are affected by, the diabetic condition.

Omega-3 Fatty Acids

A diet abundant in fish oils and flaxseed is associated with a low incidence of diabetes, heart disease, hypertension, rheumatiod arthritis and related inflammatory conditions, and other degenerative diseases. Such a diet increases insulin sensitivity, decreases the risk of type 2 diabetes, and protects against diabetic neuropathy.

This is because these foods are an abundant source of an omega-3 EFA called alpha-linolenic acid (ALA), or its two important spinoffs, eicosapentaenoic acid (EPA) and docosahexaenoic acid (DHA). EPA and DHA provide multiple health benefits. DHA nurtures the brain and has been shown to improve memory and cognitive function. More important for diabetics, however, is EPA, for in addition to its important role in healthy cell membranes, EPA lies at the top of the biochemical pathway that ends in the production of powerful chemical messengers affecting numerous systems in the body.

Most of the research on EPA has involved its effects on heart disease. This is important for diabetics, for as you know, the condition dramatically increases the risk of heart disease. It was noted years ago that Eskimos, who consume a very high-fat diet in which the fat comes primarily from fish and marine mammals, had far less heart disease than inhabitants of countries where meat from land animals was the staple food. The dominant fat in the Eskimo diet was discovered to be EPA, which explains why their high-fat diet provided such remarkable protection against heart disease.

EPA works on a number of fronts to enhance cardiovascular health. First, because it facilitates the burning of fatty acids in the liver, it lowers cholesterol and triglyceride levels. (This is also a plus for diabetics, because, as we discussed in previous chapters, excess fats in the bloodstream interfere with insulin sensitivity.) Dr. William Connor and his group at the Oregon Health Sciences University Department of Medicine gave patients with dangerously high levels of cholesterol and triglycerides supplementary EPA in the form of fish oil for four weeks. The average cholesterol level fell from 373 to 207 mg/dl, a drop of 46 percent. The triglyceride level fell even more dramatically—from 1353 to 281 mg/dl, a drop of 1072 mg/dl![39]

Second, EPA acts as a safe blood thinner by reducing the production of a substance known as thromboxane A_2. This chemical messenger causes blood platelets to stick together, forming dangerous clots that may lead

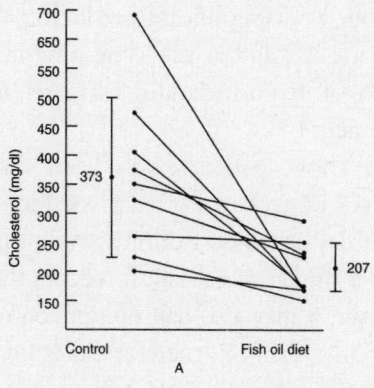

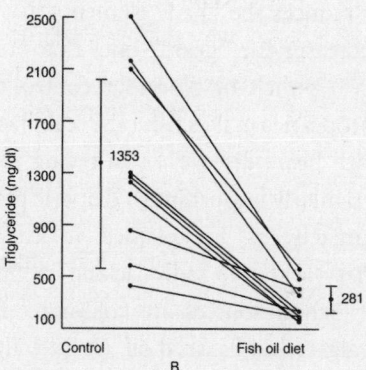

Figure 12. The effect of dietary fish oil in ten patients with elevated cholesterol and triglyceride levels.
From Connor, WE, et al. "Reduction of Plasma Lipids, Lipoproteins, and Apoproteins by Dietary Fish Oils in Patients with Hypertriglyceridemia." *New England Journal of Medicine* 312: 1210–16, 1985.

to heart attack or stroke. Howard R. Knapp, M.D., and his colleagues at Vanderbilt University in Nashville, studied 13 men with severe atherosclerosis of the arteries in the legs. They found that five capsules of fish oil daily for four weeks significantly reduced production of thromboxane A_2, and at the same time increased the production of a prostaglandin that acts as a natural blood thinner.

As you know, patients with heart disease or at increased risk of stroke are often advised to take a single aspirin per day as a blood thinner. Well, aspirin works in a manner similar to fish oil: It reduces thromboxane A_2. However, it may also halt production of beneficial prostaglandins. Fish oil, therefore, may be superior to aspirin for the prevention of cardiovascular events, as it not only reduces the "bad" elements that cause clots but also increases the "good" ones that prevent them. The one-two punch of blood-fat control and blood-thinning properties makes fish oil a real plus in treating patients with heart disease, or in trying to prevent it. This is particularly important to diabetic patients.

Unfortunately, as I explained in chapter 7, the omega-3 fatty acids are sadly lacking in the American diet. Their richest sources are cold-water fish, marine mammals, algae, and flaxseed oil. (A little algae for you? Seal, perhaps?) Therefore, deficiencies are quite common. Fortunately, supplements that contain EPA and DHA (fish oil capsules) or their precursor, ALA (whole flaxseed and flaxseed oil), are sold in every health food store.

The recommended dose of flaxseed is one to two tablespoons of flaxseed oil, or one-fourth cup of freshly ground flaxseed. The suggested dose of fish oil (which may be preferable because ALA has already been converted to the more useful EPA and DHA) is two 1000-milligram capsules per day, equaling 360 milli-grams of EPA. If your cholesterol and triglycerides are high, you may consider increasing this to four or more capsules daily. You may have read warnings that high doses of fish oil may cause elevations in blood glucose. I have heard such reports for years, although I have very rarely, if ever, seen such an effect in my patients, and I recommend fish oil capsules for almost all of them. Recent research suggests that this is an unfounded myth. A 1998 study in which 6000-milligram doses of fish oil were administered daily to type 2 diabetic men for two months showed no deleterious effects on glucose control—but it did improve their lipid profiles.[40] Furthermore, recent animal studies suggest that therapeutic doses of fish oil, rather than causing problems for diabetics, may actually improve the condition by increasing the activity of the GLUT-4 transporters.[41] At the recommended levels, fish oil is safe and quite beneficial for diabetics.

Blood Lipid and Blood Sugar Levels Often Go Hand in Hand

If you have diabetes and high cholesterol and triglyceride levels, pay attention. I want to tell you about one of my patients, David, a thirty-three-year-old man for whom fish oil supplements, along with a diet and exercise program, improved not only his blood lipids but also his diabetes. David had been bothered with obesity for most of his life. He had enormous weight swings and would actually gain or lose up to 75 pounds over a several-month period. Following one of his rapid-weight-loss regimens, he developed exceedingly high blood fat levels and elevated blood glucose. His triglyceride level measured 1047, his cholesterol level a whopping 346, and his blood sugar level had risen to 267. His general practitioner started him on Micronase, an oral drug for diabetes, and told David that he probably would have to have insulin within the year.

David came to the Institute for a second opinion. We immediately stopped the Micronase and put him on the high-fiber, low-fat diet outlined in chapters 6 and 7. We also used substantial amounts of fish oil, which has been shown to be very effective at lowering elevated triglycerides. David responded very rapidly, as predicted. Within two months, his triglyceride level had fallen to 182, his cholesterol level was 172, and his blood sugar level was a healthy normal 102.

David's story demonstrates how intimately blood sugar is associated with blood fats. One of the defining characteristics of Syndrome X and insulin resistance, as we discussed in chapter 2, is a high triglyceride level. When triglycerides are elevated, blood sugar levels often go up as well. With marked elevation in triglycerides, full-blown diabetes often ensues. Therefore, a priority for any diabetic patient with elevated blood fat levels is to get them down into the normal range. Blood sugar reductions will generally follow.

Omega-6 Fatty Acids

The most important of the omega-6 fatty acids for the diabetic is gamma-linolenic acid (GLA), which is derived from the EFA linoleic acid. GLA is integral to many functions in the body, yet diabetics are frequently deficient in this important fat. Even if they get enough linoleic acid in their diet from vegetable, nut, and seed oils, they still may exhibit deficiencies of GLA. This is because diabetics often have problems converting dietary fats to GLA.

Supplemental GLA has been found to be an effective therapy for diabetic peripheral neuropathy, which is caused by inflammation and deterioration of the peripheral nerves, usually in the legs and feet. Characterized by numbness, tingling, and sometimes severe pain, diabetic peripheral neuropathy gradually destroys the nerves, and the legs become more susceptible to ulceration, infection, and the necessity of amputation. A 1993 British study looked at the effects of 480 milligrams of GLA on 111 diabetics. Sixteen measurements were made throughout the study, and at the end of a year the subjects had significant improvements in nerve conduction velocities, hot and cold sensation, muscle strength, and reflexes. The researchers concluded, "Administration of GLA to patients with mild diabetic poly-neuropathy may prevent deterioration, and, in some cases, reverse the condition."[42]

The best GLA supplements are derived from borage oil or evening primrose oil. The recommended dose for diabetics with symptoms of peripheral neuropathy is 240 to 480 milligrams per day.

Herbal Extracts Improve Glucose Transport

Herbal medicine is the primary form of medicine for the vast majority of people on earth. In this country, however, this "unsophistocated" therapy fell out of favor decades ago when allopathic medicine with its "scientific" pills and potions came on the scene. Until a few years ago, herbal medicine was completely ignored in the U.S. However, we are now in the midst of an herbal renaissance. Time-honored herbal therapies have gained new respect in recent years as the American public and, to a lesser degree, the medical community have finally decided to accept plant-based supplements for what they are: safe, natural, and effective remedies for a variety of health challenges. Several of these compounds have been studied for their ability to lower blood sugar and improve the diabetic condition.

Gymnema Sylvestre

Gymnema sylvestre is perhaps the most powerful herbal agent for improving blood sugar control. The leaves of this climbing plant native to the forests of central and southern India have been used by practitioners of Ayurvedic (traditional Indian) medicine since the sixth century B.C. This herb works on several fronts to improve diabetes. Some studies suggest that it slows absorption of sugars in the gastrointestinal tract,[43] while others point to its revitalizing effects on the pancreas.

In fact, incredible as it may seem, *Gymnema* appears to regenerate the insulin-producing beta cells in the pancreas. In a study conducted on insulin-dependent rats, *Gymnema sylvestre* returned fasting blood glucose levels to normal after twenty to sixty days of treatment, and there was a trend toward normal blood levels of insulin. Even more remarkable, autopsies on the rats showed that the insulin-producing beta cells of the pancreas had doubled in number, compared to those of the untreated animals.

Human studies have demonstrated that *Gymnema sylvestre* has therapeutic value for both type 1 and type 2 diabetics. In one study, individuals with type 1 diabetes taking an extract of the herb for six to eight months had reductions in fasting blood sugar averaging 23 percent. Furthermore, they were able to cut their insulin dose by an average of 25 percent.[44] In a study of type 2 diabetes, patients taking 400 milligrams per day of a similar herbal extract for eighteen to twenty months also had notable reductions in blood glucose. The most impressive aspect of this study, however, was that twenty-one of the twenty-two patients involved in the study were able to significantly reduce the doses of their blood-sugar-lowering drugs, and five of them managed to discontinue their drugs altogether.[45]

I recommend that patients with diabetes try *Gymnema sylvestre* at a dose of 400 milligrams daily of a standardized extract. Because of its rather significant blood-sugar-lowering effect, you should closely monitor your blood sugars and discuss what you are doing with your physician.

Banaba Leaf

Another herb that shows great promise in the treatment of diabetes is banaba leaf (*Lagestroemia speciosa L.*). Banaba leaf contains corosolic acid, a compound that has been shown to activate glucose transport into the cells, resulting in a lowering of blood sugar. Although this herb was only recently introduced to the U.S. from Asia, early research is quite compelling. The eight human studies undertaken to date on the effects of banaba leaf on type 2 diabetics have demonstrated an average reduction in blood sugar of up to 32 percent.

In a 1998 Japanese placebo-controlled clinical trial, twenty-four diabetics were given a supplement containing banaba leaf or a placebo three times a day for four weeks. Blood sugar levels declined in the group taking banaba leaf from an average of 153.9 mg/dl to 133.1 mg/dl, while there was little change in the placebo group.[46] Other improvements were also noted in several of the studies. Blood glucose levels after meals fell more rapidly, approaching the pattern of nondiabetic individuals. Positive effects persisted even after the supplement was discontinued. Finally, and most impressive, weight loss was not uncommon. In fact, in one study, patients lost an average of 3.2 pounds after forty-five days of taking banaba leaf.

The suggested dose of banaba leaf is 48 milligrams per day of a standardized extract. Oil-based extracts seem to be the best absorbed and most effective. Banaba leaf is well tolerated and has no adverse side effects.

Bitter Melon

Bitter melon (*Momordica charantia*) is a fruit grown in tropical areas of Asia, Africa, and South America. It looks like a cross between a cucumber and a bumpy gourd and, as its name suggests, has a bitter taste. Long used by traditional healers for a variety of medicinal purposes, including the treatment of diabetes, bitter melon has been discovered to contain a number of compounds that have blood-sugar-lowering effects.

One is charantin, the effects of which have been compared to oral diabetic drugs. Another is polypeptide P, which lowers blood sugar when injected into type 1 diabetics.[47]

The juice and extracts of this bitter fruit have been demonstrated in clinical trials to lower blood sugar in patients with diabetes. In one such study that involved type 2 diabetics, 15 grams of a bitter melon extract lowered average postprandial (after-meal) blood sugars by more than 50 percent.[48] In another study, two ounces of bitter melon juice improved glucose control in 73 percent of the diabetic subjects.[49]

The recommended dose of bitter melon juice is 3–4 ounces or an equivalent amount in supplemental form. Because it too may result in significant drops in blood glucose, levels should be closely monitored.

Garlic

The oils found in garlic (*Allium sativum*) have been found to confer numerous benefits. In addition to enhancing the immune response, garlic has been shown to aid in lowering cholesterol and triglycerides and normalizing blood pressure, important concerns for individuals with insulin resistance. In addition, garlic also has ameliorating effects on blood sugar control.

The nice thing about garlic is that you don't have to take it as a supplement. You can just eat it: roasted, cooked in soups and casseroles, or minced and raw in a salad dressing. For years I have tried to find convenient ways to increase my patients' consumption of garlic. Some like my "garlic cocktail," which consists of 6 ounces of unsweetened grapefruit juice or unsalted tomato juice, one whole clove of fresh garlic, and two sprigs of parsley blended together. The resulting concoction is only 60 percent as offensive as it sounds! In fact, it is quite well tolerated, as the juices do wonders to mask the odor and taste of the garlic. One clove of garlic does not seem to be enough to create a chronically offensive breath odor, but many patients, to avoid this, drink the garlic cocktail at night.

Garlic supplements are another option. Look for a supplement that contains the equivalent of one clove of fresh garlic. Also, eat more onions, as they have many of the same beneficial compounds as garlic.

Flavonoids (from Bilberry, *Ginkgo Biloba*, and Grapeseed or *Pycnogenol*)

Another group of plant compounds that individuals with diabetes need to know about is the flavonoid family. Although these substances have only slight ameliorating effects on glucose control and insulin sensitivity, they are highly protective of the tissues that take a beating from elevated levels of glucose and insulin. They are potent antioxidants and protect the cells from free-radical damage. Equally important, flavonoids strengthen the capillaries, which are often damaged and fragile in diabetics, and thus improve blood flow to the tissues. This protective action has been noted in the capillaries of the eyes, kidneys, extremities, brain, and penis, areas that are extremely hard hit by diabetes.

Among the best-studied of the flavonoids for diabetics, and especially those with complications of the eyes, is anthocyanoside. This flavonoid is most concentrated in bilberry (*Vaccinium myrtillus*), a European cousin of blueberries. Along with other flavonoids in these berries, anthocyanosides improve circulation, strengthen collagen, and discourage inflammation in eye tissues. Bilberry was used by Royal Air Force pilots during World War II to improve nighttime vision and adjustment to darkness and glare. Studies have also confirmed its value in the treatment of cataracts and macular degeneration.

Ginkgo biloba is another flavonoid-rich herb that may benefit diabetics. Ginkgo neutralizes free radicals and increases blood flow to the tiny capillaries throughout the body. This herb improves nutrient and oxygen delivery to areas affected by both diabetic neuropathy and retinopathy. Ginkgo has also been shown to be beneficial in the treatment of erectile dysfunction and memory problems, common conditions in advanced diabetes.

Yet another favorite flavonoid is proanthocyanidin, found in extracts from grapeseeds or pine bark (*pycnogenol*). Proanthocyanidin has potent antioxidant activity. In addition, this flavonoid decreases the fragility and leakiness of the capillary walls to improve blood flow to damaged tissues.

Suggested doses of these three sources of flavonoids and indications for their use are as follows:

- Bilberry for diabetic retinopathy: 320 milligrams per day of a standardized extract containing 25 percent anthocyanidins

- *Ginkgo biloba* for circulation problems in the extremities, erectile dysfunction, and memory loss: 120 milligrams a day of a standardized extract containing 24 percent ginkgo flavone glycosides

◉ Grapeseed extract or pycnogenol for circulatory disorders: 100–150 milligrams of proanthocyanidin daily

Other Herbs for Diabetics

I have only touched on the best-known and well-studied of the herbs that benefit patients with diabetes. Be aware that there are dozens of others, which may in the future prove to be equally effective. Here is a brief overview of some of the most promising.

◉ **Fenugreek** (*Trigonella foenum-graecum*). Largely through the action of its soluble fiber, the seeds of this edible plant have been shown to lower blood sugar.

◉ **Ginseng**. Both Siberian ginseng (*Eleutherococcus senticosus*) and American ginseng (*Panax quinquefolium*) are therapeutic for patients with diabetes. Siberian ginseng enhances compromised kidney function, and American ginseng improves blood sugar regulation, particularly after meals.

◉ **Essiac**. The herbal combination of burdock root, sheep's sorrel, slippery elm, and Indian rhubarb root has been used as a therapy for cancer since the 1920s. Although it has been subjected to little formal research, tea made from essiac has also been reported over and over again to dramatically lower blood sugar and reduce the need for medication in both type 1 and type 2 diabetes.

⊙ **Stevia, Holy Basil, Cinnamon, and Cumin**. These well-known seasonings have ameliorating effects on blood glucose control.

Supplements That Facilitate Weight Loss

Obesity is a powerful predictor of future diabetes. At least twenty-eight studies have confirmed the relationship between excess weight and the risk of developing diabetes. One of the most recent, a 1999 study carried out at Johns Hopkins Medical Institutions in Baltimore, determined that for men, being overweight at age twenty-five is strongly predictive of diabetes in middle age.[50] Furthermore, weight loss is a powerful tool in the treatment of type 2 diabetes. In many cases, weight loss alone is enough to reverse the diabetic condition.

There is no magic pill you can take to ensure ideal weight. I firmly believe that the only way to achieve permanent weight control is through regular exercise and a healthy diet. However, for patients who need a little help in losing weight I recommend supplementing with nutrients that are involved in your body's natural energy-burning mechanisms. These include l-carnitine, which helps transport fat into the cells where it is burned for energy, and chromium and pyruvate, which are involved in insulin utilization and glucose metabolism.

At the Whitaker Wellness Institute we utilize a supplement that contains these three substances, as well as biotin (discussed on page 224) and hydroxycitrate (HCA, an extract from the plant *Garcinia cambogia*). Lipidox increases the burning of free fatty acids in the liver, which is key not only to weight loss but also to improvements in insulin sensitivity. It also enhances thermogenesis (the rate at which you burn energy), as well as having a dampening effect on appetite.

In a pilot study reported in *Medical Hypotheses* in 1999, sixteen obese voluteers (average baseline body fat percentage of 41 and BMI of 39.3) were placed on a low-fat diet and daily aerobic exercise, along with 12 grams calcium pyruvate, 1.5 grams HCA, 250 milligrams l-carnitine, and 600 milligrams chromium picolinate. The weekly weight and fat loss during this one-month study averaged 3.3 pounds and 5 pounds respectively, implying a weekly gain in lean muscle mass of 1.76 pounds![51] According to Mark McCarty, Research Director of NutriGuard Research, this combination of nutrients dramatically facilitates the fat-burning process in the liver—but only if used in conjunction with a low-fat diet and regular exercise.

We are having very good success with this supplement, particularly in diabetics. Because patients see results much more quickly than with exercise and diet alone, it is a wonderful motivator to stick with the program. (I'll tell you more about this unique supplement in chapter 12.)

Another helpful weight-loss aid is soluble fiber from diet and supplements (psyllium is a good source), which staves off hunger by causing a slower release of glucose. While ephedra (ma huang) and caffeine (from guarana and kola nut), common ingredients in herbal dietary supplements, suppress the appetite and increase thermogenesis, these strong stimulants may raise blood pressure and heartbeat, alter heart rhythm, and cause nervousness and insomnia in some people. I prefer milder thermogenic agents such as green tea and cayenne pepper, which can be taken as a premeal beverage or supplement.

One natural appetite suppressant I do recommend is 5-hydroxytryptophan (5-HTP), which cuts cravings, particularly for carbohydrates, by balancing serotonin levels. The recommended dose is 50–100 milligrams three times a day, 20 minutes before meals. However, the problem with any appetite suppressant—natural or prescription—is that once you stop taking it, your appetite returns, often with a vengeance. Unless you use these aids to help you get started on a better diet and a regular exercise program, you're destined to repeat the vicious loss-gain cycle that plagues so many.

DHEA Increases Sensitivity to Insulin

Although it is a hormone rather than a nutritional supplement, I want to tell you about dehydroepiandrosterone (DHEA). Your body produces more DHEA than any other steroid hormone, yet, as with other hormones, its production tapers off as we age. There is a direct correlation between low DHEA levels and the diseases of aging, including insulin resistance, diabetes, and heart disease.

As we discussed in chapter 2, elevated levels of insulin have a number of adverse effects on the body. Among them is an increase in the secretion of stress hormones such as cortisol. High levels of cortisol are a decided negative. This hormone unleashes a cascade of damaging mechanisms, including depression of DHEA production. Since low levels of DHEA are very common among diabetics, restoring levels of this protective hormone makes sense for patients with diabetes and insulin resistance. Furthermore, early research suggests that supplemental DHEA actually increases insulin sensitivity.

I routinely recommend that my patients with diabetes have their level of DHEA measured with a blood or saliva test, and, if it is low, consider supplementing with DHEA. For patients whose levels are suboptimal (below the average for a healthy young adult), I recommend a starting daily dose of 25 milligrams for women and 50 milligrams for men to bring their level up into the healthy range. DHEA is quite safe and has few side effects. Because it converts in a woman's body to testosterone, too-high doses may cause oily skin, acne, or increased facial hair growth. Cutting back on the dose immediately ameliorates these conditions. I do not recommend that men with prostate cancer take DHEA, as theoretically it may exacerbate the condition by elevating testosterone levels. In reality, the conversion of DHEA to testosterone in men is not very efficient. However, I would prefer to err on the side of caution and suggest that men with a history of prostate cancer avoid DHEA. It is sold in health food stores and does not require a prescription.

Putting Together a Supplement Program

The first step for diabetics embarking on a nutritional supplement program is to start with a multivitamin and mineral supplement that contains adequate doses (meaning for the most part above-RDA dosages) of a broad array of nutrients. As I mentioned earlier, deficiencies in water-soluble nutrients are epidemic in diabetic patients. And although I have singled out those most intimately involved in blood glucose metabolism, I strongly recommend that you cover your bases and replace all of the important vitamins and minerals.

Be aware that it is impossible for a one-a-day type of multivitamin and mineral to contain therapeutic doses of these vital nutrients. There is just no way to get all those nutrients in a single capsule. A high-potency formula will require taking several capsules or tablets per day. (The daily dose of the brand we use at the clinic, the Forward Daily Regimen, is twelve capsules, taken in divided doses.)

You should take your multivitamin and mineral supplements with meals to ensure optimal absorption and reduce the likelihood of stomach upset. You should also spread them out over the day: Take several with breakfast or lunch, and the rest with dinner. Depending on the brand you select, you may need to mix and match, adding a bit extra of this and that to meet to my recommended doses.

Here is a list of suggested doses of vitamins and minerals to look for in a multivitamin and mineral. This is what we recommend to our patients at the Whitaker Wellness Institute, and I believe that every diabetic should be on a similar basic supplement program.

Nutrient	Suggested Daily Intake
Vitamin A	5000 IU (international units)
Beta-carotene	15000 IU
Vitamin D	400 IU
Vitamin E (d-alpha tocopheryl)	800 IU
Vitamin C	2000 mg (milligrams)
Folic acid	400 mcg (micrograms)
Thiamine (vitamin B_1)	50 mg
Riboflavin (vitamin B_2)	50 mg
Niacinamide (vitamin B_3)	100 mg
Vitamin B_6 (pyridoxine)	75 mg
Vitamin B_{12} (cyanocobalamin)	100 mcg
Biotin	16 mg*
Pantothenic acid (vitamin B_5)	50 mg
Calcium	1000 mg
Iodine	150 mcg
Magnesium	1000 mg*
Zinc	30 mg
Copper	2 mg
Potassium	99 mg
Manganese	10 mg
Chromium (picolinate or polynicotinate)	400 mcg*

*Level is higher than what you will likely find in most multivitamin and mineral supplements. You may have to supplement with an additional dose.

Selenium	200 mcg
Molybdenum	125 mcg
Silica	25 mg
Bioflavonoids	100 mg
Inositol	40 mg

Do not be overwhelmed by this list. All of these nutrients are found in most multivitamin and mineral formulations. Now, the doses in many will be considerably less, but shop around, and you will be able to come up with a supplement such as my formulation, Forward, that doesn't require opening twenty bottles.

The next step in designing your supplement program for reversing diabetes is to add some of the more targeted nutrients discussed in this chapter. I am not suggesting you run out and buy everything I've talked about in this book. However, taking a good multivitamin and mineral supplement is only the first step. In the chart below, I have summarized the additional supplements that have been demonstrated in clinical studies to improve the diabetic condition. After each I have noted what aspect of diabetes they target and have given the doses that the bulk of the research has shown to be most effective.

Supplement	Action	Suggested Dose
Vanadyl sulfate	Lowers blood sugar	45–100 mg
Lipoic acid	Protects against diabetic neuropathy and lowers blood sugar	200–600 mg
Nicotinamide (niacinamide)	For new-onset type 1 diabetics only	25 mg per kilogram of body weight (see page 223 for details)
EPA (fish oil capsules—omega-3 EFAs)	Protects cardiovascular system	2–4 1000 mg capsules
GLA (evening primrose or borage oil—omega-6 EFAs)	Protects against diabetic neuropathy	240–480 mg
Gymnema sylvestre	Lowers blood sugar	400 mg
Banaba leaf	Lowers blood sugar	48 mg
Garlic	Protects cardiovascular system	1 clove or supplemental equivalent
Bitter melon	Lowers blood sugar	2–4 oz or supplemental equivalent

Supplement	Action	Suggested Dose
Bilberry	Protects eyes	320 mg of an extract standardized for 25 percent anthocyanidins
Ginkgo biloba	Enhances circulation, improves memory loss and erectile dysfunction	120 mg of an extract standardized for 24 percent ginkgo flavone glycosides
Grapeseed extract or pycnogenol	Circulatory disorders	100–150 mg of proanthocyanidin
Lipidox	Facilitates weight loss	7–9 capsules, 2–3 times per day on an empty stomach
5-hydroxytryptophan (5-HTP)	Suppresses appetite	50–100 mg 3 times per day, 20 minutes before meals

The best way to begin any supplement program is to start slow and add one or two of these nutrients at a time as you see fit. If, for example, you are having problems with blood sugar control, add vanadyl sulfate and/or chromium. If you are suffering from diabetic retinopathy, add bilberry. You will find some of these specialized nutrients in combination formulations created for diabetes. In fact, I've formulated one myself, Glucose Essentials. These combos eliminate the need to take so many separate supplements. Just make sure the doses of the various nutrients in the formula you choose approach those shown to be effective.

Important note: Remember that if you are taking any of the above-mentioned supplements whose primary action is to lower blood sugar (vanadyl sulfate, lipoic acid, *Gymnema sylvestre*, banaba leaf, or bitter melon), you should monitor your blood sugar levels carefully. These substances have the potential of driving glucose too low, particularly in patients who are also taking insulin or oral drugs. It is especially important to work with your doctor if you are giving vanadyl sulfate a try, for decreases in blood sugar may be dramatic.

Nutritional supplements are an integral part of my program for reversing diabetes. When I first began my foray into alternative medicine I thought that diet and exercise were the most powerful therapies available. As I delved into the research on nutritional supplements and started using them with my patients, I gained more and more respect for these often-neglected therapies. Today, I do not think I could practice medicine without prescribing nutritional supplements. They are among the most effective and safest therapeutic tools available.

CHAPTER 10

Additional Therapies for Diabetes

In addition to the well-known complications associated with diabetes, such as problems with the eyes, nerves, and kidneys, diabetics have much higher than average rates of high blood pressure, abnormalities in triglyceride and cholesterol levels, and increased risk of heart disease. Excess glucose in the blood damages the blood vessels and encourages the development of atherosclerosis, which leads to higher rates of heart attack and stroke. Furthermore, as I explained in chapter 2, insulin resistance, the underlying cause of type 2 diabetes, also contributes to the development of hypertension and heart disease. The high insulin level typical of insulin resistance appears to be a risk factor in and of itself for the development of these concurrent medical problems.

The beauty of the diet, exercise, and nutritional supplement program we use at the Whitaker Wellness Institute is that because it focuses on the underlying principles of health, rather than simply aiming to clear up symptoms, it is highly therapeutic for a wide variety of medical problems. Hypertension and cardiovascular disease respond to the same dietary modifications that help bring blood sugar into the normal range. Regular exercise not only heightens insulin sensitivity, but also strengthens the heart and improves circulation.

The nutritional supplements discussed in the previous chapter to target the diabetic condition are also extremely beneficial for the cardiovascular system. Antioxidants counter the damaging effects of free radicals and protect LDL cholesterol from oxidation, a primary step in the development of arterial blockages. The B-complex vitamins prevent the buildup of homocysteine, which has in recent years been discovered to be a primary cause of cardiovascular disease. Omega-3 essential fatty acids improve blood flow, and magnesium helps maintain normal heart rhythm. Therefore, when you undertake the program outlined in this book to improve your diabetes, you are also benefiting your heart, your circulatory system, and your overall health.

Try Safe Alternatives Rather Than Resorting to Drugs

Yet, as with diabetes, the conventional way of treating these associated conditions is with drugs and more drugs. Because so many medical problems can manifest in individuals with insulin resistance and diabetes, it is not uncommon for patients to be prescribed five, six, or even more medications. Once you get on the drug merry-go-round, it tends to pick up speed. More and more drugs are added, some to treat problems caused by the drugs themselves! Furthermore, certain drugs actually worsen the diabetic condition, necessitating even more intensive drug therapy.

Needless to say, the diabetic condition makes the use of drugs for lowering blood pressure, triglycerides, and cholesterol much more complicated and danger-ous. Unfortunately, the increased dangers of many commonly used drugs in diabetic patients are not gen-erally recognized. Mary E. Callsen, M.D., as an inter-nal medicine resident at Brooke Army Medical Center in San Antonio, did a small but very informative pilot study on prescription drug use in 122 subjects who had type 2, non-insulin-dependent diabetes. Of the 122 subjects, 50 were being treated with oral drugs, 47 were being treated with insulin, and 25 were receiving diet therapy alone.

Dr. Callsen found that 96 percent of the study group (117 out of 122) were taking drugs for medical prob-lems other than diabetes. The most common additional conditions for which medications were prescribed were hypertension and heart disease. Other problems included rheumatoid arthritis, gout, and gastrointes-tinal disorders. The patients who were being treated with diet alone for their diabetes were taking an aver-age of 3.3 drugs for other problems. Those on the oral pills were receiving an average of 3.8 additional drugs. Patients being treated with insulin were using an aver-age of 4.4 additional medications.

While 68 percent of all diabetic patients were taking thiazide diuretics, only a little more than half of the physicians prescribing the drugs were aware that they may have negative effects on diabetic control. Over 20 percent of the patients were taking beta-blockers, even though these drugs are associated with worsening of diabetic control. Dr. Callsen found that the more drugs a diabetic patient was taking, the worse the diabetic control. The rare patient being treated only for diabetes was found to be in the best diabetic control.[1]

Often quality of life is not considered when medications are prescribed. Sexual performance routinely deteriorates with drug therapy, particularly with certain types of antihypertensive drugs. In addition, patients often report poor concentration, decreased work performance, and significant reductions in energy. Some medications make it difficult to exercise because patients taking them report that they have neither the energy nor the inclination to become more active. Furthermore, patients often state that they "just don't feel well."

Dr. Gordon Williams, chief of endocrinology/hypertension at Brigham and Women's Hospital in Boston, recalled his experience with a thirty-two-year-old truck driver referred to him for treatment of high blood pressure. This strong and virile man could bench-press 300 pounds, and he had no health complaints. He felt great! Then a routine checkup revealed that he had hypertension. One year and five medications later, his blood pressure was normal—but he was a "fatigued, impotent wimp."[2] Unfortunately, given the potential for adverse side effects and interactions of prescription drugs, stories such as this are not uncommon.

Needless to say, drugs are sometimes required. For example, if blood pressure remains high after all natural therapies have been exhausted, a course of an antihypertensive medication may be appropriate. However, when drugs are used before any attempt is made to utilize a safer, equally effective program of diet, exercise, and nutritional supplementation, they often do more harm than good.

In this chapter I want to give you an overview of some of the powerful alternatives we utilize at the Whitaker Wellness Institute in place of drugs. These therapies are not only effective in the treatment of the direct complications of diabetes, but also in the concomitant medical problems that so often afflict patients with insulin resistance: hypertension, heart disease, and abnormal blood lipids.

I do not want you to think of these therapies as a replacement for the diet, exercise, and supplement program outlined in this book. Nor do I want you to neglect your doctor's recommendations if you are being treated for any of these conditions. However, I do want you to know about these remarkable therapies—and it is unlikely you'll hear about them anywhere else. For some of you, these innovative treatments may mean a new lease on life.

Note: Unfortunately, some of the therapies discussed in this chapter are not widely available. To obtain more information and to locate a practitioner or facility where they are administered, please see the Resources section.

Inexpensive Help for Diabetic Neuropathy

For four years G.M. literally could not feel his feet. He had no perception of touch or temperature on the soles of his feet, and walking was an ordeal. He constantly had to think about where his feet were. He also had continuous pain and aching in his lower legs, from which he could find no relief. G.M. had diabetic neuropathy, a disease that affects up to 45 percent of all diabetics.

Diabetic neuropathy often has serious consequences. In addition to pain and loss of sensation, patients may feel weak and lack muscle control and coordination. They sometimes develop ulcers on their feet, which are very slow to heal and prone to serious infection, making diabetic neuropathy the number one cause of nontraumatic amputations in the U.S. Conventional physicians prescribe nonsteroidal anti-inflammatory drugs (NSAIDs) for pain, but relief is often fleeting.

I can't remember the last time I recommended a prescription NSAID for anything, and particularly for diabetic peripheral neuropathy. At the Whitaker Wellness Institute, in addition to the supplements discussed in the previous chapter, we use two inexpensive over-the-counter therapies that have been shown to be quite effective in relieving the pain of diabetic neuropathy.

Penetran+Plus: A Unique Ointment

One is a unique topical ointment called Penetran+Plus. We use it successfully for all types of pain, from arthritis to bumps and bruises to diabetic neuropathy. Penetran+Plus contains an ammonium compound that relieves pain by normalizing the electrical currents in the cell membranes at the site of pain or injury. It is combined with methylsulfonylmethane (MSM), which acts as a carrier to rapidly facilitate absorption into the skin. In a recent study it was found to provide significant pain relief for 70 percent of study subjects with arthritis, bursitis, or tendinitis.[3]

G.M. happened to be one of the patients in this study. He experienced such dramatic relief from the pain and stiffness in his arthritic knees that he tried it on his numb feet and painful lower legs. For this patient, one application provided 10 hours of pain relief. Here's how he described his experience: "The most amazing thing happened. After just a few applications, I realized that not only was the ache gone, but I could feel the bottoms of my feet again for the first time in years."

A little dab of this inexpensive ointment rubbed into painful areas one to four times a day provides excellent pain relief for neuropathy and other types of pain. See the Resources section for information on Penetran+Plus.

Magnificent Magnets

The other therapy that has proved to be effective for relieving the pain of neuropathy is magnets. Magnets have a long history—and growing scientific support—as a therapy for pain associated with neuropathy, arthritis, post-polio syndrome (a painful condition that often strikes polio survivors years, even decades, after their bout with the disease), PMS, and other conditions. A study published in the January 1999 issue of the *American Journal of Pain Management* illustrated that magnetic insoles worn in the shoes are effective in relieving the symptoms of diabetic neuropathy. In this randomized study of twenty-four patients with neuropathy, half used magnetic foot pads and the other half placebo insoles; after four months, the groups were switched. Researchers found significant improvement in the symptoms of 90 percent of the diabetic patients using the magnetic insoles, compared to 33 percent of those using the placebo insoles. Symptoms returned when the patients stopped using the magnets.[4]

Although no one is exactly sure how magnets work, they are believed to improve blood flow, which decreases inflammation and facilitates the delivery of nutrients and oxygen to damaged tissues. They also appear to stimulate the release of pain-relieving neurotransmitters. Although magnets have not been demonstrated to actually heal damaged nerves, their ability to alleviate pain associated with neuropathy and other conditions makes them an invaluable therapy.

A Folk Remedy That Helps Heal Diabetic Ulcers

This extremely inexpensive, widely available therapy that we routinely use at the Whitaker Wellness Institute probably raises more eyebrows than just about anything else we recommend. It's sugar—and, believe it or not, it is the best antibiotic ointment around. When placed on an open wound such as a diabetic ulcer, the fluid weeping from the ulcer dissolves the sugar, forming a highly osmotic, or concentrated, dressing. While bacteria will thrive in a substance containing a low concentration of sugar, they are instantly killed in this highly concentrated solution. Furthermore, the high osmolarity of the solution draws fluid out of the wound, dramatically improving blood flow and reducing inflammation. The combination of these three things—absolute sterility, improved blood flow, and reduced swelling—stimulates healing like no other ointment I am aware of.

When I first suggested this therapy to a patient of mine named Julie, who had had diabetes for many years, she thought I was crazy. She had an ulcer on her right ankle that just would not heal. In fact, she had been told that she would require surgery to improve circulation to the area. I removed her bandages, washed away the expensive antibiotic ointment that wasn't doing any good at all, covered the ulcer with a quarter-inch-thick layer of table sugar, and rewrapped her ankle. I instructed Julie to wash the ulcer as often as she wished, as long as she loaded on more sugar and wrapped it up again. The ulcer began to heal almost immediately, and within four weeks it was completely closed.

The Whitaker Wellness Institute is not the only place using this neglected therapy. Richard Knutson, M.D., an orthopedic surgeon in Mississippi, learned about it from an elderly nurse working in the hospital where he was doing rounds. After he expressed his concerns about a patient who had developed an ulcerated bedsore the size of a softball, she suggested that he try dressing the wound with sugar. Sure enough, it resulted in complete healing. He has since treated more than 5000 patients with sugar and has eliminated the need for antibiotics and skin grafting in 97 percent of them.

It sometimes makes the sugar application easier if you build up a barrier around the edge of the wound with petroleum jelly before adding the sugar and bandaging it. Give this oldie but goodie a try. You won't believe how effective it can be.

EDTA Chelation Saves Limbs

EDTA chelation is an intravenous therapy used to treat circulatory disorders. EDTA (ethylenediaminetetraacetic acid) is a synthetic protein that, when slowly infused into the bloodstream, binds to metal ions in the blood vessels and arteries. These heavy metals are then carried to the kidneys and excreted. Initially used to remove heavy metals such as lead (it remains the premier therapy for lead poisoning), chelation has gained popularity as a treatment for vascular problems. By restoring the health of the blood vessels, it improves blood flow and the vast number of conditions related to decreased circulation: diabetic neuropathy, heart disease, hypertension, intermittent claudication (leg pain caused by poor circulation), and memory loss.

Chelation also promotes the healing of wounds caused by inadequate blood flow, which is a problem for many diabetics. Ulcers on the lower extremities often become infected, sometimes so severely that amputation is required. This is the state one of my patients, J.J., a high school teacher with a thirteen-year history of diabetes, found himself in several years ago. For almost three years he had been plagued with persistent diabetic ulcers on the bottom of his left foot that never completely healed, in spite of several hospital stays for massive doses of antibiotics. He was told that his only option was amputation, so he was admitted to the hospital for amputation of his left leg and the fitting of a prosthesis.

On the morning of the day he was scheduled for surgery, J.J. called the substitute teacher who would be handling his classes to tell him that he would be out for the rest of the semester to undergo physical rehabilitation. By a stroke of luck, this teacher had heard of EDTA chelation therapy and how it benefited circulatory disorders. He also knew that it was administered at the Whitaker Wellness Institute, and he advised J.J. to call the clinic and check it out. His comment to J.J. was (no pun intended), "What have you got to lose?"

Against his physician's advice, J.J. checked out of the hospital and came to the clinic. He was given a full course of thirty treatments consisting of three-hour sessions once or twice a week. In addition, his wound was treated with topical dressings of sugar as described previously, and he was started on the diet and supplement program outlined in this book. Today, J.J. is walking around on his own two feet and living a full and active life teaching and coaching softball.

Chelation is also beneficial for patients with heart disease and circulatory problems. A retrospective study published in 1989 of the effects of chelation therapy on 2870 patients with various conditions revealed that of the 844 patients with heart disease enrolled in the study, after twenty to thirty treatments, 76.9 percent had marked improvement. Stress tests that had previously been abnormal reverted to normal, and symptoms such as chest pain disappeared. Furthermore, some patients who had been taking medications for their heart were able to discontinue them. Of the

1130 patients with peripheral vascular disease (caused by poor circulation to the extremities), 91 percent reported marked improvement. They were able to walk five times their pretreatment distance without pain in the legs, and Doppler ultrasound studies, which evaluate blood flow to the legs, returned to normal.[5]

EDTA chelation therapy is exceptionally safe and easy to administer. Infusions are given in a doctor's office once or twice a week over a two-and-a-half- to three-hour period, for an average of thirty to forty treatments. It is also relatively inexpensive. J.J.'s amputation, prosthesis, rehabilitation, and disability would have cost $150,000 to $200,000. The course of chelation therapy that saved his leg cost $4000. Ironically, his insurance company was ready to cover the cost of cutting his leg off and giving him a prosthesis, but when he presented the much smaller bill for chelation, which had resulted in a healthy leg, he was turned down. I encouraged J.J. to sue the insurance company for reimbursement and suggested that as evidence he take off his shoe and wiggle his toes.

An IV Therapy for Diabetic Retinopathy

Another intravenous therapy we often recommend for diabetics at the Whitaker Wellness Institute targets the eyes. Unfortunately, many diabetic patients suffer from vision problems, for they are more prone to cataracts and glaucoma than are people with normal blood sugar metabolism. However, the primary cause of vision loss among diabetics—and indeed the leading cause of blindness among all Americans under the age of seventy-four—is diabetic retinopathy. As we discussed in part I, elevated levels of glucose and insulin damage the small blood vessels that nourish the eyes. Over time, this may lead to severe deterioration and ultimately loss of vision. Although the condition can be retarded with laser therapy, it is usually progressive, and the prognosis is often dire. Yet impaired vision is not an inevitable part of being diabetic. Even patients with diagnosed diabetic retinopathy can retard, stop, and sometimes reverse this insidious condition.

Let me tell you about Vic, a longtime patient from South Carolina. Vic has had diabetes for years and in 1994 was diagnosed with diabetic retinopathy with macular involvement. (The macula is a small focal area inside the eye that conveys visual messages to the optic nerve.) Within eighteen months of diagnosis, Vic's failing vision necessitated five laser treatments, and he was on a downward spiral. At that point, he decided to explore his options. He had heard about the Institute through my monthly newsletter, and he and his wife paid us a visit.

I started Vic on the diet, exercise, and nutritional supplement program discussed in the previous chapters. Because his diabetic retinopathy was well under way, I also recommended a course of intravenous nutrients aimed at the eyes, including high does of vitamin C, B-complex vitamins, the amino acid taurine, magnesium, and other minerals. Intravenous administration allows for a much more concentrated dose of nutrients than can be taken orally, and ensures that they are absorbed and delivered to the targeted tissues.

This IV drip is often used in conjunction with chelation therapy, which by improving overall circulation further enhances nutrient delivery.

We've had a lot of success with this protocol, not only for diabetic retinopathy but also for macular degeneration, and Vic is one of our shining stars. After he returned home he continued to receive periodic IV treatments from a physician in his area, and he stuck with the overall program. Since he began our program in 1996, he has only required five additional laser treatments (compared to five in the first eighteen months!). Vic credits his nutritional program and IV therapies with a dramatic slowing in the progression of his disease. His ophthalmologist concurs.

Hyperbaric Oxygen Therapy Facilitates Circulation and Wound Healing

You can live months without food and days without water, but if you are deprived of oxygen for more than a few minutes, you'll die. Yet some of our tissues exist in a state of relative oxygen deprivation. Stroke, circulatory disorders, heart disease, some types of memory loss, and all types of wounds are seemingly unrelated conditions that have one thing in common: The affected area is just not getting enough life-sustaining oxygen.

There is an excellent therapy, hyperbaric oxygen therapy, that delivers much-needed oxygen to tissues. When 100 percent oxygen is administered in a pressurized environment, virtually every cell of your body, including those with a poor blood supply, is flooded with massive amounts of healing oxygen.[6] Exposure to this pressurized infusion of oxygen results in remarkable benefits that cannot be achieved by any other therapy.

More than 30,000 scientific studies have been published on this therapy over the past sixty years. Hyperbaric oxygen has been demonstrated to be beneficial for almost two hundred diverse conditions, from stroke recovery and memory loss to bone infections and carbon monoxide poisoning. Of particular interest to diabetics are improvements in diabetic neuropathy and memory loss that is due to inadequate blood flow to the brain. In addition, because wound healing is greatly accelerated, slow-healing, oxygen-starved diabetic ulcers respond particularly well. Hyperbaric oxygen reduces inflammation, encourages new tissue growth, and dramatically curtails infection. Oxygen actually kills many types of anaerobic bacteria that thrive in the absence of oxygen. Many a limb destined for amputation has been saved by hyperbaric oxygen.

Hyperbaric oxygen is administered in a specially designed chamber in which pressure is slowly increased to 1.4 to 3 times that of the normal atmosphere. Most people notice increased pressure in the ears, a feeling similar to that experienced during an airplane takeoff or landing, but there is no other discomfort. A typical session lasts 45 minutes to 2 hours, after which the pressure is slowly returned to normal. Sessions may be repeated, depending on the condition, anywhere from five to forty times.

EECP Dramatically Improves Circulation

Enhanced external counterpulsation (EECP) is an innovative therapy that diabetic patients who suffer with heart disease or hypertension should know about. It was developed by Harry Soroff, M.D., at Harvard University almost fifty years ago as a treatment for angina pectoris, the chest pain associated with heart disease. EECP is a remarkable therapy that dramatically increases blood flow through the arteries of the heart and improves circulation throughout the body. It also accelerates the growth of collateral circulation, the additional avenues of blood that open up around arterial blockages, making it nature's equivalent to heart bypass surgery.

It is a particularly powerful therapy for eliminating angina. In one study, twelve patients with serious heart disease underwent a course of EECP. At the study's onset, they reported an average of 3.9 episodes of chest pain per day, rating the pain at 2.9 out of 4. After a full EECP course, the pain episodes were reduced to an average of 0.1 per day (one episode every ten days) with an intensity of only 1.7 out of 4. All of the patients reported improvements in their ability to work, energy level, and sense of well-being.[7]

EECP is also beneficial for other conditions involving impaired circulation, including hypertension, peripheral neuropathy, and diabetic neuropathy. It has even proven useful in memory loss and vision problems associated with inadequate blood flow.

Here's how it works. You lie on a flat or slightly elevated surface, and what looks like a wet suit is strapped onto your lower extremities from ankles to the waist. Then, timed with each beat of your heart, the device contracts, forcing blood up the extremities through the veins back to the heart. One treatment session lasts about an hour, and, aside from the squeezing sensation, there is no discomfort or danger. A usual course is thirty-five one-hour treatments, given twice a day. In three or four weeks—far less time than it takes to recuperate from a bypass—chest pain is often eliminated and circulation restored.

Quick-Start Diet for Hypertension

More than 50 percent of all type 2 diabetics also have hypertension. Too often they are placed on drugs that may actually cause a worsening of the diabetic condition. As I mentioned above, thiazide diuretics, which may decrease glucose control and increase the risk of heart attack, are often the first-line treatment for elevated blood pressure.[8] And another common type of antihypertensive drugs, beta-blockers, has also been shown to cause a worsening of diabetes.

Lying dormant in the archives of every medical library is the work of Dr. Walter Kempner of Duke University, who demonstrated that a high-potassium, low-sodium diet, consisting primarily of rice, vegetables, and fruit, is quite effective in lowering blood pressure, even in the most difficult cases of hypertension.[9] When diet is used to replace drugs, quality of life is dramatically enhanced. All that is required is for the physician and the patient to give vigorous diet therapy a chance.

The following patient story illustrates how temporary use of Dr. Kempner's diet can be helpful in both hypertension and diabetes. G.M. came to our clinic with a fifteen-year history of type 2 diabetes and high blood pressure, as well as heart disease with angina pectoris (chest pain) that she had developed two years previously. A recent angiogram showed significant blockages in her coronary arteries, and although one cardiologist had enthusiastically recommended bypass surgery, another had been much less certain. Therefore, she chose a conservative route and enrolled in our Institute to see if we could help. Until this time she had not altered her diet a great deal but had been following the earlier recommendations of the American Diabetes Association, whose regimen at that time consisted of excessive calories derived from fat.

G.M. had been treated with drug therapy exclusively. When she arrived she was taking an ACE inhibitor (Capoten), a thiazide diuretic (hydrochlorothiazide), a beta-blocker (Tenormin), and a calcium channel blocker (Procardia). She wore a nitroglycerin patch and had been directed to use a nitroglycerin sublingual (under-the-tongue) spray when needed for chest pain. She was receiving insulin by a continuous infusion pump. The pump delivered one unit every hour (24 units per day), and she gave herself an additional 42 units daily, divided between three meals and a bedtime snack. This was a lot of insulin (66 units a day), considering that she weighed only 152 pounds.

We put G.M. on a diet of brown rice, vegetables, and fruit to lower her blood pressure rapidly and reduce her need for so much medication. After ten days she was shifted to the regular diet program outlined in this book. Her insulin pump was stopped because her new diet almost certainly would have caused significant hypoglycemic reactions, and she was put on doses of 5 to 10 units of insulin before each meal. Her blood pressure medications were gradually reduced and then discontinued without significant elevation in her blood pressure. In addition, the frequency of her angina attacks was reduced from three to four times per day to one a day, which occurred while she was exercising mildly. (She had not been exercising before her arrival. In fact, she had been totally inactive for the last eight months.)

At the end of two weeks she was taking only one heart medication, Procardia, and insulin, 20 units in divided doses before meals. She wore a nitroglycerin patch delivering 5 milligrams a day and used a nitroglycerin spray when needed. Over this time her blood pressure—after discontinuing her antihypertensive medications—remained in the normal range. Her cholesterol fell from 233 to 188, and her protective HDL cholesterol went from 51 to 55, resulting in a favorable cholesterol to HDL ratio of 3.4. Triglycerides, uric acid, BUN—all returned to the normal range. And her fasting blood sugar? Her initial fasting glucose test, taken while she was on 66 units of insulin, was 193. The day she left the Whitaker Wellness Institute on 20 units of insulin, it was 125.

More dramatic was the rapid transformation in the way G.M. felt. On arrival she was despondent to the point of hopelessness. At the end of only twelve days she was hopeful and had experienced a dramatic increase in her energy level. She went from no exercise to walking five and a half miles a day as a part of her exercise regimen.

The positive experience of this patient is not uncommon for the many diabetic patients who go through the Institute. We place great emphasis on a dietary regimen, exercise, and nutritional supplementation. When patients make a concerted effort to follow this program, in many cases they simply no longer require medication.

In the next chapter I'll tell you more about the Whitaker Wellness Institute and share with you some success stories of patients who by following this program for reversing diabetes have regained control of their lives.

CHAPTER 11

Reversing Diabetes Success Stories

Now I want to share with you some patient success stories, for they are what make this all worthwhile. These are patients who have either come through the Whitaker Wellness Institute Back to Health program (which I will describe in detail at the end of this chapter) or have read about the program for reversing diabetes in this book or in my monthly newsletter, *Health & Healing*. They have followed the program outlined in *Reversing Diabetes*, and, as you will see, it has not only improved their diabetes, but also many other aspects of their health.

Paul Zimmerman

My husband was deteriorating right before my eyes. We'd been married over forty years, built a successful business together, enjoyed "the good life." But for years I'd been helplessly watching him go downhill. He'd had a heart attack at the age of forty-five, surgery to replace arteries in his legs at fifty-one, four bypass operations before fifty-seven, and his diabetes had worsened to the point where now, at age sixty-five, he was taking 55 units of insulin by injection every day.

The surgery improved the circulation in his legs for several years, but the pain had returned, and now Paul could walk no farther than fifty yards. Another catheterization and special X-rays were done. They showed that his arteries and even the grafts were rapidly closing up with fat and cholesterol. Another operation would not help, his doctor said; he had no choice but to send us home. We expected gangrene to set in, and that a surgeon would have to amputate Paul's legs. Diabetes and its terrible complications had a stranglehold on my husband. We had both lost hope.

Then I read an article by Julian Whitaker, M.D., about how a diet, exercise, and vitamin and mineral program can be used to treat the very problems that were killing my husband. We were skeptical. Paul had been under medical supervision for ten years, and he was getting worse. But we had nothing to lose. We went to California to see Dr. Whitaker and enter his clinic.

During our time there we experienced the specialized diet and the vitamin and exercise program and learned how to do them at home. In four weeks, Paul was completely off insulin with normal blood sugars. In six weeks, he had lost twenty-two pounds and was able to walk three to four miles a day, nonstop, without pain. Even the pins-and-needles sensations in his feet, so common with diabetics, had improved.

His blood cholesterol (we now understand how

important this test is) had dropped from 196 to 148. After eight weeks on this program, his doctor at home repeated the studies of circulation in his legs and found a 66 percent improvement in the right leg and a 42 percent improvement in the left leg. He told us he'd never seen such rapid improvement, and that Paul would probably not lose his legs.

What more can be said? During our stay, Dr. Whitaker and his staff made sure we understood exactly how to follow the program once we were home. Now, eight months later, Paul is closely following the program that saved his life, and he's improving every day. He recently passed a new milestone: Now he's completely off all heart medication!

Six months after Paul Zimmerman left the Institute, I received a letter from his vascular surgeon, along with copies of his last two peripheral vascular studies that showed dramatic improvement in his diabetic neuropathy since he started on the program for reversing diabetes. He wrote:

I am sure that you will agree with me that this is not only a very pleasant surprise, but solid proof that improvement can be made in these patients with diet and exercise. You may feel free to use our studies for any use that you may wish to put them to.

Parenthetically, I should add that Paul still feels well and keeps up his diet and exercise program. I told him that if he continues, in the next three to six months, he should be able to go up to the mountains and do the trout fishing that he enjoys so much. He sends along his best regards, as do I.

Sincerely yours,
Dr. D.C.

Marjorie Atwood

I do believe that my participation in Dr. Whitaker's program has saved my sight. When I arrived at his clinic I was fifty-six years old and had been a diabetic for eighteen years. I had been treated for the first four years with an oral drug, and I have been on insulin ever since. Like most diabetics, my insulin requirement gradually and slowly increased until I was taking 55 units when I entered. I did not get off of insulin completely, but reduced my insulin from 55 units to 20 units a day.

Before I entered Dr. Whitaker's Wellness Institute, I had been having bleeding episodes in my eyes and had had laser treatments. When I arrived at the Institute, my cholesterol level was 240, my triglycerides were 852, and my blood sugar was 187. When I left the Institute my cholesterol had dropped to 236, my triglycerides were down to 203, and, on much less insulin, my fasting glucose was 126. For a year and a half after that, and up to the present, I have not had any more bleeding in my eyes. In addition, my cholesterol level has stayed lower and my very high triglycerides have also stayed low.

My ophthalmologist is baffled as to what happened. Prior to my going to Dr. Whitaker's Institute, he had mentioned that it was a good idea, but it was likely too late for me as the eye problems would probably continue. After a year and a half of no further damage, he was pleasantly surprised and told me to "keep doing whatever you are doing."

Since that time I am now able to drive, and I'm back in business as a real estate agent doing better than ever. I couldn't be happier or more satisfied with the result.

Glenora and Don Baker

We feel so great. We have excess energy and our mental outlook has been reversed completely. We look forward to another glorious day, which always seems too short for all the things we want to do. We are truly alive. Between us, we have lost eighty pounds in six months— Glenora has lost fifty and I have lost thirty. In addition, my wife has not had an insulin shot in six months, whereas she had been on insulin daily for eight years and was taking 65 units when we arrived at the Institute in California.

People ask: What do we eat? My reply: We eat anything we want to. However, if you think for one minute we would eat red meat, fats, sugar, salt, or dairy products, except for skim milk and a few other things, you are out of your mind. The benefits my loving wife and I have received by deleting these foods from our diet are so great that we will continue it for the rest of our lives. In addition, we will also stay on the vitamin program designed by Dr. Whitaker that complements this diet, and we will continue to exercise on a regular basis as well.

Of interest to me is that we require so much less sleep now. I used to get up about 8:00 A.M., go to work, and be so tired that I would need a nap every afternoon before going back to work until 6:00 P.M. After work I would go home, sit in a lounge chair and watch a little TV before going to bed around 9:00 P.M. I then would get up at 8:00 A.M. to repeat the cycle.

Now, I do not need an afternoon nap and if I go to bed before 11:00, I am up by 5:00 A.M., ready to do anything and everything. Our children and employees now say, "Stay out of the way, here comes Dad, he will run you over." We get things done and love it. Our attitude continues to spiral upward. Many people who knew us have seen this remarkable change in our mental attitude. We were at times quite depressed. Now we truly glory at being alive.

We also love to share our experience with others in our shop and our personal lives. Actually, Glenora's doctors had been telling both of us that diet and exercise were powerful and could get Glenora off of insulin, but the program was simply not implemented. I guess they expected us just to figure out how to do it ourselves. We share with our friends and family how valuable the experience at the Institute has been. We never would have believed such good things could happen to us without the time we spent there, following through completely on the program designed for us. I guess it all seems so simple now. If you want a program of vigorous diet and exercise, go to where they teach diet and exercise, not to places that simply say it might work.

Dr. Whitaker, we truly thank you.

Leland P. Robinson

Your program has been of great benefit in bringing about a new feeling of well-being. I feel well and sleep well. I have suffered no ill effects from the new lifestyle. I'm particularly pleased that I have been able to stay off the oral diabetic medication since attending your Institute. My weekly blood sugar measurements are averaging about 130 and I expect these will reduce even more with the added exercise and reduced weight.

My doctor now considers me a miracle. He never believed that your diet program would work and said that I would always need medicine. He now tells me to "keep doing whatever you are doing."

Thank you very much for your help.

Sigmund Czarnecki

Your program has changed my life—all for the better. My weight is under control, having lost fifteen pounds, and I no longer have blood pressure problems or require blood pressure medication. My attitude and stamina have greatly improved. My blood sugar levels have been in line, perhaps a bit on the high side, but much better than before the program. My "quality of life" is at a much higher level than prior to this program.

Thank you very much.

Vasken Imasdounian

When I arrived at your office I had been on insulin for approximately six months. My blood sugar at the time of diagnosis was found to be 287 and it went to 300-plus. My glycohemoglobin was approximately 16. Shortly after starting on insulin, I began having significant hypoglycemic reactions. My glycohemoglobin fell rapidly, but I was continued on insulin.

When I came to your clinic, you and I were both concerned about the hypoglycemic reactions, so we decided, under close control, to go without insulin. It has been nine months now and I have not gone back on insulin. I am very happy that my glycohemoglobin and blood sugar levels stay within normal limits and that I have measurements of C-peptide that show my body is producing insulin.

I truly love the dietary regimen and exercise. I feel so much healthier, vibrant and alive. You have no idea how happy I am to be off of daily injections. I know, as you have told me, that I will most likely have to have insulin down the road. However, I have been happy for the past nine months, and frankly, I see no end in sight to my improved health. Somehow—and I know there is no proof of this—I think the vitamins and minerals are contributing to my improved status.

I will always be grateful for your attention, concern, and help.

Ray and Ad Kimball

Even though I was taking 130 units of insulin and seventeen prescription pills every day of my life, I was surprised to be at the Whitaker Clinic. After reading about Dr. Whitaker and the Institute in Prevention *magazine, my wife had recommended we go. For the past two years she had literally begged me to go.*

But I was not easily persuaded. As a "workaholic" who can't remember missing a day's work in the last thirty-five years, except for a one-night stay in the hospital after the removal of a melanoma mole, I wanted to try everything else first. And I did!

When I was diagnosed with early-onset diabetes, my reaction was perhaps typical. Trying to forestall the traditional insulin, I ran the gamut on oral drugs. I even cheated by taking more than the doctor prescribed, hoping to avoid the needle. But the blood sugar levels kept rising, so I finally gave in and started on a modest level of insulin injections.

For nine months I had dutifully gone to the hospital twice a week for two blood tests. These automatically resulted in an increase of insulin intake until I reached the 30-units-per-day mark. In answer to my question, "Will this situation ever be better?" the doctor just flatly told me, "No." At this time I was also taking medication for high blood pressure and atrial fibrillation, resulting in a daily intake of the seventeen prescription pills. While I'm grateful for the limited number of doctors who have literally saved my life in specific situations—Dr. Whitaker tops that list—I've surely had my share of medical kiss-offs of the "keep taking your present medications and call me if you need help" type!

When I finally arrived at the Whitaker Clinic I was taking 130 units of insulin per day (44 of humulin R and 86 of humulin NPH) for diabetes; two hydrochlorothiazide, eight "micro K" potassium pills, and two Midamor (another diuretic) for high blood pressure; plus one digoxin and four verapamil tablets for atrial fibrillation control.

Diet had hardly been mentioned at all during this buildup of my "pathological museum." We had been told to use salt sparingly, and we cut out all sugar, thinking it was the culprit. What a shocker we received at the Whitaker Institute. Dr. Whitaker placed me on a low-fat diet and increased my exercise schedule. In two days I was totally off insulin, and within a week I had discontinued all prescription pills. My blood sugar levels were, for the first time in years, safely within the desired range of 80–120, my blood pressure remained at the same, or lower, levels than I had achieved under medication, and my pulse was normal. At the end of the first week I had dropped six pounds. I really was a new person!

The clinic's low-fat diet, personally prepared by a professional chef, was simple, adequate, and, best of all, understandable. Taking time to exercise was a scheduled luxury, and a totally new lifestyle was formulated— health, attitude, and commitment being the keys.

We will be forever grateful for the Whitaker Institute and the wonderful people associated with it.

About the Whitaker Wellness Institute

Although the Whitaker Wellness Institute is a place where people come to get well, it is not a hospital and is not designed to look or feel like one. Patients stay at a nearby deluxe hotel, where lectures are held, meals are eaten, and exercise classes are conducted. What is accomplished in this environment could not be done in the usual hospital setting. Hospitals deal with crisis intervention and use the tools necessary to rescue patients from disaster. As such, they are quite impersonal and are often uncomfortable places charged with fear. As its name implies, the Whitaker Wellness Institute deals with creating health, so the environment is comfortable, personal, pleasant, and charged with hope and enthusiasm.

The Institute was founded on the concept of nutritional healing. Our primary therapies are diet and nutritional supplements, along with regular exercise and stress management. The food here is unprocessed, whole, natural, loaded with fiber, and low in cholesterol and fat. We exercise on a daily basis, and our patients are prescribed a personalized program of nutritional supplements for their specific health concerns. The one-week Back to Health program of medical evaluation, treatment, and education is designed to create health. In order to get a feel for how the Institute functions, it might be helpful for me to describe a typical day.

A Typical Day at the Institute

◉ 7:30 A.M. Patients weigh in, have their blood sugar, blood pressure, and pulse recorded, and give a history of the previous day—how far they walked, the pulse rate attained during exercise, and a rundown of any symptoms experienced. These daily reports help us evaluate progress and alter medication dosage.

◉ 8:00 A.M. to 9:00 A.M. Breakfast is prepared by our own gourmet chef, who has worked with me for the past twenty years. It may be egg-white omelets, oatmeal, French toast, or even tofu scramble (which is delicious, despite its scary name), along with fresh fruit, hot drinks, and vitamin and mineral supplements.

◉ 9:00 A.M. to 10:00 A.M. Seminar. These seminars, conducted by our professional support staff, help patients get a handle on the nuts and bolts of the program. They are designed to inform and motivate patients to follow the program at home. Some of the sessions deal with food selection and preparation, so that, in addition to receiving printed recipes and menus, patients clearly understand the mechanics of following this program at home. Other sessions explain the ins and outs of nutritional supplementation, or how to get started on—and stay on—a personalized exercise program. All the morning sessions are recorded on tape and every patient is given the complete series of taped lectures. This provides reinforcement and program recall after they return home.

- 10:30 A.M. to 11:30 A.M. Scheduled exercise. We encourage patients to exercise throughout the day, but we also have group exercise classes. Our certified personal trainer makes sure every patient understands the basics of stretching, warming up and cooling down, taking a pulse reading accurately, and exercising at an appropriate level according to their own personal exercise prescription.

- 12:00 A.M. to 1:00 P.M. Lunch. Back to the dining room for a healthy lunch. Salads, soups, even the Whitaker Wellness version of quiche may be on the menu.

- 1:00 P.M. to 4:00 P.M. The afternoons are left open for physician visits, nutritional consultations, and additional therapies. Every patient is evaluated by his or her physician twice during the week. Each patient is given an individualized nutritional supplementation regimen that addresses all of their health concerns. Medications are often lowered and in many cases eliminated. Insulin and diabetic drugs are almost always reduced in a gradual manner, as are the numerous heart and blood pressure drugs used by so many patients before they enter the Institute. Our physicians spend a lot of time with each patient, discussing all of the health problems, diagnoses, laboratory test results, and treatment recommendations. We believe that patient education and open discussion about all aspects of treatment are essential to the practice of medicine. Many patients also opt for a private session with our nutritionist to fine-tune their diet.

Optional therapies include hyperbaric oxygen, EDTA chelation therapy, and enhanced external counterpulsation, discussed in the previous chapter, as well as acupuncture, chiropractic, massage, and reflexology. These unique therapies are particularly beneficial for diabetics who already suffer from poor circulation and damage to the vascular system.

- 5:00 P.M. to 6:00 P.M. Seminar. Patients meet back at the hotel for another lecture. Each day a specific subject is presented by one of the Whitaker Wellness physicians, followed by a question-and-answer session with the physician.

Subjects include diabetes, heart disease and bypass surgery, hypertension, natural hormone replacement therapy, arthritis, immune function, mood, and memory. It is during these seminar sessions that patients get an in-depth explanation of their medical problems as well as the role that diet, exercise, and nutritional supplementation play in their improvement.

◉ 6:00 P.M. Dinner. This is a time to enjoy the end of a day of accomplishment. Salmon and couscous, chicken and rice, vegetarian lasagna, and other delectable, healthful meals are served in the dining room. These delicious meals are enjoyed with good fellowship and leisurely conversation.

◉ 7:00 P.M. The evenings are free. Some patients enjoy getting out in beautiful Newport Beach, while others prefer to hit the sack early.

Obviously, the days are full and active. For perhaps the first time in their lives, patients spend the whole day doing things specifically designed to improve their health. Many accomplished and disciplined people, experts in their own field, limp into the Institute riddled with diabetes, high blood pressure, heart disease, and other serious problems. For many, this is a unique experience in making their health the top priority.

My Observations

Having watched thousands of patients since 1979 attend this program, I have observed some general trends.

First day: Almost everyone is a little skeptical. After all, a medical program housed in a nice hotel may not match their expectations. However, most are convinced that this approach makes a lot of sense and have decided before arrival to give it a try. There is a lot of testing the first day—including a complete physical examination, blood tests, and, for most patients, an exercise stress test. Patients meet the other members of the group and often talk about why they came and what they hope to get out of the program. They begin to make friends rapidly. Everyone is in the same boat, going in the same direction, with the same goal: to regain their health.

Second and third days: The mood is considerably lighter. Information presented in the seminars convinces patients of the benefits of a healthier lifestyle. For a few, improvements have already begun—a little less angina, more physical endurance, or fewer insulin and drug requirements. Friendships are becoming stronger and a group spirit begins to form. Even though each patient comes from a different walk of life and will return to such, they're all learning the same thing: how to alter their lifestyle in key areas to regain and maintain their health. This is fertile ground for camaraderie.

Fourth and fifth days: The routine of activities, exercise, meals, and relaxation has been established and patients now concentrate on improvements. Many symptoms are ameliorating. Patients who had never walked more than a few blocks without difficulty and considered such a feat impossible are covering reasonably long distances. Blood sugar levels have stabilized, blood pressures are down, and many patients have lost some excess weight. Seminars continue to give more information and serve to reinforce each patient's commitment to the program. Most are already planning how to handle life in the "real world"—grocery shopping, dining out, and the logistics of exercise. For the most part, patients are continually surprised at how pleasant the food is—even tofu scramble. By the time everyone packs up and leaves the next day, significant strides have been made. Medications have been discarded, new goals have been set, and close friendships have been formed. Our patients report that they not only feel better physically, but they also have new hope and confidence that their health will continue to improve.

For more information on our clinic and this one-week program, which attracts people from all over the country, plus quite a few from outside the U.S., please contact us at: The Whitaker Wellness Institute, 4321 Birch Street, Newport Beach, CA 92660; (800) 488-1500; www.whitakerwellness.com.

I hope I have made clear in these last six chapters, which detail my program for reversing diabetes, that drugs are not the only answer. If patients with a recent diagnosis of type 2, insulin-resistant diabetes embrace this lifestyle regimen, they can improve their body's sensitivity to insulin and likely avoid drug therapy altogether. And as the stories above make clear, even patients with a history of years of prescription drug dependency are often able to obtain good blood glucose control naturally and reduce or eliminate their need for drugs.

In part IV, we will leave theory behind and jump into the nuts and bolts of the program: how to begin and stay on an exercise program and how to make the transition to a healthy diet. Let's get started.

Putting the
Program into
Practice

Let's Get Moving

I f all the benefits of exercise were available in a prescription drug, it would be the world's most widely prescribed medication. Everyone would be on it, diabetic or not! The resistance to using exercise on the part of both doctors and patients is innately human: Exercise requires effort. However, the effort need not be unpleasant. For patients who successfully start an exercise program and persevere until it becomes established in their daily lives, physical activity becomes a joyful release of tension rather than a tedious chore.

Getting an exercise program firmly implanted in your daily life is like taking an airplane ride. The hardest part is getting off the ground and up to cruising altitude.

The Stress Test: A Vital Precaution

Before anyone with diabetes (or anyone over age forty, for that matter) begins an exercise program, he or she should have an exercise stress test. During a stress test, the patient exercises on a treadmill or a stationary bicycle while an electrocardiograph (EKG) machine monitors the activity of the heart. The patient exercises at gradually increasing work levels, and as the heart rate increases, the EKG monitor picks up any abnormalities in the heart that are present only when it is working hard. For example, some EKG patterns indicate that arteries may be blocked. Such blockages could prevent the heart from getting enough blood at certain levels of exertion. This test will also reveal any tendency toward arrhythmia, or skipped beats, brought on by exertion.

The stress test you obtain prior to starting an exercise program contains vital information that your doctor needs to create your personalized exercise prescription. It allows your doctor to determine how much you are to exercise, what type of excercise is appropiate for you, and what your heart rate should be during the activity. You should treat your exercise prescription with the same respect and discipline you treat prescriptions for drugs.

Your Exercise Heart Rate

One of the guidelines that your exercise prescription will contain is your training heart rate. When you exercise, your pulse rate increases as your heart beats faster to pump more blood to the working muscles. It has been determined that the benefits of exercise are best achieved when your heart reaches a certain rate. Below that, you're not working your heart hard enough to get the cardiovascular benefits of exercise. Above that, and you may be putting yourself in jeopardy.

What should your heart rate be during exercise? Well, it depends. Again, the best thing you can do is work with your doctor to determine the exercise intensity that is appropriate for you. Short of this, you can use this commonly accepted formula. First, determine your *maximum heart rate* (the safe upper limit) by subtracting your age from 220. For instance, if you are twenty, your maximum heart rate at exercise is 200 (220 minus 20 equals 200). If you are sixty, it is 160 (220 minus 60 equals 160), and, as a rule, you should never let your exercising pulse climb above this rate. Then, depending on your fitness level, select a *training heart rate:* the pulse rate to strive for in exercise sessions. Usually the recommended training rate is between 65 and 85 percent of the maximum calculated heart rate. As a rule, beginning exercisers should stay in the lower range, while more fit individuals may aim for the higher end. However, having done thousands of exercise stress tests on patients, I consider this to be only a general guideline. Individual training heart rates can vary substantially, depending on level of fitness and overall health. This is yet another reason for having an exercise stress test done by a professional and getting your own personalized exercise prescription before you start your program.

While you are exercising, monitor your pulse rate periodically to make sure you are working at an appropriate intensity. First, find your pulse by placing your middle and index fingers on the large artery on either side of your neck. (An alternative pulse point is inside your wrist, just below your thumb.) Once you feel the pulse, count the number of beats during a ten-second interval, then multiply it by six. This tells you how many times your heart is beating per minute.

Your age	Minimum heart rate	Maximum heart rate	10-second pulse (minimum-maximum)
20–29	120	151	20–25
30–39	114	143	19–24
40–49	108	135	18–22
50–59	102	127	17–21
60–69	96	120	16–20
70+	90	112	15–19

Figure 13. Target ranges for training heart rate

Types of Exercise

The primary type of exercise I prescribe as a treatment for diabetes is aerobic conditioning exercise designed to elevate the heart rate and sustain that elevation for a minimum of 20 minutes—and preferably 30 minutes or more. Types of aerobic exercise include brisk walking, bicycling, swimming, slow jogging, or any other exercise that moves the body through space at a rate that permits a sustained elevated pulse rate. Regular walking is an activity I often recommend because almost everyone can do it. And it definitely helps. A 1999 study conducted at Deakin University in Australia found that when women with type 2 diabetes were put on a walking program consisting of an hour-long walk at a moderate pace five days a week, fasting blood glucose levels improved.[1]

The value of resistance or muscle-building exercise has also been recognized in recent years. As I stated in chapter 8, the more muscle or lean body tissue you have, the less resistant your cells are to insulin. Therefore, exercise that builds up muscle tissue is highly therapeutic for the type 2 diabetic. Resistance exercise such as weight lifting, push-ups, chin-ups, sit-ups, and crunches is also known as anaerobic exercise because it involves muscle fibers that utilize little oxygen but large amounts of glucose—a plus to the diabetic. However, the greatest benefit of resistance exercise is building muscle that improves insulin sensitivity over the long term.[2]

Frequency and Duration of Exercise

Many patients contend that their daily activities are already filled with exercise. Some feel that doing housework, walking up and down stairs, or working in the garden is adequate. Others think that their work provides more than enough exercise, particularly if it includes a lot of walking. The idea of "short-burst" activity—ten minutes here, five there, as long as they add up to at least 30 minutes a day—has gained favor in the past decade. And recent studies suggest that simply making a conscious effort to fit in 30 minutes of physical activity during the day is effective in achieving and maintaining weight loss.

In a 1999 study published in the *Journal of the American Medical Association*, researchers at Johns Hopkins University School of Medicine placed forty sedentary, obese women, ages twenty-one to sixty, on a low-fat, restricted-calorie diet. They were then enrolled in either a lifestyle activity group and encouraged to exercise on their own during the course of their daily activities, or a structured aerobic exercise group. Although women in both groups lost similar amounts of weight during the initial sixteen-week period, after one year those in the structured exercise group had regained some of the weight, while those in the lifestyle group had maintained their weight loss.[3]

Although I do suggest that my diabetic patients take a short, brisk walk—8 to 12 minutes—after meals, the bulk of the research suggests that for patients with diabetes, more sustained exercise is preferable. I suggest you work with a health professional to put together a program consisting of aerobic exercise (at least 20 minutes at your training heart rate, with 5 to 10 minutes each of warm-up and cool-down). Ideally, these sessions would be interspersed with resistance (weight) training.

For years experts recommended that exercise training take place at least four days per week and at most six days, with rest days spaced in between. However, the most recent recommendation of the American College of Sports Medicine is to engage in at least 30 minutes of exercise most every day.

If you are doing particularly vigorous exercise of longer duration, four or five times per week with a day or two of rest in between may be more appropriate. Vigorous exercise programs deplete the muscles of stored carbohydrates (glycogen), the primary fuel of the muscles, and occasional days of rest allow glycogen stores to be replenished. Otherwise exercise may become very difficult and unpleasant.

Ready, Get Set, Go

After a stress test has determined your targeted heart rate during exercise, and your doctor has written your exercise prescription, you and your doctor need to sit down and work out the "what," "when," "where," and "why" of your program.

- *What* will it be? Walking? Stationary bicycling? Cycling? Weight lifting? Swimming? Of course, you can vary your activities, and I suggest you add a couple of weight training sessions every week. But the most important thing is to decide on something.

- *When* will you be doing it? This is very important! The program will not start until you have designated some time during the day for the activity. Though this seems obvious, I have had many patients who kept putting off exercise because they just couldn't seem to find the time. Make it a priority by writing in your calendar or on a tracking form like the one on page 303 precisely when you plan to exercise.

- *Where* is all this activity going to take place? In areas of the country where the weather does not permit year-round outdoor activity, you must make plans to continue your exercise program during inclement weather. You may decide on walking in a shopping mall, swimming in an indoor pool, working out in a heated gym or athletic club, or exercising at home on a treadmill or exercise bicycle.

- *Why?* Never lose sight of why you are exercising: to improve your health. Set specific goals, such as getting your blood sugar into the normal range, cutting back or eliminating medications, losing weight, reducing your risk of heart disease and other diabetic complications, and just feeling better. When the going gets rough, reflect on these things. It may be just the motivation you need to stay on an exercise program.

If you are just beginning an exercise regimen I suggest you get some instructions in the basics. Attend classes at your local gym or spend a session or two with a personal trainer. Ask a knowledgeable friend to "coach" you so you'll get started right. Or get a book or video from your library or bookstore that provides detailed instructions in the ins and outs of exercise.

Learn the proper way to stretch and warm up your muscles before exercise, and how to gradually cool down and stretch out after exercise. Make sure you understand how to exercise at a proper intensity—hard enough to obtain benefits but not so hard that you could endanger your health. (Your respiration and pulse rates should go up, but you should not exert yourself to the point that you are unable to carry on a conversation while exercising.) Get some help in the proper mechanics of weight lifting. Even if you decide to purchase some hand weights to use at home, rather than going to a gym, it is imperative that you do these exercises correctly to avoid the possibility of injury.

An Exercise-Weight Loss Strategy

Taking a short, brisk walk after meals does wonders for lowering blood sugar, and I recommend this activity for all diabetics. However, if you are a type 2 diabetic and weight loss is one of your primary goals, the best time to do your most prolonged exercise session is in the morning before eating. (Important: If you are a type 1 diabetic or a type 2 diabetic being treated with insulin or oral drugs, please see "A Word of Warning" on page 191. This is not recommended for these patients.)

Before eating is the optimal time for burning fat. If you exercise after you eat, you'll burn the food you just ate—which is good, but it doesn't do much to reduce body fat. On the other hand, if you exercise in the morning on an empty stomach, after being in a fasting state for several hours during sleep, you're much more likely to mobilize fat stores. Glucose levels are low (assuming that you don't wake up in the night and raid the refrigerator!), so the body will revert to its next-favorite energy source: fat.

To further facilitate fat burning, drink one or two cups of coffee before you begin exercising. Caffeine increases the body's ability to release fat from storage. This provides the muscles with a quick and ready source of energy and improves endurance. Caffeine has long been recognized to enhance athletic performance—so much so, in fact, that the International Olympic Committee for the 2000 Olympics limited blood levels of caffeine in athletes to no more than that found in three to six cups of coffee.

If you want to see results more quickly, consider trying Lipidox after drinking your coffee and before you begin exercising. As I explained in chapter 9, this supplement enhances the burning of free fatty acids in the liver. Then exercise aerobically (walking at a fast pace is fine) for at least 40 minutes. While shorter periods of time are certainly beneficial, only with prolonged exercise do all the factors involved in fat burning come into play. If you refrain from eating carbohydrates for a few hours after you exercise—provided that your blood sugar doesn't drop too low—you will continue to burn fat. (Believe it or not, this is easy to do, for this supplement suppresses appetite as well.) This combination of caffeine, Lipidox, and prolonged morning exercise before eating is ideal for fat burning.

If you do not need to lose weight—or if morning exercise just doesn't work for you—then schedule it for anytime during the day. The most important thing is that you get active.

How to Stay on Track

So now you have an exercise prescription from your doctor. You know your target heart rate and how to monitor your exercise intensity, and you are aware of the special precautions you must take during exercise. You've decided on the type of exercise you're going to do, and you have figured out how to fit it into your schedule. You recognize the rewards, and you are committed to your exercise program. You blast out of the starting blocks the first week and hit all of your exercise goals. The second week you only miss a day or two, but by the third week the temptation to stay in your warm bed rather than get up and hit the pavement grows stronger and stronger.

Don't despair. This is normal, and there is a solution. I have been utilizing exercise as a primary therapy for diabetes and other conditions for more than twenty-five years now, and most of the patients I see at the Whitaker Wellness Institute face a similar crisis.

During their week at the clinic, it's easy. They are in a healthy, encouraging environment, exercising daily under the supervision of a certified exercise instructor with like-minded, enthusiastic people. Many report that this week is the jump-start they needed to finally implement a regular exercise program, which they've always known they should do and wanted to do but just couldn't seem to get underway. They leave the clinic armed with information and enthusiasm.

The flip side of this is that after they've been home for a while, slugging it out on their own, trying to fit exercise into their busy schedules (and being challenged by restaurant menus, dinner parties, and people who think they're "health nuts"), motivation again becomes a problem. The truly committed work through the expected ups and downs, climbing back on board after setbacks. The less diligent may give up altogether. After all, exercising and avoiding steak and ice cream are not the path of least resistance.

Now, if these patients could follow up with us every week or two for encouragement and monitoring of their progress, I am confident that most would stay on track. However, because they come from all over the country (and more than a few from Canada and other countries), this isn't possible. Therefore, I have developed a planning and tracking system that, patients report, has made it much easier to comply with their program. This system works very well for the Whitaker Wellness Institute patients who are not able to return to the clinic regularly, and it will work equally well for readers of this book who may never visit the clinic.

This will require some time and effort on your part.

You will be expected to write down your daily goals, specifying when, for how long, and what type of exercise you plan to engage in. I have found that the best way to do this is to take it one week at a time, writing on your calendar or a form like the one on the next page your specific plans. Once your weekly schedule is in place, all that remains is to just do it. In my opinion, tracking forms such as this are invaluable, for they are a constant reminder of what you need to do and when you need to do it. Keep your exercise log handy, and make notes after you've completed your day's activity. Jot down how you feel before and after your exercise sessions. Record your blood sugar measurements every time you take them, as well as your weight and BMI (see page 40), on a weekly or biweekly basis. Include comments on your diet, and use this form as a reminder to take your nutritional supplements.

I cannot overemphasize the importance of tracking. First, it is a concrete reminder of your goals. Stick it on your fridge or your calendar—someplace where you can't escape it. Second, it keeps you honest. No more kidding yourself about how compliant you really are. And most important, it is a great motivator. By tracking your progress, you will have a record of objective improvements—lower blood sugar levels, weight loss, more endurance and energy. This alone can be a huge inspiration to continue on the program.

I suggest that you make several copies of the form on the next page and promise to diligently monitor yourself for one month. Then recommit for another month, then another. Most of my patients report that after a few months the program becomes more or less routine and the need for daily surveillance eases up.

Whitaker Wellness Institute Exercise Log

Date & Time	Exercise Duration & Frequency	Comments How do you feel? How was your diet today? Did you take your supplements? Record blood sugar, weight, etc.
	Goal Attained	
Sun.		
Mon.		
Tues.		
Wed.		
Thurs.		
Fri.		
Sat.		

Just Do It—No Excuses

Regardless of how much planning you do with your doctor, and how thoroughly you map out your exercise program, it won't do you any good unless you just do it. And the blunt truth is that most people *don't* do it. Fewer than two out of ten adults exercise regularly, and three out of ten get absolutely no physical activity. We use our cars for 93 percent of all trips and log a mere 1.4 miles per week (350 yards per day) of walking. Is it any wonder that we're more overweight and out of shape than ever?

The good news is that exercise needn't be painful or prolonged to produce measurable improvements in your overall health and wellbeing. So before you revert to your favorite excuse (believe me, I've heard every one in the book—in fact, I've used a fair number of them myself!), let's discard the most common reasons for avoiding exercise.

- **"I'm too busy."** For many folks, fitting exercise into an already overpacked schedule seems almost impossible. But it takes less time than you think. How much time do you really need to invest to reap the benefits of exercise? To get the 30 minutes a day recommended by the American College of Sports Medicine and the Centers for Disease Control and Prevention, all you have to do is replace half an hour of TV a day with moderate physical activity and you're there.

- **"I'm too tired."** Paradoxical as it may seem, physical activity actually increases your energy. It does this in two ways. First, as I explained earlier, it strengthens your heart, lungs, and blood vessels. With regular, sustained exercise, your heart pumps more blood with each beat, your lungs supply more oxygen to your blood, and your arteries deliver more blood to your tissues. The result is a body that does more work with less effort, which means more endurance and energy for you. Second, exercise acts directly on the brain to relieve depression, anxiety, and stress—all of which drain your energy. The magical effects of exercise on mood result largely from its ability to promote the release of "feel-good" endorphins, which we discussed in chapter 8. Endorphin production begins after about 20 minutes of brisk activity and continues for hours thereafter. People who exercise regularly benefit from a natural and energetic "high" throughout the day.

◉ **"I'm too old."** One of the surest ways to feel old before your time is to be sedentary. And one of the simplest antidotes to aging is physical activity. According to an eight-year study conducted at Tufts University, men and women in their forties who were inactive and out of shape were as likely to report limitations in daily activities as active men and women in their sixties. In other words, the fit sixty-year-olds were functionally as young as unfit people twenty years their junior.[4] Exercise benefits extend well into old age. In a recent Hawaiian study, men aged seventy-one to ninety-three who were free of heart disease at the study's onset were followed for two to four years. At the end of the study, men who walked a mile and a half per day were half as likely to have had a heart attack as those who walked less than half a mile per day.[5] If a ninety-three-year-old man can walk a mile and a half a day, we "youngsters" have no excuse to retire to our La-Z-Boy recliners.

To close this chapter I want to reiterate the exercise caveats diabetics must be aware of. Before starting an exercise program, you should be examined by a physician and given an exercise prescription. Then ease into your program slowly, always following the recommended guidelines.

Insulin-dependent diabetics should closely monitor blood sugar levels when exercising, and adjustments in food and medication intake may be required. Patients taking oral sulfonylurea drugs should take similar heed. (For more on this, see pages 192–193.) It is imperative that these patients recognize and know how to manage an insulin reaction. They should always carry with them glucose tablets or another form of carbohydrate with them. Poorly controlled diabetics should never exercise alone. Patients with diabetic retinopathy or other conditions involving fragility of the blood vessels should avoid strenuous exercise; moderate exercise is fine. All diabetics should pay special attention to how their shoes fit and practice scrupulous foot hygiene. And don't forget to drink lots of water before and after exercise and during long workouts.

By following these few precautions, rest assured that you are exercising sanely and safely, and you will reap great rewards for your efforts.

CHAPTER 13

How to Implement the Diet for Reversing Diabetes

Now let's talk about something that everyone loves to do: eat! The diet for reversing diabetes that we will detail in chapters 13 and 14 was put together by Diane Lara, M.S., certified nutritionist at the Whitaker Wellness Institute. Diane expanded upon the meal plan and recipes from the first edition of this book, which were developed by Barbara Tancredi, former chef at the Institute, and incorporated recipes created by our current chef, Idel Kelley. Each and every recipe included has been tested on family and friends, and many are used here at the Institute as well.

We have tried to make this program as easy to follow as possible and have included detailed instructions, down to describing exactly what is needed in kitchen utensils and shopping requirements. At first glance, these diet changes may appear to be overwhelming.

However, with time and practice you will find that this way of eating and cooking becomes easier and easier. As with any kind of change you make in your life, practice and experience eliminate the rough spots.

Our Purpose

The purpose of this chapter is to help you succeed in preparing a healthy dietary regimen from readily available, common foods, using uncomplicated recipes to produce familiar, tasty dishes. The meal plan is designed to contain high-quality, fiber-dense, low-fat, moderate-protein foods, with minimal sodium and sweeteners.

You can do it! Just follow the step-by-step instructions on these pages. Don't skip anything. For example, if you neglect to obtain the basic kitchen equipment, you may find yourself frustrated when trying to whip up many recipes. You'll be defeated before you even begin. We have deliberately kept the required equipment and pantry stock down to a minimum. You will be relieved to know that you don't have to own every spice and herb known to man to succeed with these recipes.

The recipes in the next chapter conform to the requirements not only of health but also of taste! Too many recipes concocted by nutritionists boast no fat, no sugar, no salt, and frankly, we find most have no taste either. So we insist that our recipes undergo strict taste tests, because we recognize that if the food doesn't taste good, you aren't going to stick with the program.

STEP ONE: Obtaining the Necessities

Start out your new dietary regimen by obtaining the necessities. When your kitchen is fully and properly equipped with cookware, baking supplies, serving and storage dishes, spices, and food staples, you will be ready to begin. Then when you start to prepare that first recipe and find that every ingredient is at your fingertips—success! When the food you're cooking doesn't stick to your griddle and skillets—success! All because you took the time to prepare.

Use our kitchen equipment and food staples lists like a shopping guide. You probably have most of the items already. What you don't have you might obtain from a friend or relative to cut costs, or you may find secondhand in a thrift store. However, as you will see, you don't need that many items to begin with. So take the time to stock up. Plan to begin your new regimen after your cupboards and pantry are stocked with the items on our lists. It will be well worth the effort.

Healthy Sweeteners

As we discussed in chapter 6, most sweeteners, both traditional (sugar, etc.) and "healthy" (molasses, honey, maple syrup), are not recommended for people with diabetes or insulin resistance, as they all cause rapid rises in blood sugar. The three sweeteners we use at the Whitaker Wellness Institute, stevia, xylitol, and brown rice syrup, are acceptable for diabetics because they do not wreak havoc with blood sugar levels. They are each unique in their own way.

Stevia is a noncaloric herbal extract with an intensely sweet flavor. It comes in several forms. The unrefined, dark extract is probably the healthiest way to go. It has even been shown in studies to improve blood sugar control. However, this thick black extract doesn't look like we want our sweeteners to look. Most people prefer stevia in the form of a refined clear liquid extract or a white powder that looks like sugar. Although these may lack some of the medicinal benefits of the whole herb, they are perfectly adequate for use as a sweetener. Because refined stevia is two to three hundred times sweeter than sugar, a few drops or sprinkles in your cereal or coffee are all you need. Stevia may also be used in cooking, but it does require some recipe modifications in baking. You can use as much of this unique sweetener as you would like. It will not raise your blood sugar levels, and, if you use the unrefined extract, may actually lower them.

Xylitol is a sweetener obtained from birch trees. Although it looks and tastes pretty much like white sugar, its similarities end there. Rather than causing a rapid spike in blood sugar, it is slowly absorbed and broken down, making it acceptable for diabetics. Furthermore, it contains about 40 percent fewer calories than sugar. Xylitol makes a great sweetener for cereal and beverages, and because it looks like sugar and is used in similar quantities, it lends itself well to substitutions for sugar in recipes. Xylitol is rather pricy, and large amounts cause loose stools in some people, so it is best not to overdo it.

Brown rice syrup is, as its name suggests, syrupy. Unlike other syrups, including pure maple syrup, it is slowly metabolized and thus causes no dramatic rises in blood sugar. Brown rice syrup makes a nice topping for French toast and pancakes, and a drizzle also perks up a fruit salad or hot cereal. It may also be used in cooking, as you will see in the recipes that follow.

Although you won't likely find these sweeteners in your grocery store, they are readily available in many health food stores, or they can be ordered as described in the Resources section on page 481. All three may be used in cooking, although their substitutions may require some recipe modifications. We have included several recipes utilizing these sweeteners in chapter 14 and have listed a few cookbooks in the Resources section.

Low-Sodium Seasonings and Salt Substitutes

The number one reason why people fail in a low-sodium regimen is that without salt, food for many just doesn't taste good. We must find a suitable replacement, because no matter how much garlic, herbs, Tabasco, or spices you pour on a dish, nothing perks up food like salt. While various herbs and spices are wonderful, they are an addition to salt, not its replacement. Therefore, we aren't asking you to give up salt altogether. Instead, we're going to ask that you do two things. First, when you see salt used for boiling pasta or baking cookies, cakes, and the like, scratch it off completely and leave nothing in its place. It isn't necessary and you won't miss it. Second, when you see salt in a recipe, cut back on it dramatically or replace it with one of the low-sodium substitutes we use at the Whitaker Wellness Institute.

Vegetable Seasoning

One option is "vegetable seasoning." Such seasonings are produced from dehydrated vegetables, grains, and even fruits—but with no added salt. They do contain some natural sodium, about 240 milligrams per teaspoon, but this is nothing compared to the more than 2000 milligrams in a teaspoon of salt. They taste salty because of the combination of natural ingredients used. Vegetable seasoning is used to season foods and can also be made into a broth or bouillon (it makes an excellent soup base). When it is used in place of salt, the general rule of thumb is to use two to three times as much vegetable seasoning as you would salt.

Several brands of vegetable seasoning are available, and you will need to experiment to find which ones you prefer. We recommend Bernard Jensen's Vegetable Seasoning very highly. It's the best we've found so far. It has a superior taste without the aftertaste that some vegetable seasonings have. In fact, most of our patients don't miss salt one iota when they use this seasoning. It is found in many health food stores. A mail-order source is listed in the Resources section.

Vegetable seasoning is used in a number of the recipes in this book. However, regardless of how flavorful it is, you may miss the taste of good old salt and reach for the salt shaker anyway. Therefore, I want to tell you about two other salt options that we use at the clinic.

Potassium Chloride (Nu-Salt and NoSalt)

Nu-Salt and NoSalt are salt substitutes available in most grocery stores. They contain potassium chloride (about 500 milligrams of potassium per ⅛ teaspoon) and absolutely no sodium. While sodium is associated with elevations in blood pressure and other health problems, potassium helps balance levels of sodium and other important minerals, protecting against high blood pressure, heart disease, and stroke. This is the salt substitute of choice for patients with hypertension whose blood pressure elevates whenever they eat any sodium. When a recipe calls for salt, I suggest that these patients substitute potassium chloride.

Most of our patients love these salt substitutes because they taste similar to salt and satisfy their salt cravings, while boosting protective levels of potassium. Others, however, complain of a bitter taste associated with the potassium.

Cardia Salt

Another option is Cardia Salt, a patented product developed in Finland that truly tastes just like real salt. This is because it does contain sodium—135 milligrams per ⅛ teaspoon (compared to 295 milligrams for an equal amount of salt). However, it also contains potassium (90 milligrams per ⅛ teaspoon), magnesium (7 milligrams) and l-lysine monohydrochloride, an amino acid that takes the bite off the bitterness some people perceive with potassium.

I am quite intrigued by Cardia Salt. Several clinical

studies have demonstrated that when substituted for regular salt, it lowers blood pressure in patients with mild to moderate hypertension. In one of these studies, systolic blood pressure fell an average of thirteen points and diastolic pressure an average of eight points over six months when table salt was replaced by Cardia Salt.

Cardia Salt is a little harder to find. If you can't find it in your pharmacy, a mail-order source is listed in the Resources section. Remember, it does contain sodium, so use just enough to satisfy your "salt tooth." And again, if you have salt-sensitive hypertension, stick with potassium chloride.

Food Staples: Always Have These on Hand

Herbs and spices

Basil
Black pepper
Cardia Salt (optional)
Cinnamon
Cloves
Garlic powder
Nu-Salt or NoSalt (optional)
Onion powder
Oregano
Parsley
Vegetable seasoning

Extracts

Vanilla

Baking supplies

Arrowroot
Baking soda
Carob powder (unsweetened)
Tapioca
Whole wheat flour (stone-ground)
Yeast (active dry yeast keeps longer)

Beans and grains

Dried beans (any kind—select your favorites)
Grains (your choice from the list on page 338)
Oatmeal, long-cooking
Pasta (whole-grain or high-protein preferable;
    any kind acceptable; your choice
    of type)

Nuts and seeds (store in freezer)

Almonds, raw
Flaxseed, whole, raw (not necessary to store in
    freezer)
Pumpkin seeds, raw
Sesame seeds, raw
Sunflower seeds, raw

Canned goods

Beans (Garbanzo beans and soybeans have the
    lowest glycemic index of the canned beans.
    Other varieties have a lower glycemic index
    when cooked from dried beans and are
    better for diabetics.)
Mushrooms (or keep fresh on hand)

Spaghetti sauce (low-fat, low-sodium spaghetti
    sauce with no added sugar—or homemade
    and frozen—see recipe on page 367)
Tomatoes, whole
Tomato paste
Tomato puree

Miscellaneous

Catsup (preferably low salt and low sugar)
Flaxseed oil (store in refrigerator or freezer)
Mayonnaise (low fat, no sugar)
Mustard, American and Dijon
Olive oil
Olive oil pan spray
Parmesan cheese, grated (store in refrigerator)
Pickles, dill
Salsa (low sodium)
Soy sauce (low sodium)
Tabasco sauce
Vinegar (flavored if desired; balsamic, rice, and
    white wine vinegar are all good)

Sweeteners (available in health food stores or mail order from sources on pages 482–483)

Brown rice syrup
Stevia
Xylitol

Kitchen Equipment

While you truly don't need much in quantity, you do need to pay attention to the quality of what you use in the kitchen. One example is your waffle iron. If it does not have a nonstick surface, you will meet with disaster. Until we got wise we spent more than a few precious moments scraping waffles off a nonstick iron. The same goes for pancakes. They must be cooked on a nonstick griddle.

- **Pots and pans.** You will use sizes ranging from ½ quart up to 8 quarts. The best pots and pans are stainless steel. Look for a waterless type of cookware if you want the very best. These are designed with tight-fitting lids and have a bottom and core that allows even heat throughout the pan, creating an "oven" effect. This cooks the food evenly instead of burning the bottom.

- **Casseroles and baking dishes.** Any type—clear glass, Corningware, or stoneware—is fine. You'll use from 1-quart up to 4-quart casseroles, square or rectangular baking dishes to cook lasagna and similar dishes, and a pie pan.

- **Nonstick cookware.** You will need a nonstick griddle: a flat, square, or rectangular pan to be used for cooking pancakes and French toast and grilling sandwiches. It may be heated on the stove, or you may use an electric griddle. If you like waffles, you also need a waffle iron that has a nonstick coating. Your bakeware needs to be nonstick coated too. Try to have a bread-loaf pan, a muffin pan, one or two cookie sheets, and a round cake pan (usually 8½ inches round and 1½ inches deep). Finally, you'll need small and large nonstick skillets. When you sauté without much fat, these skillets are a necessity.

- **Blender or food processor.** Be sure that you get the 1-cup jars (usually glass or plastic) that come with many blenders. These are used for grinding small quantities of nuts, vegetables, and fruits. You can see through the jar to monitor the progress, and using the little jars leaves the large blender jar clean for something else. Some people prefer a food processor, and this is also acceptable. You won't need both.

- **Hand mixer.** If you have a large mixer, don't toss it out. But if you don't have anything along this line, just get a small hand mixer. It will be needed for beating egg whites stiff, mixing batters, and more.

- **Colander.** Make sure you have a colander to drain pasta, thaw food by running hot water over it, rinse salt off canned foods, and rinse off fruit and vegetables.

- **Teakettle.** You will use a teakettle to heat water for hot drinks.

- **Thermos.** A one-quart thermos is handy for preparing grains overnight to be eaten as hot cereal.

- **Bowls.** You will need 2-, 4-, and 6-quart bowls for making large salads, and for mixing batters. The best are stainless steel, glass, or stoneware.

- **Knives.** A good set of knives is invaluable, especially considering the number of vegetables you will be cutting up. A paring knife is best for peeling. A large serrated knife is handy for cutting tomatoes, onions, green peppers, eggplant, and other slippery things. A chef's knife is good for chopping, and a cleaver is handy if you've got a lot of chopping to do. Don't forget to have a large cutting board on hand.

- **Utensils.** Make sure you have the following utensils:

  - Spatula for flipping pancakes and similar tasks. It must be made out of a material that won't scratch nonstick surfaces.

  - Wooden spoons for stirring sauces.

  - Ladle for dishing up soups, sauces, and syrups. Get stainless steel.

  - Slotted and regular large spoons for dishing up vegetables, casseroles, cereals, and more.

  - Tongs for lifting things out of hot water.

  - Rubber spatulas for scraping out bowls and other dishes to get every last drop.

- **Measuring cups and spoons.** The minimum you'll want to have handy is a 1-cup measuring cup (Pyrex is best because it withstands any temperature), and 1-teaspoon and 1-tablespoon measuring spoons. But if you want to add more, have a second measuring cup so you can have one for wet and one for dry and the whole set of spoons from ⅛ teaspoon up to 1 tablespoon.

If you don't find it on this list, you probably don't need it. But if you've got it already, keep it. Use it if you can.

STEP TWO: Review of General Guidelines

Let's review the general guidelines from chapters 6 and 7 for making healthy food selections.

Base Your Diet on Diabetes-Friendly Carbohydrates

The best carbohydrates for general good health are vegetables, fruits, beans, and whole grains, especially those in their natural, unprocessed state. They contain an abundance of fiber and a plethora of vitamins, minerals, and phytonutrients that engender health.

The best carbohydrates for the diabetic are those that cause the smoothest and steadiest release of blood sugar. These are, in most cases, fiber-rich, unprocessed vegetables, fruits, beans, and whole grains. However, there are a few exceptions. Some vegetables, most notably starchy root vegetables such as potatoes, cause the blood sugar to rapidly rise and precipitously fall. Certain fruits, particularly many tropical fruits, have a similarly negative effect on the blood sugar. And some of the grain-based foods that you've been taught are natural and healthy are dietary disasters for diabetics: cold cereals, rice cakes, and most breads. All of these foods have a high glycemic index rating—they drive up blood sugar—and should largely be avoided by diabetics. (See chapter 6 for the full scoop on the glycemic index. The lists we consulted in making our food recommendations were compiled by Rick Mendosa from his Web site http://www.mendosa.com/gilists.htm.)

You should make low-glycemic-index carbohydrates the foundation of your diet to reverse diabetes. All of the foods for reversing diabetes listed in this chapter have a low to moderate glycemic index. As we go through the various categories of food, I will explain which ones you can eat with abandon, what you should eat in moderation, and which foods you should save for very, very rare occasions. Healthy low-glycemic-index carbohydrates should comprise about 60 percent of your total caloric intake.

Eat Lots of Fiber

Fiber is found in fruits, vegetables, nuts, seeds, grains, beans, and other plants. It is absent in meat and other animal products. Fiber has been found to help prevent cancer, protect against heart disease, aid in weight loss, and lessen a diabetic's need for medication. It lowers blood sugar by slowing down and smoothing out the absorption of glucose. There are two primary types of fiber. *Insoluble fiber* includes lignans and cellulose, which give plants their structure. *Soluble fiber* is the gelatinous type of fiber that is particularly important for the diabetic. It includes pectin, found in citrus fruits, apples, strawberries, some vegetables, and gums, found in legumes and some grains.

Unfortunately, when foods are processed, their fiber is often removed. When you squeeze the juice out of an orange and discard the pulp, you're depriving yourself of pectin and other soluble fibers. When you buy white flour and baked goods made with white flour, you are getting zero fiber—regardless of how "enriched" the product may claim to be. Try to eat a bare minimum of 30 grams of fiber every day. This will take a concerted effort, as most Americans' fiber intake is less than half of that. However, by following the meal plan in *Reversing Diabetes*, you will easily get this recommended amount, and more. And your diabetes and overall health will improve as a result.

Avoid Unhealthy Fats

Fats in the bloodstream interfere with the effectiveness of insulin. That is bad enough by itself, but that's not all fat does. Saturated fats from animal sources like meat, butter, milk, and egg yolks and trans fatty acids from highly processed oils also contribute to the risk of stroke and heart attack. A lot can be said about fat. In fact, entire books have been written about it. Let it suffice to say that fatty foods should play a supporting role in your diet—but not be the main attraction.

However, this is far from a fat-free diet. About 20 percent of your total calories will be from fat, but the emphasis here is on *quality* of fats. Stay away from the sources of saturated fat listed above, and even farther away from chemically altered trans fatty acids, which are found in margarine, shortening, and anything made with hydrogenated oils. If you are ever faced with choosing between margarine and butter, go with butter. But save it for very special occasions and make it organic. Also avoid most of the polyunsaturated vegetable oils sold in grocery stores, as their healthful properties have been dramatically diminished during the extraction and refinement process.

So what are you going to use in their place? The best cooking oil is olive oil because, unlike most vegetable oils, it can tolerate heat. Flaxseed oil, a rich source of omega-3 essential fatty acids, is good for salad dressings, but it must never be heated. Other vegetable oils are acceptable only if they are expeller-pressed, as several health food store brands are. These oils may be damaged by heat and light and should be stored in the refrigerator.

To coat your nonstick pans, use a vegetable cooking spray, such as Pam. This can take the place of oil, butter, or margarine on baking pans, griddles, and waffle irons. Pan sprays are used in such minute amounts compared to the oil, butter, or margarine you might otherwise use that their fat content is insignificant. We particularly recommend the olive oil pan sprays, since that is the healthiest of the cooking oils. Another option is to purchase a kitchen sprayer and fill it with virgin olive oil.

To flavor your food with that good old butter taste, try Butter Buds Brand Natural Butter Flavored Mix or a similar product found in your grocery store. And for an occasional bread spread, substitute for butter or margarine an old Italian trick: Dip your bread in a little olive oil. This is even tastier when mixed with a little balsamic vinegar.

Include Moderate Amounts of Protein

As I explained in chapter 7, moderate amounts of protein—about 20 percent of total calories—are very important in a healthy diet. Focus on quality: Avoid fatty red meat and instead eat lots of fish (salmon and other cold-water fish are particularly healthful), moderate amounts of skinless poultry and low-fat dairy products, a wide range of protein-rich soy products, and other beans and legumes.

Don't Count Calories—But Watch Your Portions

We are a nation obsessed with calories. Yet little good it is doing us, considering that over half of all Americans are overweight. One of our patients' biggest complaints about the diets recommended for diabetics is that they are too darn complicated. Counting calories, figuring out exchanges and food groups, calculating percentages of this and that leaves them so confused that they often throw up their hands in dismay.

Therefore, we have simplified our approach to food. We avoid the use of the word "diet" altogether, as it conjures up visions of deprivation and cravings. Rather than insisting that our patients count calories, we teach them how to make healthy food selections and monitor portion sizes. If you are eating the right types of carbohydrates (those that do not cause surges in your blood sugar) and lean protein sources that are low in saturated fats, and you are avoiding junk food laden with white flour, sugar, salt, and trans fatty acids, the exact number of calories you eat isn't so critical. People don't get fat on salad, zucchini, and salmon. Their blood sugar doesn't soar after a bowl of vegetable soup or an egg-white omelet.

Of course, you can't go hog-wild, especially if you're trying to lose weight—a critical step for most type 2 diabetics. If you want to achieve your ideal weight you must focus on quantity as well as quality. Rather than counting calories, however, we instruct our patients in portion control. Learn what size piece of chicken, for example, constitutes a reasonable serving. (Believe me, it is not the monster portions we are served in many restaurants.) Here are the general guidelines we teach our patients to help keep caloric intake within reason without having to subject each meal to mathematical scrutiny.

Recommended Daily Intake and Portion Sizes

Carbohydrates (60 percent of total calories)

- ◉ Vegetables: 5–8 servings from list below—includes almost all vegetables except for starchy root vegetables (white potatoes, turnips, etc.), which should be limited for diabetics. 1 serving = 1 cup raw (about the size of a tennis ball) or

½ cup cooked vegetables. If you're going to overeat, eat foods from this category. They are the healthiest and least calorie dense.

⦿ Fruit: 2–3 servings from list below—includes almost all fruits except for most dried fruits, tropical fruits, and some melons. 1 serving = 1 medium whole fruit or ¾ cup sliced fruit.

⦿ Starches and grains: 3–4 servings from the bread, cereal, pasta, and grain categories. Pay close attention to the recommended breads, cereals, and grains. Starches and grains are among the most problematic of all carbohydrates for diabetics because they cause the most dramatic increases in blood sugar. 1 serving = 1 slice of bread, ½ bagel or ¾ cup cooked cereal, pasta, or grain. Try to not exceed this number of servings.

Protein (20 percent of total calories)

⦿ 3–4 servings of lean protein. Always include some protein with each meal. Remember, protein doesn't have to come from meat.

⦿ Fish or poultry: 1 serving = 4 ounces—about the size of a deck of cards.

⦿ Beans: 1 serving = ¾ cup cooked beans.

⦿ Soy products: 1 serving = 4 ounces tofu, 1 cup soy milk, ½ cup soy protein.

⦿ Raw nuts and seeds: 1 serving = 2 tablespoons nuts, seeds, or nut butter.

- Dairy: 1 serving = ½ cup nonfat cottage cheese or 1 cup plain, nonfat yogurt.

- Eggs: 1 serving = 3 egg whites, 2 egg whites mixed with 1 yolk, or ½ cup Egg Beaters or another frozen egg product.

Fat (20 percent of total calories)

- Limit added fat to 1–2 tablespoons olive or flax-seed oil (with occasional use of other expeller-pressed oils). The remainder of the fat in your diet will come from that naturally present in foods. Strictly avoid fried foods and those made with hydrogenated oils (including margarine), as they contain the most harmful types of fat.

For those of you who care to track such things, we have also provided nutritional breakdowns of the rec-ommended foods and recipes, including calories and grams of fat, protein, and carbohydrate. However, I want to stress that what we emphasize in the education program for diabetes at the Whitaker Wellness Institute is not numbers and calculations but quality of food and portion size.

STEP THREE: Foods for Reversing Diabetes

We have compiled a comprehensive list of the foods that will help you get your diabetes under control. The good news is that, as you will see in the next few pages, you have many, many choices. The bad news is that there are some foods you really should avoid. We have attempted to make this list as complete as possible, even going so far as to name brand names in a few cases. If something is not on this list, it is likely off limits to people coping with diabetes.

Commit this list to memory. It will make shopping, cooking, and eating out much simpler. If it is not on this list, use in moderation on very special and rare occasions. We have included the nutritional breakdown for the serving size of each food. These were calculated by Mark Wettler of Wettler Information Services using the U.S. Department of Agriculture Standard Reference, Release 13 (1999), which contains nutritional data for over 6,200 foods.[1] Also useful was the 2000 update of *The Complete Book of Food Counts* by Corrine T. Netzer.[2]

Vegetables

Make vegetables the foundation of your meals. Cooked or raw, they are loaded with fiber, vitamins, minerals, and protective phytonutrients. Snack on raw vegetables with a tasty dip, have a large salad with a variety of vegetables at every meal, and explore the possibilities of vegetarian entrees. You'll find that vegetables are anything but boring.

Most vegetables are perfectly suited for a diet for reversing diabetes. The few exceptions that you will not find on this list of recommended foods are starchy root vegetables. They have a very high glycemic index, and if you have diabetes you should stay away from them.

These include white potatoes (red potatoes have a lower glycemic index and may be eaten occasionally), parsnips, and turnips.

The following nutritional information pertains primarily to fresh vegetables. Frozen vegetables are also acceptable, but many canned vegetables contain added sugar and salt, so read labels carefully. Note again that the average serving size is 1 cup of raw vegetables, which typically translates into ½ cup cooked. Notice how few calories and how little fat the majority of these vegetables contain. Most of you can eat them to your heart's content. Even if you are trying to lose weight, if you're going to eat too much of anything, make it vegetables.

Food	Portion	Calories	Carbohydrate	Protein	Fat	Fiber
Alfalfa sprouts, raw	¼ cup	2.39	0.31	0.33	0.06	0.21
Artichoke, whole	1 avg.	60.00	13.42	4.18	0.19	6.48
Asparagus, cooked	¾ cup	32.40	5.71	3.50	0.42	2.16
Avocado	½ avg.	153.11	5.98	1.83	14.99	4.24
Bamboo shoots, raw	¼ cup	42.94	1.98	0.99	0.11	0.84
Beet greens, cooked	½ cup	29.16	5.90	2.78	0.22	3.13
Broccoli, raw	1 cup	24.64	4.61	2.62	0.31	2.64
Broccoli, cooked	¾ cup	32.76	5.92	3.49	0.41	3.39
Brussel sprouts, cooked	1 cup	60.84	13.53	3.98	0.80	4.06
Cabbage, raw	1 cup	17.50	3.80	1.01	0.19	1.61
Cabbage, cooked	¾ cup	24.75	5.02	1.15	0.48	2.59

(Continued)

Food	Portion	Calories	Carbohydrate	Protein	Fat	Fiber
Cabbage, red, raw	1 cup	18.90	4.28	0.97	0.18	1.40
Carrot, raw	1 cup	55.04	12.97	1.32	0.24	3.84
Cauliflower, cooked	¾ cup	21.39	3.82	1.71	0.42	2.51
Celery, raw	1 cup	19.20	4.38	1.32	0.24	3.84
Chard, cooked	¾ cup	26.25	5.43	2.47	0.11	2.76
Chives, chopped	1 tbsp.	0.30	0.04	0.03	0.01	0.03
Collards, cooked	¾ cup	37.05	6.98	3.01	0.51	3.99
Cucumber, peeled, raw	1 cup	15.96	3.33	0.76	0.21	0.93
Dandelion greens, cooked	¾ cup	25.99	5.04	1.58	0.47	2.28
Eggplant, cooked	¾ cup	20.79	4.93	0.62	0.17	1.86
Endive, raw	1 cup	4.25	0.84	0.31	0.05	0.78
Garlic, raw	1 clove	4.47	0.99	0.19	0.02	0.06
Green beans, raw	¾ cup	25.58	5.89	1.50	0.10	2.79
Lettuce, Boston	1 cup	7.15	1.28	0.71	0.12	0.55
Lettuce, iceberg	1 cup	6.60	1.15	0.56	0.10	0.77
Lettuce, loose leaf	1 cup	10.08	1.96	0.73	0.17	1.06
Lettuce, romaine	1 cup	7.84	1.33	0.91	0.11	0.95
Mung bean sprouts, raw	¼ cup	31.20	6.17	3.16	0.19	1.87
Mushrooms, sliced, raw	1 cup	17.50	2.86	2.03	0.23	0.84
Mustard greens, cooked	¾ cup	15.75	2.21	2.37	0.25	2.10
Okra, cooked	¾ cup	38.40	8.65	2.24	0.20	3.00
Olives, green	6 med.	33.00	0.40	0.40	3.60	0.70

Food	Portion	Calories	Carbohydrate	Protein	Fat	Fiber
Olives, ripe	6 med.	20.24	1.10	0.15	1.88	0.56
Onions, raw	¼ cup	15.20	10.36	1.39	0.19	2.16
Onions, cooked	¾ cup	69.30	15.99	2.14	0.30	2.21
Onions, green	¼ cup	25.63	5.48	0.59	0.46	0.88
Parsley, chopped, raw	¼ cup	5.40	0.95	0.45	0.12	0.50
Peas, cooked	¾ cup	100.80	18.77	6.43	0.26	6.60
Peas, edible pods, raw	1 cup	41.16	7.41	2.74	0.20	2.55
Peppers, green, raw	½ cup	20.12	4.79	0.66	0.14	1.34
Peppers, red, raw	½ cup	20.12	4.79	0.66	0.14	1.49
Pimientos, canned	1 tbsp.	20.00	3.00	1.00	0.00	0.00
Potatoes, new	½ cup	67.86	15.70	1.46	0.07	1.40
Radishes, raw	5 med.	4.50	0.81	0.14	0.12	0.36
Shallots	1 tbsp.	7.20	1.68	0.25	0.01	0.00
Spinach, raw	1 cup	6.60	1.05	0.86	0.11	0.81
Spinach, cooked	½ cup	20.70	3.38	2.67	0.23	2.16
Squash, summer, cooked	¾ cup	27.00	5.82	1.23	0.42	1.89
Tomato	1 med.	25.83	5.71	1.05	0.41	1.35
Tomato sauce	1 cup	73.50	17.59	3.25	0.41	3.43
Tomato paste	1 tbsp.	13.45	3.17	0.60	0.09	0.67
Tomato puree	1 cup	100.00	23.90	4.23	0.40	5.00
Turnip greens, cooked	½ cup	14.40	3.14	0.82	0.17	2.52
Water chestnuts	4 avg.	34.92	8.62	0.50	0.04	1.08
Watercress, raw	1 cup	3.74	0.44	0.78	0.03	0.51
Zucchini, cooked	¾ cup	28.43	5.95	1.91	0.22	2.17

Beans and Legumes

Beans and legumes are good sources of fiber, protein, vitamins, and minerals. They are particularly abundant in the type of fiber that lowers blood sugar levels, and therefore deserve a prominent place in a diabetic's diet. Make beans the basis of your soups, and throw a handful into every salad. Eat them as a side dish, or puree them as a sandwich spread. Soybeans deserve a special mention, as, in addition to being one of the best sources of protein, they are also an excellent source of isoflavones, phytonutrients that have been demonstrated to protect against cancer. Do yourself a favor and eat soybeans, tofu, or products made with soy protein several times a week.

The best beans are those you purchase dried. To prepare dried beans, cover them with water (three to four inches above the top of the beans), and let soak overnight. The next day, drain the water, add more water to cover, and bring to a boil. To cut down on a common side effect of eating beans (you know what I'm talking about), drain the water a second time after the beans have come to a boil. Add more water, and continue cooking. Different beans require different boiling times, so cook as directed on the package.

Frozen beans are acceptable, but canned beans often have a much higher glycemic index than those you cook from dried. The canned beans with the lowest glycemic index are soybeans. Garbanzo beans (chickpeas) and pinto beans are acceptable—but dried are preferred.

Food	Portion	Calories	Carbohydrate	Protein	Fat	Fiber
Black-eyed peas, cooked	¾ cup	120.38	25.16	3.92	0.47	6.19
Butter beans, cooked	¾ cup	156.00	30.15	8.70	0.45	6.75
Garbanzo beans, cooked	¾ cup	123.75	20.56	6.65	1.94	5.70
Kidney beans, cooked	¾ cup	168.59	30.28	11.51	0.66	8.50
Lentils, cooked	¾ cup	172.26	29.91	13.40	0.56	11.73
Lima beans, cooked	¾ cup	162.15	29.45	11.00	0.54	9.87
Navy beans, cooked	¾ cup	117.00	22.50	10.61	1.22	0.00
Pinto beans, cooked	¾ cup	175.70	32.90	10.53	0.67	11.03
Soybeans, cooked	¾ cup	223.17	12.80	21.47	11.57	7.74
Split peas, cooked	¾ cup	173.46	31.03	12.26	0.57	12.20
Tofu	4 oz.	94.24	2.33	10.02	5.93	0.37

Fruits

Some say that fruit is nature's perfect food, and it does have many healthful components: fiber, antioxidants and other vitamins and minerals, and scores of phytonutrients. Because of its relatively high sugar content, however, diabetics should go easy on fruit and limit servings to two or three per day. Get into the habit of substituting fruit for sugar-laden desserts and snacks. It will satisfy all but the most ardent sweet tooth.

Most fruits are acceptable for diabetics. Exceptions are most tropical fruits and many (but not all) dried fruits, as they have a very high glycemic index and can drive up your blood sugar. Frozen fruits are fine, but

Food	Portion	Calories	Carbohydrate	Protein	Fat	Fiber
Apple, raw (with peel)	1 med.	81.42	21.05	0.26	0.50	3.73
Applesauce, unsweetened	½ cup	52.46	13.77	0.21	0.06	1.46
Apricots, dried	¼ cup	77.35	20.07	1.19	0.15	2.93
Blackberries, raw	¾ cup	56.16	13.78	0.78	0.42	5.72
Blueberries, raw	¾ cup	60.90	15.37	0.73	0.41	2.94
Boysenberries, raw	¾ cup	49.50	12.07	1.09	0.26	3.86
Cherries, raw	¾ cup	78.30	18.00	1.31	1.04	2.50
Grapefruit, raw	½ med.	36.80	9.29	0.72	0.12	1.27
Grapes, raw	¾ cup	46.23	11.83	0.44	0.24	0.69
Lemon juice, unsweetened	1 tbsp.	6.71	1.98	0.14	0.10	0.12
Lime juice, unsweetened	1 tbsp.	6.47	2.06	0.08	0.07	0.12
Nectarine, raw	1 med.	66.64	16.02	1.28	0.63	2.18
Orange, raw	1 med.	59.29	14.39	1.26	0.36	3.03
Peach, raw	1 med.	42.14	10.88	0.69	0.09	1.96
Pear, raw	1 med.	97.94	25.09	0.65	0.66	3.98
Plums, raw	2 med.	72.60	17.16	1.04	0.82	1.98
Raspberries, unsweetened	1 cup	60.27	14.23	1.12	0.68	8.36
Strawberries, raw	¾ cup	45.60	10.67	0.93	0.56	3.50
Tangerine, raw	1 med	36.40	9.40	0.53	0.16	1.93

beware of canned fruits with added sugars. Note that fruit juices are not included on this list as they are a very concentrated source of fiberless sugar.

Nuts and Seeds

Nuts and seeds have a bad reputation because they are so high in fat. However, if those nuts and seeds are in their natural state, their oils are among the most healthful. Too bad we have a preference for roasted nuts, for once they are heated their delicate oils are damaged. The same goes for nut butters. Although most brands of peanut butter you'll find in the grocery store are made with roasted nuts and then hydrogenated, resulting in harmful trans fatty acids, there's nothing wrong with eating modest amounts of raw nut butter. You'll find these in your health food store.

Enjoy a small handful of nuts and seeds as a snack, in your salad, or as part of your breakfast. Just make sure they're raw. It's easy to get carried away with nuts, so remember that the recommended serving size is about two tablespoons.

Food	Portion	Calories	Carbohydrate	Protein	Fat	Fiber
Almonds	2 tbsp.	69.36	2.37	2.55	6.08	1.42
Almond meal	2 tbsp.	116.00	8.20	11.20	5.20	2.14
Brazil nuts	2 tbsp.	185.98	3.63	4.07	18.77	1.53
Cashews	2 tbsp.	162.73	9.27	4.34	13.14	0.85
Coconut, unsweetened	2 tbsp.	159.30	6.85	1.50	15.07	4.05
Filberts	2 tbsp.	178.04	4.73	4.24	17.22	2.75
Peanuts	2 tbsp.	161.60	4.49	7.41	14.06	2.69
Pecans	2 tbsp.	195.90	3.93	2.60	20.40	2.72
Pumpkin seeds	2 tbsp.	153.37	5.05	6.96	13.00	1.11
Sesame seeds, hulled	2 tbsp.	47.63	0.76	2.14	4.44	0.94
Sunflower seeds, hulled	2 tbsp.	175.49	5.84	4.88	16.10	3.26
Walnuts	2 tbsp.	185.41	3.89	4.32	18.49	1.90

Breads and Baked Goods

Most of us love bread and baked goods, and we eat way too much of them. Unfortunately, most of these starchy carbohydrates drive up blood sugar as quickly as sugar. This doesn't mean you have to avoid breads and baked goods altogether, but you will have to eat them sparingly and be much more selective in which ones you eat. When eating out, ask that you be served a salad or a plate of raw vegetables in place of bread. Warm, crusty rolls are much too tempting when they are right under your nose. When you have a sandwich, make it open-faced, on one slice of bread. And forget about snacking on goodies like pretzels, cookies, and chips. They will wreak havoc with your blood sugar.

The best bread for the diabetic is sprouted-grain bread (sometimes called Ezekiel bread). A few whole grain breads are acceptable in moderation. Read labels. Look for breads that are truly whole grain. Many breads contain white flour and have been colored (usually with caramel coloring), even though the label says "whole wheat." But even the best breads are still in the moderate glycemic index range. Limit total servings of bread *and* other starches such as pasta and cereal to three or four per day.

Food	Portion	Calories	Carbohydrate	Protein	Fat	Fiber
Sprouted-grain bread	1 slice	80.00	16.00	4.00	0.5	3.00
Sprouted-grain bagel	½ bagel	160.00	33.00	11.00	1.00	2.00
Whole wheat pita	1 small round	160.00	30.00	7.00	2.00	1.00

Food	Portion	Calories	Carbohydrate	Protein	Fat	Fiber
Rye bread (100% rye flour)	1 slice	82.88	15.46	2.72	1.06	1.86
Rye crackers	3 small	47.34	11.40	1.36	0.13	3.25
Sponge cake (for an occasional treat)	1 ounce	81.93	17.32	1.53	0.77	0.16
Whole wheat crackers (100% whole)	1 ounce	125.59	19.45	2.49	4.88	2.98
Whole wheat tortilla	1 med.	120.00	20.00	4.00	3.00	3.00

Grains, Cereals, and Pasta

This is another category you must approach with caution. Because these foods are such a major part of the American diet, we don't want to restrict them altogether. However, you should strictly limit both your portion size and number of servings of grains, cereals, and pasta. Interestingly—and counterintuitively—pasta, even white pasta, is a better choice for the diabetic than some of the grains we often think of as healthier. The best pasta is protein-enriched, and it has a much lower glycemic index. However, all pasta is acceptable. All rice has a relatively high glycemic index. The type with the lowest is long-grain brown rice, but it is still up there. Eat rice in moderation.

Likewise, most cold breakfast cereals are off the chart when it comes to the glycemic index. I know you've been told that they are low in fat and high in fiber, and some are. But even the sugar-free cereals—the flakes, squares, pops, squares, and puffs—cause dramatic spikes in blood sugar. There are a limited number of acceptable cold cereals, which you will see on the list below. Better choices are slow-cooking oatmeal or some of the other accepted grains cooked up and served with skim milk or soy milk and a healthy sweetener. A serving size is about ¾ cup.

Food	Portion	Calories	Carbohydrate	Protein	Fat	Fiber
All-Bran cereals	¾ cup	118.80	34.16	5.49	1.40	14.54
Barley, pearl, cooked	¾ cup	144.83	33.23	2.66	0.52	4.47
Bulgur, cooked	¾ cup	113.30	25.36	4.20	0.33	6.14
Lasagna noodles, cooked	¾ cup	200.00	41.00	7.00	0.50	2.00
Macaroni, cooked	¾ cup	148.05	29.76	5.01	0.70	1.37
Oatmeal, long-cooking, cooked	¾ cup	366.00	80.94	12.48	2.82	13.20
Rice bran	¾ cup	278.91	43.98	11.81	18.45	18.59
Rice, brown, long-grain, cooked	¾ cup	162.34	33.58	3.77	1.32	2.63
Rye, cooked	¾ cup	424.61	88.42	18.71	3.17	18.51
Spaghetti, cooked	¾ cup	148.05	29.76	5.01	0.70	1.79
Spaghetti, protein-enriched, cooked	¾ cup	172.20	33.24	8.48	0.22	1.79
Spaghetti, whole wheat, cooked	¾ cup	130.50	27.90	5.25	0.45	4.73

Dairy, Meat, and Other Protein Sources

Protein is an important part of your diet, but as I made clear in chapter 7, we eat entirely too much of it. You need to rethink portion size when it comes to protein. The average serving, the one listed in all the food composition charts, is a mere three to four ounces. For us Americans who grew up on 16-ounce steaks, that takes some getting used to. The easiest way to gauge an appropriate serving of meat, poultry, or fish is to compare it to a deck of cards.

I have left red meat off this list because of its high saturated fat content. An occasional piece of lean, trimmed red meat is acceptable—but don't kid yourself that prime rib is lean. Make fish, particularly salmon, tuna, and other cold-water fish, your protein source several times a week. Also explore tofu and other soy protein products. You'll be surprised by all the selections in your health food store—and many are creeping into grocery stores as well. Boca Burgers, "chicken breasts," "fish fillets," and soy protein granules you can add to chili and other dishes have come a long way in taste and appearance.

Food	Portion	Calories	Carbohydrate	Protein	Fat	Fiber
Dairy						
Cottage cheese, fat free	½ cup	80.00	4.00	15.00	0.00	0.00
Milk, fat free	½ cup	45.16	6.15	4.37	0.31	0.00
Yogurt, fat free, no sugar	1 cup	124.85	22.47	7.72	0.45	0.00
Poultry						
Chicken breast, without skin (approx. 1 small, ½ large)	4 oz.	141.90	0.00	26.67	3.07	0.00
Chicken breast, ground	4 oz.	190.00	0.00	19.00	13.00	0.00

(Continued)

Food	Portion	Calories	Carbohydrate	Protein	Fat	Fiber
Turkey breast, ground	4 oz.	169.86	0.00	19.90	9.42	0.00
Turkey	4 oz.	88.40	0.00	15.25	2.58	0.00
Fish						
Cod and other fish	4 oz.	87.13	0.00	18.92	0.71	0.00
Salmon	4 oz.	194.44	0.00	21.14	11.53	0.00
Shrimp	4 oz.	105.19	0.00	22.22	1.15	0.00
Tuna	4 oz.	153.00	0.00	24.79	5.21	0.00
Tuna, canned, water packed	4 oz.	123.25	0.00	27.10	0.87	0.00
Eggs						
Egg	1 medium	65.56	0.54	5.50	4.41	0.00
Egg white	2 medium	30.38	0.63	6.39	0.00	0.00
Egg Beaters	¼ cup	95.89	1.92	6.77	6.67	0.00
Soy						
Boca Burger	1 patty (2.5 oz.)	100.00	9.00	13.00	2.00	4.00
Soy milk	½ cup	40.43	2.22	3.37	2.34	1.59
Soy protein (dry)	¼ cup	95.82	2.09	22.88	0.96	1.59
Tofu	4 oz.	94.24	2.33	10.02	5.93	0.37

Condiments and Seasonings

Here is the nutritional breakdown on some of the condiments and seasonings that you will come across in the recipes in the next chapters.

Food	Portion	Calories	Carbohydrate	Protein	Fat	Fiber
Brown rice syrup	1 tbsp.	42.50	10.50	0.00	0.00	0.00
Mustard	1 tbsp.	0.99	0.12	0.06	0.05	0.05

Food	Portion	Calories	Carbohydrate	Protein	Fat	Fiber
Parmesan cheese, grated	1 tbsp.	22.79	0.19	2.08	1.50	0.50
Salsa	2 tbsp.	2.00	2.00	0.41	0.08	0.51
Soy sauce, low sodium	1 tbsp.	10.80	1.00	1.89	0.02	0.14
Spaghetti sauce, unsalted, no sugar	½ cup	71.25	10.28	1.78	2.58	2.00
Stevia	2 drops	0	0	0	0	0
Tapioca granules	1 tbsp.	32.00	7.80	0.10	0	0
Vegetable seasoning	1 tsp.	10	2	2	0	<1
Vinegar	1 tbsp.	2.10	0.89	0.00	0.00	0.00
Whole wheat flour	½ cup	203.40	43.54	7.72	1.12	7.32
Xylitol	1 tsp.	9.6	4	0	0	0

Beverages

The beverage of choice for everyone, diabetic or not, is water. Drink eight to twelve 8-ounce glasses of water, preferably filtered, every day. (If your kidney function is compromised or you have congestive heart failure, do not increase your fluid intake without running it by your doctor.) Jazz it up with a lemon or lime slice or diluted herbal tea. If you want to use skim milk on your cereal or in cooking, fine, but I do not recommend milk as a beverage. (See chapter 7 for more on this.)

Coffee does not affect the diabetic condition per se. However, caffeine increases levels of stress hormones, which is what gives you the mental perk-up you get with a cup of coffee. One or two 8-ounce cups is fine for most people, but if you drink coffee all day, these hormones remain elevated and may have negative effects on sleep, mood, and memory. A healthier wake-up drink is green tea. It contains enough caffeine to get you going (about half that of coffee), but it also provides a cupful of protective flavonoids and other phytonutrients.

Although many diabetes experts recommend sugar-free sodas, I strongly suggest that you avoid these chemical-laden brews. True, they have no calories or sugar, but most are sweetened with aspartame (Nutra-Sweet), an artificial sweetener that has been linked to scores of health problems, from headaches to seizures.

Food	Portion	Calories	Carbohydrate	Protein	Fat	Fiber
Coffee (decaf best)	I cup	4.74	0.95	0.24	0.00	0.00
Green tea	I cup	2.37	0.71	0.00	0.00	0.00
Herbal tea	I cup	2.37	0.47	0.00	0.00	0.00
Soy milk	½ cup	40.43	2.22	3.37	2.34	1.59
Tea	I cup	2.37	0.71	0.00	0.00	0.00
Water (filtered, sparkling, seltzer, etc.—no added sugar)	I cup	0.00	0.00	0.00	0.00	0.00

Snacks

Any food plan that does not incorporate snacks is destined to fail. The beauty of these foods for reversing diabetes is that because they do not cause sharp rises in blood sugar—followed by dramatic drops—you will likely feel fairly satiated all day long. It's when your blood sugar gets low that you have the ravenous hunger that drives you to eat anything in sight. Still, there will be times when you want to reach for a snack. Unfortunately, the most popular snack foods, such as pretzels, chips, cookies, most crackers, rice cakes, and candy, are off limits for diabetics. Instead try these yummy, easy-to-prepare snacks.

- Almonds, sunflower seeds, pumpkin seeds, and other nuts and seeds, raw (2 tablespoons total)

- Apple slices with raw almond butter (1 apple, 1 tablespoon almond butter)

- Cottage cheese, nonfat, with or without fruit (½ cup cottage cheese, ½ serving fruit)

- Fruit (1 serving from recommended list)

- Rye crackers with avocado slices (4 small crackers, ¼ avocado)

- Sandwich (1 slice sprouted-grain bread plus ¼ cup of one of the following: chicken, turkey, tuna, or scrambled egg whites; 1 tablespoon raw almond butter with 1 teaspoon brown rice syrup; ½ avocado; plus mustard, low-fat, low-sugar mayo, sprouts, tomatoes, etc., as desired)

- Smoothie (see recipe on page 458)

- Sugar-free protein drink

- Soybeans, raw in pod (edamame) (½ cup)

- Vegetables, raw, 1 cup (dip in 2 tablespoons of a fat-free, sugar-free dressing)

- ◉ Yogurt, plain, with added fruit and sweetened with stevia (1 cup yogurt, ½ cup fruit, 3+ drops stevia, to taste)

- ◉ Whitaker Wellness Health & Nutrition Bar

The Whitaker Wellness Health & Nutrition Bar

One of the most frequent complaints we hear from our diabetic patients at the Whitaker Wellness Institute is this: "I eat well at home. I've learned how to order healthy meals in restaurants. But there are times when I need to eat on the run. Help!"

Because virtually all of the "health bars" targeted as energy boosters, meal replacements, or weight-loss aids contain unhealthy fats and sweeteners, our nutritionist Diane Lara took matters into her own hands. She got together with a food chemist and spent two years perfecting a formula that is now the Whitaker Wellness Health & Nutrition Bar. This bar was designed specifically for patients with diabetes and insulin resistance. It is sweetened with brown rice syrup and xylitol, which have a low glycemic index, and contains almond oil that is stabilized with antioxidants. In addition, it contains a number of vitamins and minerals, including 100 percent of the RDA for chromium, vitamin C, vitamin E, and vitamin A, nutrients which, as stressed in chapter 9, have been demonstrated to improve the diabetic condition.

A small, unpublished double-blind study was conducted to determine the glucose and insulin response to this bar. Patients with type 1 or type 2 diabetes ate, on separate days, equal amounts of (1) the Whitaker bar, (2) a candy sweetened with sugar, and (3) sugar-free candy (sweetened with sorbitol). Blood samples were taken from each patient in a fasting state before they ate the samples, then at 30, 60, and 120 minutes. Bars 2 and 3 caused a sharp rise in blood sugar at 30 minutes, which continued to climb at 60 minutes, then gradually fell over the next hour. After two hours, average readings remained high: an average of 38.7 mg/dl over the fasting level in bar 2 and 35.8 mg/dl in bar 3. However, when the patients ate the Whitaker Wellness Health & Nutrition Bar (sweetened with xylitol and brown rice syrup), blood sugars measured an average increase over fasting levels of only 10 mg/dl at 30 minutes, and at 60 minutes they had fallen to just above fasting levels. After one hour they were below fasting levels. These findings are highly significant for patients with diabetes.

These bars have become a favorite at the Institute. One of our employees, in an effort to lose weight, ate the bars for lunch for six weeks. He lost twenty pounds during that time. They are also popular with people who don't like to eat breakfast and as mid-morning and mid-afternoon snacks. Best of all, the bar seems to really tide people over. When I have one for lunch on a day I am too busy to sit down to eat, I find that I breeze through the rest of the day without feeling hungry. Furthermore, unlike many of the food bars on the market, it tastes good. The Whitaker Wellness Health & Nutrition Bar comes in two chocolate-coated flavors, almond nougat and chocolate almond. See the Resources section if you would like to give the bars a try.

STEP FOUR: How to Alter Your Favorite Recipes

Now that you are familiar with the foods that will allow you to maintain good blood sugar control and those that will not, you should be able to more easily evaluate recipes. However, if you have a favorite cookbook, don't despair. Many recipes can be altered to make them healthier and equally tasty. Here are some guidelines for altering recipes.

- **Eliminate.** If an ingredient isn't essential, don't use it. Leave out salt or oil when cooking pasta and grains. Forget the sugar listed in recipes for sauces and dressings. Omit the sour cream topping in recipes. Try making a quiche or pie without the crust.

- **Reduce.** Less is best. If you can't leave something out altogether, reduce it. Cut back on the amount of oil, salt, or sweetener called for. Use half the seasoning packet that comes with some boxed, ready-to-prepare foods.

- **Substitute.** When a recipe calls for sugar, substitute stevia or xylitol. If it requires salt, try vegetable seasoning or a salt substitute. Use olive oil in place of butter, margarine, and vegetable oils, and unsweetened applesauce in place of oil and butter when baking.

Here is an example of how this can be done.

Tacos (traditional recipe)

- l lb. ground beef
- l teaspoon salt
- l cup vegetable oil
- l dozen corn tortillas
- 2 cups cheddar cheese, grated
- 2 cups lettuce, chopped
- 2 tomatoes, chopped
- l small onion, chopped
- l cup salsa
- l cup sour cream

Per Serving:

799.69 Cal (80.10% from Fat, 16.00% from Protein, 3.89% from Carb)

32.20 g Protein
71.63 g Tot Fat
- 23.81 g Sat Fat
- 20.72 g Mono Fat
- 22.63 g Poly Fat
7.83 g Carb
1.31 g Fiber
935.88 mg Sodium
124.41 mg Cholesterol

Brown the ground beef in a medium skillet until cooked through; drain excess grease. Season with the salt. Heat the oil in a medium saucepan over medium high heat. Add one tortilla at a time, turning once with tongs as tortilla softens. Remove from oil and drain on paper towels. Cover to keep warm. Continue with remainder of tortillas, adding more oil if necessary. Spoon ¼ cup meat onto each tortilla, add cheese and vegetables, and top with about 1 tablespoon each salsa and sour cream.

Serves 6

Tacos (altered recipe)

- I lb. ~~ground beef~~ ground turkey breast
- I teaspoon ~~salt~~ vegetable seasoning (or salt substitute to taste)
- ~~I cup vegetable oil~~
- I dozen ~~corn tortillas~~ small whole wheat tortillas
- ~~2 cups cheddar cheese, grated~~ ½ cup low-fat cheese, grated
- 2 cups lettuce, chopped
- 2 tomatoes, chopped
- I small onion, chopped
- I cup salsa
- ~~I cup sour cream~~

Per Serving:

354.14 Cal (28.00% from Fat, 26.70% from Protein, 45.30% from Carb)

23.38 g Protein
10.92 g Tot Fat
- 3.14 g Sat Fat
- 4.54 g Mono Fat
- 2.09 g Poly Fat
39.73 g Carb
3.18 g Fiber
945.19 mg Sodium
34.82 mg Cholesterol

Brown the ~~ground beef~~ turkey in a medium skillet until cooked through; ~~drain excess grease~~. Season with the ~~salt~~ vegetable seasoning. ~~Heat the oil in a medium saucepan over medium high heat. Add one tortilla at a time, turning once with tongs as tortilla softens. Removed from oil and drain on paper towels.~~ Soften tortillas by heating in an unoiled skillet over medium heat for about one minute on each side. Cover to keep warm. Continue with remainder of tortillas, ~~adding more oil if necessary~~. Spoon ¼ cup ~~meat~~ turkey onto each tortilla, add cheese and vegetables, and top with about 1 tablespoon ~~each~~ salsa ~~and sour cream~~.

Serves 6

In the altered recipe, we have replaced corn tortillas (which have a very high glycemic index) with whole wheat flour tortillas. Flour tortillas do not require oil. Quick heating in an unoiled skillet will make them soft and pliable. We have swapped beef for turkey breast, which eliminates lots of saturated fat, and salt for vegetable seasoning. We have eliminated the sour cream and cut back dramatically on the amount of cheese—and made that a low-fat variety.

The two recipes do not taste identical. This is not our goal. Our goal is to use our favorite recipes to our advantage. We end up with tacos, but a different version: a healthy, lower-fat, lower-glycemic-index, lower-salt version. And while they don't look the same or taste exactly the same, they are both delicious. So why not choose the healthy version?

Now let's move on to the meal plans and recipes.

CHAPTER 14

Three Weeks of Meal Plans and Recipes

H ere's where we really get down to business. This chapter contains three weeks of meal plans and recipes that constitute a therapeutic diet for people with diabetes and insulin resistance. If adhered to reasonably closely, this diet can have an ameliorating effect not only on glucose control, but also on cholesterol and triglyceride levels, blood pressure, weight, and other parameters of diabetes and heart disease.

The best way to approach this diet for reversing diabetes is to follow it to the letter for three weeks. During this time you will become familiar with the principles of the diet. You will get a feel for what foods will likely improve your condition and what ones will make it worse. You will learn how to cook in a healthier way and how to gauge appropriate portion sizes. Strict adherence to the diet will also give you firsthand experience in the power of this diet. Three weeks is plenty of time to notice improvements in blood sugar levels, especially if you are exercising and taking appropriate nutritional supplements at the same time. This will likely motivate you to continue with the program.

To get started, read through the meal plans for each week and take a look at the menus. Shop for all that you need by using the shopping guide provided. If you are unable to obtain some of the ingredients in the recipes, use your judgment and make healthy substitutions. For example, if you cannot find xylitol, use brown rice syrup or stevia; if you can't get ahold of vegetable seasoning, use a salt-free or low-sodium salt substitute.

If you find that you are hungry between meals, you may select snacks from the suggestions in the previous chapter or warm up leftovers. If you feel you are not getting enough to eat at meals, fill up on additional vegetables and salad. Drinking a glass of water 15 to 30 minutes before meals also helps you feel fuller, as does eating more slowly.

These menus are designed to generate the least amount of frustration on your part. We have deliberately avoided specifying fruits, for example, due to the unavailability of all types of fruit year round. Nor did we think it necessary to give the specifics on side-dish salads or vegetables.

We have not listed any beverages in these meal plans— the choice is up to you from the accepted drinks listed in the previous chapter. Water is the most important beverage, and you should get in the habit of drinking a minimum of eight glasses of filtered water every day.

After the end of the initial three-week period, you can pick and choose among the recipes that you like and begin incorporating your own modified recipes. You may end up fixing your favorites repeatedly. That's fine. There is nothing wrong with enjoying the same healthy foods again and again as long as they are getting you toward your goal of reversing diabetes. You can also repeat the three-week meal plans indefinitely as is or with modifications, such as switching days around, adding another ingredient to a recipe, or making up your own meals using the recipes in this chapter as a springboard.

Fruit, Green Salad, Vegetables, and Bread

Not every menu item has a recipe. When you see the following items on your menu, refer back to these guidelines:

***Fruit.** Select one serving of fruit (for example, one medium apple or orange, or ¾ cup of berries). Stick to the fruits from the recommended list in the previous chapter. You can jazz fruit up by slicing it and drizzling with two teaspoons of brown rice syrup or a dollop of plain, nonfat yogurt sweetened with stevia. Served in a parfait dish or wineglass, this makes an elegant, healthy dessert.

Green salad. Any salad made with lettuce, spinach, or other greens and added vegetables from the list in chapter 13 can be eaten liberally. (Use up the leftover vegetables in your refrigerator to give your salads more variety.) For most people, 1 cup of lettuce or spinach plus lesser amounts of other vegetables is plenty. However, if you want more, feel free. These vegetables are low in calories and contain a powerhouse of nutrients. They may be served with store-bought fat-free, sweetener-free dressings, or you can make your own. The standard rule of thumb for salad dressing is one part oil (flaxseed or olive oil) and one to two parts vinegar (balsamic and white wine vinegar are tasty) or lemon juice. Garlic, pepper, salt substitutes, and vegetable seasoning give dressings a nice flavor. Limit oil to one tablespoon for two people; there is no limit on the amount of vinegar or seasonings.

*****Vegetables.** When a menu item is listed simply as "vegetables," select ¾ to 1 cup of your favorites, fresh or frozen, lightly steamed or cooked in a microwave, if available, until just tender. Vegetables may be seasoned with vegetable seasoning, salt substitutes, low-sodium soy sauce, lemon juice, or other herbs and spices of your choice.

******Bread.** Breads are among the most restricted of foods for people with diabetes. The only breads that have a reasonable glycemic index are sprouted-grain breads and breads made from 100 percent rye or barley. One serving means one slice of bread, one roll, one English muffin, half a bagel, or one pita round. Crackers made with 100 percent whole wheat or rye with no added sugar (four or five small crackers) or one small whole wheat tortilla are acceptable substitutes.

To review once again, the percentage of carbohydrate desirable in your diet should be around 60 percent, give or take a little, with the remaining 40 percent divided more or less equally between protein and fat. Please do not become obsessed with these percentages. You will even notice that the percentages of carbohydrate, protein, and fat in our recipes and daily meal plans do not always fit into these exact specifications. We are following general principles here, not mathematical formulas. Never forget that quality is more important than quantity. Rest assured that even the "high-fat" recipes contain healthful fats. Please note that if you are using low-sodium seasonings and sauces and rinsing and draining canned beans, the sodium content in some of the recipes will be even lower than the calculations suggest.

The dishes on the menus for which there are recipes are printed in capital letters. Most of the recipes are designed for two people, although quite a few serve four and a few serve even more. The leftovers make a great snack or second meal, if you are in a hurry. The soups and some of the other dishes may also be frozen for later use. If the recipe says that it serves four, each person is to be served one-fourth of the entire recipe. Of course, you may halve or double the recipe. The recipe breakdowns were computed with AccuChef (V5.09h/32, 1999 version) from Sivart Software (www.AccuChef .com). Though every attempt was made to be accurate, we apologize for any minor discrepancies.

Week One Shopping List

- Is your pantry stocked with the staples on pages 314–316?

- Do you have all the ingredients listed below you'll need this week? Amounts listed will feed two people. Several of the recipes serve four and make great leftovers or snacks.

▶ Vegetables

Alfalfa sprouts, I container
Bean sprouts (mung), ¼ pound
Broccoli, I bunch
Cabbage, I small head
Carrots, I small bunch
Cauliflower, I head
Celery, I small bunch
Cucumber, I
Eggplant, 3 medium
Ginger root, I small piece (or powdered)
Green beans, ½ pound
**Lettuce, your choice, romaine or Boston preferred (3–4 heads, depending on size, should be enough for your salads for the week)
Mushrooms, 3 pounds (or canned)
Parsley, I bunch
Peppers, green, 2
Onions, yellow, 6
Onions, green, I large bunch
Spinach, 2 bunches
Summer squash, 3 small
Tomatoes, 5–6
Zucchini, 9 small to medium
***Vegetables (You will need 2 extra side dishes of vegetables per person this week. Choose from accepted list—includes most vegetables)

▶ Fruit

Apples, pippin, Granny Smith, or other cooking apples, 4

Lemon, I
*Fruit of your choice from acceptable fruit list
   (enough for I I servings per person for the
   week)

▶ Canned Foods

Applesauce, unsweetened, I jar
Garbanzo beans (several cans)
Mushrooms, 4 small cans (or fresh)
Pimientos, 2-ounce jar
Soybeans, I5-ounce can
Water chestnuts, I small can

▶ Bakery

Rye crackers, I box
Sprouted grain bread, I loaf
Sprouted grain hamburger buns, I package (freeze
   what you don't use)
****See notes on bread. (You will need enough for
   about ten servings per person of bread for
   the week.)

▶ Frozen Foods

Blueberries, unsweetened, 2 large (I-quart) bags
Peas, I large (I-quart) bag
Strawberries, unsweetened, I small bag

▶ Dried/Packaged Foods

All-Bran cereal, I box
Barley, pearled, I bag
Lasagna, I box
Lentils, I small bag
Lima beans, I small bag

Macaroni (whole grain preferred but optional),
1 package
Rice, brown, long grain, 1 small package
Rotelli (spiral pasta), 1 package
Spaghetti (whole grain or high protein preferred
but optional), 1 package

►Meat, Eggs, and Dairy

Chicken breasts, boneless and skinless, 3 pounds
Cottage cheese, low fat, 1 container
Eggs, 1½ dozen
Milk: soy milk or nonfat milk, small container
Ricotta cheese, nonfat, two 8-ounce containers
Salmon, fresh or frozen, two 4-ounce pieces
Tofu, firm, 1 container
Tuna, water packed, 1 small can
Turkey breast, ground, 1½ pounds
Yogurt, plain, nonfat, 4 cups

►Staples

(If you stocked up on the basics as suggested in
the previous chapter, you should have these
staples on hand.)
Almonds, raw
Baking powder
Basil
Bay leaves
Brown rice syrup
Cinnamon
Cloves
Flaxseed oil
Flaxseed, whole

Garlic, fresh and powdered
Mustard, Dijon and American
Nu-Salt, NoSalt, or Cardia Salt
Oatmeal, long-cooking
Olive oil
Olive oil pan spray
Onion powder
Oregano
Parmesan cheese
Pepper
Pickles, dill
Salsa
Sesame seeds
Soy sauce, low sodium
Spaghetti sauce, low sugar, low fat (or homemade),
      2–3 jars
Stevia
Sunflower seeds, raw
Tapioca
Tomato paste
Tomatoes, canned, whole
Vanilla extract
Vegetable seasoning
Vinegar
Whole wheat flour (stone-ground preferred)
Xylitol

Day One Menus

▶ Breakfast

*Fruit
Poached or soft-boiled eggs (2)
****Bread

▶ Lunch

GARDEN SOUP
****Bread

▶ Dinner

**Green salad
BARLEY RAFFAELE
BROILED SALMON STEAKS
*Fruit

Garden Soup

5 cups water
½ cauliflower head, diced
1 cup peas, fresh or frozen
1 carrot, scrubbed and diced
1 small yellow onion, diced
¼ small head of cabbage,
   chopped (approximately
   1 cup)
1 small tomato, diced
1 apple, peeled and diced
4 ounces rotelli (spiral pasta)
½ cup cooked garbanzo beans
1 tablespoon olive oil
1 tablespoon vegetable
   seasoning
⅛ teaspoon pepper

Per Serving:

164.44 Cal (21.60%
from Fat, 13.40% from
Protein, 65.00% from
Carb)

5.81 g Protein
4.17 g Total Fat
 • 0.56 g Sat Fat;
 • 2.61 g Mono Fat
 • 0.62 g Poly Fat
28.19 g Carb
5.84 g Fiber
169.12 mg Sodium
0.00 mg Cholesterol

Start the water boiling as you prepare the vegetables. Add the vegetables and apple to the pot one by one as they are ready. Add the pasta and beans, cover the pot, and cook for 10 minutes. Then add the oil and seasonings and simmer 3–5 more minutes.

Serves 4

Barley Raffaele

½ small onion, chopped

8 ounces fresh mushrooms, chopped

1 large green pepper, chopped

4 small zucchini, sliced and quartered

1 tablespoon olive oil

2 tablespoons tomato paste

1 cup water

2 tablespoons mild salsa

¼ teaspoon oregano

½ teaspoon salt (or a salt substitute to taste)

½ teaspoon onion or garlic powder

3 cups cooked pearl barley

Per Serving:

221.33 Cal (16.80% from Fat, 9.90% from Protein, 73.30% from Carb)

5.82 g Protein
4.40 g Tot Fat
• 0.65 g Sat Fat
• 2.58 g Mono Fat
• 0.75 g Poly Fat
43.05 g Carb
7.44 g Fiber
495.98 mg Sodium
0.00 mg Cholesterol

Sauté the onion, mushrooms, green pepper, and zucchini in the olive oil. Add the tomato paste and water and stir. Add the remaining ingredients except the barley and simmer for 15 minutes. Stir in the barley and heat through for 5 more minutes.

Serves 4

Broiled Salmon Steaks

2 4-ounce salmon steaks (may substitute other favorite fish)

¼ teaspoon salt (or salt substitute to taste)

2 teaspoons olive oil

Parsley

Lemon wedges

Per Serving:

248.37 Cal (62.30% from Fat, 37.20% from Protein, 0.51% from Carb)

22.62 g Protein
16.82 g Tot Fat
• 3.08 g Sat Fat
• 7.70 g Mono Fat
• 4.84 g Poly Fat
0.31 g Carb
0.10 g Fiber
362.04 mg Sodium
66.91 mg Cholesterol

Preheat the broiler to high and set the oven rack so the top of the fish will be two inches from the heating element. Dry the fish with paper towels. Season by rubbing with salt or salt substitute and half of the olive oil. Broil for about 2 minutes, brush with additional oil, and broil for another 5 minutes or so. It will be ready when it lightly springs to the touch, yet is still moist. (When in doubt, cut into the fish to see if it is done.) Garnish with parsley and lemon before serving.

Serves 2

Day Two Menus

▶Breakfast

Yogurt, plain, nonfat, sweetened with stevia
*Fruit (add to yogurt)
APPLE PANCAKES

▶Lunch

PEA AND CUCUMBER SALAD
EGGPLANT GINA
****Bread

▶Dinner

**Green salad
CHICKEN-BROCCOLI PASTA
COMPANY BLUEBERRY-APPLE COBBLER

Apple Pancakes

1 ½ cups water
1 tablespoon olive oil
¾ cup whole wheat flour
1 teaspoon cinnamon
1 teaspoon baking soda
2 egg whites, stiffly beaten
2 drops stevia
½ large apple, grated

Per Serving:

250.12 Cal (26.40% from Fat, 14.80% from Protein, 58.70% from Carb)

9.77 g Protein
7.73 g Tot Fat
  • 1.08 g Sat Fat
  • 5.09 g Mono Fat
  • 0.95 g Poly Fat
38.65 g Carb
6.71 g Fiber
691.93 mg Sodium
0.00 mg Cholesterol

Put the water and oil in a blender. While it is running, add the dry ingredients. Pour into a bowl and fold in the egg whites, stevia, and the grated apple. Bake on a hot griddle sprayed with olive oil. Serve with unsweetened applesauce or berries sweetened with xylitol or stevia.

Serves 2

Pea and Cucumber Salad

- ½ cucumber, peeled, sliced thin, and quartered
- 2 green onions, chopped
- 1 small tomato, chopped
- 1 cup peas, thawed
- 2 tablespoons white wine vinegar (with tarragon nice but optional)
- 1 tablespoon olive oil
- ½ teaspoon oregano
- ¼ teaspoon salt (or salt substitute to taste)

Per Serving:

147.07 Cal (44.50% from Fat, 14.40% from Protein, 41.10% from Carb)

5.28 g Protein
7.22 g Tot Fat
 • 1.01 g Sat Fat
 • 5.01 g Mono Fat
 • 0.78 g Poly Fat
15.01 g Carb
5.08 g Fiber
49.77 mg Sodium
0.00 mg Cholesterol

Mix all of the ingredients together and serve on a bed of lettuce.

Serves 2

Eggplant Gina

1 medium eggplant, peeled
and sliced lengthwise into
approximately 12 slices
16 ounces fresh mushrooms,
sliced, or 8 ounces canned,
rinsed
1 small onion, chopped
8 ounces spaghetti sauce
(homemade—recipe
follows—or canned, low
sodium, no sugar)
2 tablespoons sesame seeds
1 tablespoon vegetable
seasoning

Per Serving:

183.64 Cal (12.00%
from Fat, 18.70% from
Protein, 69.30% from
Carb)

10.02 g Protein
2.85 g Tot Fat
  • 0.38 g Sat Fat
  • 0.46 g Mono Fat
  • 1.27 g Poly Fat
37.10 g Carb
10.78 g Fiber
646.54 mg Sodium
0.00 mg Cholesterol

Layer the ingredients in a 9-by-13-inch casserole in
the order given, ending with a sprinkling of vegetable
seasoning. Cover and bake at 400° F for 45 minutes.

Serves 2

Healthy Spaghetti Sauce Recipe

Because many of our recipes call for spaghetti sauce, we suggest you make up a pot of this healthy sauce and then freeze it in 1- or 2-cup portions. Remove the sauce from the freezer the night before you need to use it and keep it in the refrigerator. You may also purchase a natural, low-sodium spaghetti sauce with no added sugar.

6 cups chopped canned tomatoes or tomato puree (two 28-ounce cans)
½ cup tomato paste
2 cups minced green pepper
2 cups fresh minced onion (approximately 1 medium onion)
4 teaspoons oregano
2 tablespoons vegetable seasoning (or salt substitute to taste)
8 cloves garlic, minced or pressed in garlic press (or less, to taste)

Per Serving:

48.83 Cal (7.53% from Fat, 14.90% from Protein, 77.60% from Carb)

2.15 g Protein
1.01 0.48 g Tot Fat
• 0.07 g Sat Fat
• 0.07 g Mono Fat
• 0.20 g Poly Fat
11.21 g Carb
2.35 g Fiber
49.13 mg Sodium
0.00 mg Cholesterol

Combine all of the ingredients in a large pot and simmer slowly for 1 hour. You may add more tomato puree for thickness or more water if you desire your sauce less thick. The amount of vegetable seasoning (or salt substitute) may be increased to taste.

Makes 8 ½ cups

Note: If you are using this sauce for pasta and want it to be ready to serve, you may add 1–2 cups chopped mushrooms, 1–2 cups browned lean ground turkey, and/or 1 cup low-sodium soy protein substitute, and increase the seasoning to 4 tablespoons of vegetable seasoning.

Chicken-Broccoli Pasta

- 1 large head broccoli (2 cups), cut into 1-inch pieces
- 1 pound boneless chicken breasts, cut into ½-inch-thick slices
- 1 teaspoon olive oil
- 1 clove minced garlic (or ½ teaspoon garlic powder)
- ½ teaspoon onion powder
- ½ teaspoon salt (or a salt substitute to taste)
- 8 ounces spaghetti (whole grain or protein-enriched preferred but optional)
- 1 tablespoon olive oil
- 2 tablespoons parsley, chopped
- 4 tablespoons Parmesan cheese

Per Serving:

332.31 Cal (30.80% from Fat, 50.60% from Protein, 18.50% from Carb)

40.82 g Protein
11.04 g Tot Fat
 • 3.03 g Sat Fat
 • 5.35 g Mono Fat
 • 1.54 g Poly Fat
14.94 g Carb
0.09 g Fiber
499.70 mg Sodium
120.02 mg Cholesterol

Lightly steam the broccoli until tender-crisp and set aside. Brown the chicken in 1 teaspoon olive oil in a large skillet pan until cooked through, 5–10 minutes, adding the garlic and seasonings during the last minute. Add the steamed broccoli to the chicken. Meanwhile, cook the spaghetti until just tender (aldente) following package directions. Toss the cooked pasta with the chicken and broccoli mixture and 1 tablespoon olive oil. Stir over low heat until heated through. Add the parsley and cheese, stir well, and serve.

Serves 4

Company Apple-Blueberry Cobbler

1 quart frozen blueberries
2 large apples, peeled and cut
   into chunks
¼ cup almonds
¼ cup uncooked oatmeal
½ teaspoon cinnamon
1 cup water
4 drops stevia
1 teaspoon vanilla
2 teaspoons tapioca granules

Per Serving:

88.57 Cal (30.10% from
Fat, 9.19% from Protein,
60.70% from Carb)

2.15 g Protein
3.14 g Tot Fat
• 0.28 g Sat Fat
• 1.64 g Mono Fat
• 0.89 g Poly Fat
14.22 g Carb
3.22 g Fiber
3.11 mg Sodium
0.00 mg Cholesterol

Preheat the oven to 350° F. Pour the blueberries and chunks of apple into a 9-by-13-inch baking dish. In the blender, chop the almonds, oatmeal, and cinnamon and set aside. Mix the water, stevia, vanilla, and tapioca and stir into the berries and apples until well mixed. Sprinkle with the dry mixture. Bake for 30 minutes. Let cool. Serve either warm or cold with Cream Sauce (see page 474 for recipe).

Serves 8

Day Three Menus

▶Breakfast

*Fruit

EGG-WHITE SCRAMBLE OVER TOAST

▶Lunch

HIGH-FIBER SALAD

APPLE MUFFINS

▶Dinner

**Green salad

SPINACH LASAGNA

*Fruit

Egg-White Scramble Over Toast

½ yellow onion, chopped
1 zucchini, sliced and
  quartered
4 ounces fresh mushrooms,
  sliced
½ green pepper, chopped
1 teaspoon olive oil
2 tablespoons mild salsa
¼ teaspoon salt
¼ teaspoon pepper
4 egg whites
4 slices sprouted-grain bread,
  toasted

Per Serving:

248.71 Cal (17.60%
from Fat, 24.30% from
Protein, 58.10% from
Carb)

15.85 g Protein
5.09 g Tot Fat
  • 0.89 g Sat Fat
  • 2.65 g Mono Fat
  • 0.96 g Poly Fat
37.84 g Carb
6.29 g Fiber
506.18 mg Sodium
0.00 mg Cholesterol

In a nonstick skillet, sauté the onion, zucchini, mushrooms, and green pepper in the olive oil. Add the salsa, salt, and pepper. While the mixture simmers, beat the egg whites with a fork and pour onto the mixture, stirring while it cooks to keep it from sticking. (Use a utensil that is safe for nonstick surfaces.) Cook until the eggs set but are still moist. Spoon over the toast.

Serves 2

High-Fiber Salad

- 2 teaspoons olive or flaxseed oil
- 2 tablespoons vinegar
- ¼ teaspoon seasoned salt (or a salt substitute to taste)
- ¼ teaspoon pepper
- ½ head lettuce, washed and dried (romaine or Boston preferred)
- 1 tomato, chopped
- ¼ cup chopped green onions
- 1 cup cooked garbanzo beans (if canned, rinse before using)
- ¼ cup freshly ground flaxseed

Per Serving:

399.27 Cal (41.50% from Fat, 14.00% from Protein, 44.50% from Carb)

14.65 g Protein
19.38 g Tot Fat
 • 2.04 g Sat Fat
 • 6.33 g Mono Fat
 • 9.82 g Poly Fat
46.71 g Carb
17.52 g Fiber
392.54 mg Sodium
0.00 mg Cholesterol

Mix the oil, vinegar, and seasonings together and set aside. Tear the lettuce into bite-size pieces, then add the remaining vegetables and beans. Toss with the dressing, sprinkle on the flaxseed, and serve on dinner plates.

Serves 2

Apple Muffins

¾ cup whole wheat flour
⅓ cup finely ground almonds
1 tablespoon baking powder
¼ cup finely grated apple
2 stiffly beaten egg whites
½ cup water
1 tablespoon olive oil
⅓ cup xylitol

Per Muffin:

81.50 Cal (34.80% from Fat, 17.20% from Protein, 48.00% from Carb)

3.76 g Protein
3.39 g Tot Fat
- 0.29 g Sat Fat
- 2.06 g Mono Fat
- 0.83 g Poly Fat
10.51 g Carb
2.10 g Fiber
208.40 mg Sodium
0.00 mg Cholesterol

Sift the dry ingredients together and set aside. Mix the apple, beaten egg whites, water, oil, and xylitol. Gently stir into the dry ingredients until just moist. Pour into a muffin pan that has been sprayed with olive oil spray. Fill each muffin cup two-thirds full. Bake in a preheated 375° F for 20 minutes or until done.

Serves 8

Spinach Lasagna

12 lasagna noodles
½ pound ground turkey breast
½ teaspoon minced garlic or garlic powder
½ teaspoon onion powder
2½ cups spaghetti sauce (low sodium or homemade; see recipe on page 367)
1½ cups fat-free ricotta cheese
1 small eggplant, thinly sliced
4 tablespoons Parmesan cheese
1 large bunch fresh spinach, washed and stems removed
12 ounces fresh mushrooms, sliced

Per Serving:

559.57 Cal (18.20% from Fat, 29.20% from Protein, 52.60% from Carb)

38.04 g Protein
10.50 g Tot Fat
  • 7.69 g Sat Fat
  • 5.15 g Mono Fat
  • 2.62 g Poly Fat
68.40 g Carb
10.77 g Fiber
434.13 mg Sodium
95.89 mg Cholesterol

Precook the lasagna noodles until just tender. Drain immediately and separate. Meanwhile, brown the ground turkey with the garlic and onion powder in an olive oil-sprayed pan. Add to spaghetti sauce. Spray a 9-by-13-inch baking dish with olive oil. Layer in this order: ½ cup of the spaghetti sauce, one layer of the noodles (4 noodles), ½ cup ricotta cheese, and eggplant. Spread this with ½ cup of spaghetti sauce and sprinkle with 1 tablespoon Parmesan cheese. Now add a second layer of lasagna noodles. Spread another ½ cup of ricotta over the noodles. Heap the spinach over this second layer, about 4 leaves thick. Add another ½ cup sauce, and then a third layer of lasagna noodles, followed by the last ½ cup of ricotta and another table-spoon of Parmesan. Top with the mushrooms, 1 more cup of spaghetti sauce, and 2 tablespoons of Parmesan, being careful to sprinke it lightly so that it will cover the top. Cover with foil and bake at 350° F for 45 minutes. Cut into squares to serve. You may layer two squares so it will be thicker.

Serves 4

Day Four Menus

▶Breakfast

Yogurt, plain, nonfat (sweetened with stevia)
FRENCH TOAST with STRAWBERRY SYRUP

▶Lunch

LIMA BEAN SOUP
****Bread
*Fruit

▶Dinner

**Green salad
GINGER SESAME CHICKEN
***Vegetable
POACHED PEARS

French Toast

- 1 whole egg
- 1 egg white
- 2 tablespoons soy milk or skim milk
- ½ teaspoon vanilla
- ½ teaspoon cinnamon
- 4 slices sprouted-grain bread

Per Serving:

211.01 Cal (21.10% from Fat, 21.20% from Protein, 57.70% from Carb)

11.33 g Protein
5.01 g Tot Fat
- 1.31 g Sat Fat
- 1.95 g Mono Fat
- 0.94 g Poly Fat
30.78 g Carb
4.40 g Fiber
370.27 mg Sodium
106.32 mg Cholesterol

Use a wire whisk to blend the first five ingredients. Dip bread into the egg batter. Brown both sides in a hot skillet or griddle, lightly sprayed with olive oil spray. Do not overcook—toast should remain moist. Serve with strawberry syrup (recipe follows).

Serves 2

Strawberry Syrup

1 cup mashed fresh or frozen
  strawberries
2 teaspoons tapioca granules
½ cup water
2–6 drops stevia (to taste)

Per Serving:

22.80 Cal (9.84% from
Fat, 7.21% from Protein,
83.00% from Carb)

0.46 g Protein
0.28 g Tot Fat
  • 0.02 g Sat Fat
  • 0.04 g Mono Fat
  • 0.14 g Poly Fat
5.34 g Carb
1.75 g Fiber
2.53 mg Sodium
0.00 mg Cholesterol

Cook the combined ingredients in a saucepan,
bringing to a bubble and stirring constantly until
thickened, about 5 minutes.

Remove from heat and serve with French Toast or
waffles.

Serves 2

Lima Bean Soup

- 1 cup small lima beans
- 1½ quarts water
- 2 thinly sliced onions
- 1 clove garlic, minced
- 2 cups chopped tomatoes, canned
- 4 stalks thinly sliced celery
- 1 bay leaf
- 2 whole cloves
- 1 tablespoon lemon juice
- ¼ teaspoon pepper

Per Serving:

96.49 Cal (4.00% from Fat, 16.80% from Protein, 79.20% from Carb)

4.42 g Protein
0.47 g Tot Fat
- 0.09 g Sat Fat
- 0.06 g Mono Fat
- 0.21 g Poly Fat
20.85 g Carb
4.88 g Fiber
505.74 mg Sodium
0.00 mg Cholesterol

Soak the beans overnight in 3 cups of water. Drain, rinse, and bring to a boil with 1½ quarts water. Add the remaining ingredients. Reduce heat, cover, and simmer for 3 hours or until beans are tender. Remove the bay leaf before serving.

Serves 4

Ginger Sesame Chicken

2 small chicken breasts or
one large, halved (4 ounces
each)
1 tablespoon olive oil
1 cup plain nonfat yogurt
1 tablespoon brown rice syrup
¼ cup toasted whole grain
bread crumbs
1 teaspoon freshly grated
ginger (or ¼ teaspoon
ginger powder to taste)

Per Serving:
211.41 Cal (36.20% from Fat, 53.30% from Protein, 10.60% from Carb)
27.26 g Protein
8.22 g Tot Fat
• 1.30 g Sat Fat
• 5.33 g Mono Fat
• 0.90 g Poly Fat
5.40 g Carb
0.02 g Fiber
76.83 mg Sodium
68.44 mg Cholesterol

Brown the chicken in the olive oil over medium heat in a skillet. Do not cook completely. Mix the yogurt, brown rice syrup, bread crumbs, and grated ginger. Arrange the chicken in a single layer in an oven-safe dish, and spread the yogurt mixture over the surface of each piece of chicken. Place uncovered in a 325° F oven and bake for 30 minutes or until the chicken is tender.

Serves 2

Poached Pears

2 firm pears, peeled, cored, and
  halved
2 cups water
¼ teaspoon cinnamon
4–6 drops stevia, divided use
Dash cinnamon
4 tablespoons yogurt, plain,
  nonfat

Per Serving:

124.79 Cal (5.52% from
Fat, 2.41% from Protein,
92.10% from Carb)

0.84 g Protein
0.85 g Tot Fat
 • 0.05 g Sat Fat
 • 0.18 g Mono Fat
 • 0.20 g Poly Fat
32.03 g Carb
5.32 g Fiber
7.25 mg Sodium
0.00 mg Cholesterol

Put the pear halves, cut side down, in a large saucepan. Cover with water (2 cups or enough to cover).
Add the cinnamon and 2–3 drops stevia. Bring to a
boil, then turn down heat to a simmer, cover and cook
until just tender, about 10 minutes. Remove the pears
with a slotted spoon to serving dishes. Add 2–3 drops
stevia and a dash of cinnamon to the yogurt. Top the
pear halves with 1 tablespoon of yogurt on each.

Serves 2

Day Five Menus

►Breakfast

*Fruit
All-Bran cereal
Soy milk or nonfat milk
CINNAMON TOAST WITH SYRUP

►Lunch

Boca Burger on sprouted-grain bun (with lettuce,
tomato, pickles, onion, mustard, and catsup)

►Dinner

**Green salad
STUFFED ZUCCHINI
***Vegetables
*Fruit

Cinnamon Toast with Syrup

2 slices sprouted-grain bread
2 teaspoons brown rice syrup
½ teaspoon cinnamon

Per Serving:

95.65 Cal (11.20%
from Fat, 13.00% from
Protein, 75.80% from
Carb)

3.22 g Protein
1.23 g Tot Fat
• 0.26 g Sat Fat
• 0.49 g Mono Fat
• 0.30 g Poly Fat
18.80 g Carb
2.36 g Fiber
155.99 mg Sodium
0.00 mg Cholesterol

Toast one side of the bread under the broiler. Turn over and drizzle 1 teaspoon of brown rice syrup over each slice, then sprinkle lightly with cinnamon. Place toast under the broiler for another minute or so. Watch carefully so that it doesn't burn.

Serves 2

Stuffed Zucchini

½ cup tofu, cut into small cubes

1 clove garlic, minced

1 teaspoon olive oil

1 teaspoon low-sodium soy sauce

2 medium zucchini

¼ teaspoon dried basil (optional)

¼ cup nonfat ricotta cheese

1 egg, slightly beaten

1 tablespoon Parmesan cheese

Per Serving:

185.01 Cal (49.00% from Fat, 35.20% from Protein, 15.80% from Carb)

15.09 g Protein
9.35 g Tot Fat
• 3.78 g Sat Fat
• 4.41 g Mono Fat
• 2.43 g Poly Fat
6.78 g Carb
1.64 g Fiber
308.43 mg Sodium
125.83 mg Cholesterol

Sauté the tofu and garlic in the olive oil until browned. Add the soy sauce. Cut the zucchini in half lengthwise and carefully hollow out the flesh to within ¼ inch of the skin. Set the shells aside. Chop the zucchini flesh, then press with the back of a wooden spoon to extract as much juice as is possible and drain it away. Preheat the oven to 400° F. Combine the zucchini flesh, tofu mixture, basil, ricotta cheese, and egg until thoroughly blended. Arrange the zucchini shells skin side down in a shallow baking pan sprayed with olive oil spray. Stuff with the tofu mixture and sprinkle with the Parmesan cheese. Bake for 20–30 minutes or until the top is brown.

Serves 2

Day Six Menus

▶Breakfast

*Fruit
CINNAMON APPLE OATMEAL
Soy milk or nonfat milk

▶Lunch

TUNA MACARONI SALAD

▶Dinner

**Green salad
LENTIL STEW
****Bread
*Fruit

Cinnamon Apple Oatmeal

1 ¾ cups water
¾ cup oatmeal (not instant)
¾ teaspoon cinnamon
½ cup apple, chopped

> **Per Serving:**
>
> 127.10 Cal (16.30% from Fat, 15.00% from Protein, 68.60% from Carb)
>
> 5.18 g Protein
> 2.50 g Tot Fat
> • 0.45 g Sat Fat
> • 0.79 g Mono Fat
> • 0.94 g Poly Fat
> 23.64 g Carb
> 5.27 g Fiber
> 7.93 mg Sodium
> 0.00 mg Cholesterol

Bring the water to a boil. Stir in the oatmeal and cook for 5 minutes. Add the cinnamon and apple and remove from heat. Serve with ½ cup nonfat milk or soy milk. Sweeten with 2–3 drops of stevia, if needed. (You may sprinkle ¼ cup freshly ground flaxseed on cooked oatmeal for additional fiber.)

Serves 2

Tuna Macaroni Salad

- 1 cup uncooked macaroni (high-protein whole wheat preferred but not required)
- 2 tablespoons flaxseed or olive oil
- 2 tablespoons vinegar
- 1 teaspoon prepared mustard
- 2 teaspoons vegetable seasoning
- 1 cup cooked peas
- 4 tablespoons chopped pimientos (optional)
- 2 hard-cooked egg whites, chopped
- 2 tablespoons minced dill pickles
- 1 can water-packed tuna, drained

Per Serving:

331.19 Cal (30.40% from Fat, 28.20% from Protein, 41.50% from Carb)

23.89 g Protein
10.68 g Tot Fat
- 1.80 g Sat Fat
- 7.17 g Mono Fat
- 1.71 g Poly Fat
35.19 g Carb
5.75 g Fiber
343.28 mg Sodium
24.08 mg Cholesterol

Cook the macaroni according to the package directions. Drain, rinse, and immediately toss with the oil to prevent sticking. Mix together the vinegar, mustard, and vegetable seasoning and toss with the macaroni. Add the remaining ingredients in the order given, tossing lightly. Serve on a bed of lettuce.

Serves 3

Lentil Stew

- 4 cups water
- 1 cup uncooked lentils
- ½ whole cauliflower, cut into bite-size pieces
- 2 stalks celery, cut into bite-size pieces
- 1 tablespoon tomato sauce
- 1 tablespoon vegetable seasoning

Per Serving:

166.88 Cal (2.46% from Fat, 31.90% from Protein, 65.60% from Carb)

14.10 g Protein
0.48 g Tot Fat
  • 0.07 g Sat Fat
  • 0.08 g Mono Fat
  • 0.22 g Poly Fat
28.99 g Carb
14.93 g Fiber
97.86 mg Sodium
0.00 mg Cholesterol

Bring the water to a boil and add the lentils. Turn down the heat and simmer for 15 minutes. Add the cauliflower and celery and cook for 30 minutes more. Add the remaining ingredients and cook for an additional 10–15 minutes.

Serves 4

Leftovers suggestion: Soften a whole wheat tortilla by heating on each side for 30–60 seconds in an ungreased frying pan. Place 2 tablespoons of warmed, drained lentils in center of tortilla, along with 1 teaspoon or more of salsa. Roll and eat.

Day Seven Menus

▶Breakfast

*Fruit
TOFU SCRAMBLE WITH SPINACH
****Bread

▶Lunch

**Green salad
HEARTY SUMMER SOUP
****Bread

▶Dinner

ORIENTAL DINNER
Yogurt with BLUEBERRY SAUCE

Tofu Scramble with Spinach

1 cup chopped onion
1 tablespoon olive oil
½ container firm tofu
1 teaspoon onion powder
1 cup fresh spinach, cleaned
  and chopped
2 tablespoons grated Parmesan
  cheese

Per Serving:

126.57 Cal (60.70% from Fat, 12.50% from Protein, 26.80% from Carb);

4.10 g Protein
8.83 g Tot Fat
  • 2.14 g Sat Fat
  • 5.55 g Mono Fat
  • 0.69 g Poly Fat
8.76 g Carb
1.98 g Fiber
135.57 mg Sodium
4.92 mg Cholesterol

Sauté the onions in the olive oil until tender. Crumble the tofu and add to the onions, sprinkle with onion powder, and blend well. Continue cooking for 2–3 minutes. Add the spinach and stir just until it is wilted. Sprinkle on the cheese and cover 1–2 minutes until cheese melts.

Serves 2

Hearty Summer Soup

6 cups water
1 15-ounce can soybeans
¼ small head cabbage, chopped
1 cup green beans, chopped in one-inch pieces
1 tablespoon tomato paste
3 yellow summer squash
2 tablespoons vegetable seasoning
½ teaspoon pepper

> **Per Serving:**
>
> 168.12 Cal (32.70% from Fat, 31.80% from Protein, 35.50% from Carb)
>
> 15.13 g Protein
> 6.93 g Tot Fat
> • 0.81 g Sat Fat
> • 1.30 g Mono Fat
> • 3.26 g Poly Fat
> 16.88 g Carb
> 6.15 g Fiber
> 154.90 mg Sodium
> 0.00 mg Cholesterol

Combine all the ingredients in a large pot and simmer until the vegetables are tender-crisp, about 30–45 minutes.

Serves 4

Oriental Dinner

- 1 large chicken breast, thinly sliced and cut into 1-inch pieces
- 1 tablespoon olive oil
- ½ large green pepper, sliced
- 1 stalk celery, chopped
- 4 ounces fresh mushrooms, sliced
- ¼ pound mung sprouts
- ½ teaspoon each garlic and onion powder
- 1¼ cups water
- 1 tablespoon arrowroot
- 1 tablespoon low-sodium soy sauce
- ½ of an 8-ounce can sliced water chestnuts
- 1 cup cooked long-grain brown rice

Per Serving:

393.90 Cal (19.60% from Fat, 20.50% from Protein, 59.90% from Carb)

20.74 g Protein
8.79 g Tot Fat
- 1.36 g Sat Fat
- 5.46 g Mono Fat
- 1.24 g Poly Fat
60.42 g Carb
7.68 g Fiber
438.06 mg Sodium
34.22 mg Cholesterol

In a skillet, sauté the chicken slices in 1 teaspoon olive oil over medium heat until just cooked; remove from the skillet. Add the rest of the olive oil to the skillet, then add the vegetables in this order, stirring constantly and cooking a minute or so before adding the next one: green pepper, celery, mushrooms, and sprouts. Return the cooked chicken to the pan, along with the garlic and onion powder, and cook until the vegetables are tender yet crisp and the chicken is warm. This will take 5–10 minutes. Mix ¼ cup water with the arrowroot and stir into skillet. Combine 1 cup of water with the soy sauce, add to the skillet and stir until thickened. Add the water chestnuts. Serve over rice (½ cup rice per person).

Serves 2

Blueberry Sauce

1 cup blueberries, fresh or
  frozen
3 tablespoons tapioca granules
1 cup water
5–6 drops stevia, or to taste

Per Serving:

22.80 Cal (9.84% from Fat, 7.21% from Protein, 83.00% from Carb)

0.46 g Protein
0.28 g Tot Fat
  • 0.02 g Sat Fat
  • 0.04 g Mono Fat
  • 0.14 g Poly Fat
5.34 g Carb
1.75 g Fiber
2.53 mg Sodium
0.00 mg Cholesterol

In a saucepan, cook all the ingredients, mashing the blueberries with a fork. Cook until bubbly and thickened, about 5 minutes. Remove from heat. Serve over nonfat yogurt. *Note*: A nice presentation is to serve alternating layers of sauce and yogurt in a parfait or wineglass. Also good on pancakes or waffles.

Makes 2 cups

Week Two Shopping List

- ⦿ Do you need to replenish any of your staples from last week?

- ⦿ Do you have all the items on the shopping list you'll need this week? The amounts listed will feed two people. Several of the recipes serve four and make great leftovers or snacks.

▶ Vegetables

Alfalfa sprouts, 1 container

Asparagus, ½ pound

Avocados, 2

Basil, 1 bunch

Bean sprouts, 1 cup

Cabbage, 1 head

Celery, 1 bunch

Cucumber, 1

Eggplant, 1

Ginger, 1 small piece (you will probably have some left over from last week)

Green beans, 1 pound

Green peppers, 4

Leeks, 1 small bunch

**Lettuce, your choice, romaine or Boston preferred (3–4 heads, depending on size, should be enough for your salads for the week)

Mushrooms, 1 pound

Onion, 8 medium

Onions, green, 2 bunches

Parsley, 2 bunches

Tomatoes, 5

Zucchini, small, 4

***Vegetables (You will need one extra side dish of vegetables per person this week; choose from suggested list.)

▶ Fruit

Apples, 4

Blueberries, 2 small packages (fresh preferred, frozen acceptable)

Lemon, 4 small

Lime, I

Oranges, 3

Peach (or nectarine), I

Pears, 2

Raspberries, I small package (fresh preferred, frozen acceptable)

Strawberries, I small package (if fresh are unavailable, choose another type of acceptable fruit)

*Fruit of your choice from acceptable fruit list (enough for I I servings per person for the week)

▶ Canned Foods

Applesauce, unsweetened, I small jar

Butter beans (or frozen or made from dried), I can

Black-eyed peas (or frozen or made from dried), I can

Garbanzo beans (or frozen or made from dried), 3 cans

Green beans (or fresh or frozen), I can

Pinto beans (or frozen or made from dried), 1 can

Soybeans (or frozen or made from dried), 1 can

▶Bakery

Sprouted-grain bread, 1 loaf

Sprouted-grain pita bread, 1 package (freeze what you don't use for later use)

Whole wheat tortillas, small, 1 package (freeze what you don't use for later use)

****See notes on bread. (You will need enough for about eight servings of bread per person for the week.)

▶Frozen Foods

Blueberries, 1 small package (may have enough left from last week)

▶Dried/Packaged Foods

All-Bran cereal, 1 box (likely have enough left from last week)

Barley, 1 package (likely have enough left from last week)

Barley flakes (not instant)

Fettuccini or linguini, 8 ounces

Rye flakes (not instant)

Split peas, 1 small package

Wheat berries, 1 small package

▶Meat, Eggs, and Dairy

Chicken breasts, skinless, 2 large or 4 small (1 pound total)

Eggs, 2 dozen

Fish fillets (cod, halibut or bass), 2 4-ounce fillets

Goat cheese, 2 ounces
Ground turkey breast, 2 pounds
Milk: soy milk or nonfat milk, small container
Ricotta cheese, 8 ounces
Shrimp, 1 pound fresh or frozen
Swiss cheese, low fat, 4 ounces
Tofu, firm, 2 packages
Yogurt, plain, nonfat, 5 cups

▶Other

Miso (found in Asian markets and health food
stores)
Sesame oil, untoasted
Tahini (sesame butter)

▶Staples

(Do you need to replenish anything?)
Almonds, raw (you will need about a cup)
Baking powder
Basil
Brown rice syrup
Chili powder
Cinnamon
Flaxseed oil
Flaxseed, whole
Garlic, fresh and powder
Mustard, Dijon and American
Oatmeal, slow cooking
Olive oil
Olive oil pan spray
Onion powder
Oregano

Parmesan cheese
Pepper, black
Pepper, red
Pickles, dill
Pumpkin seeds, raw
Salsa
Sesame seeds, raw
Soy sauce, low sodium
Spaghetti sauce, low sugar, low sodium (or home-made from recipe on page 367)
Stevia
Sunflower seeds, raw
Tomato paste
Tomatoes, whole (2 cans)
Vanilla extract
Vegetable seasoning
Vinegar (rice preferred)
Whole wheat flour
Xylitol

Day Eight Menus

▶Breakfast

    *Fruit
    All-Bran cereal
    Soy milk or nonfat milk
    BLUEBERRY MUFFINS

▶Lunch

    THREE-BEAN SALAD
    ****Bread

▶Dinner

    GREEN BEANS À LA FRANÇAISE
    BROILED FISH FILLETS
    STUFT MUSHROOMS
    *Fruit

Blueberry Muffins

1 orange, peeled and
  sectioned
1 small apple, chopped
1 cup water
1 teaspoon vanilla
2–3 drops stevia
½ cup xylitol
1 teaspoon cinnamon
1 tablespoon olive oil
1 tablespoon baking powder
1 cup whole wheat flour
¾ cup ground almonds
1 cup blueberries (fresh or
  frozen)
2 egg whites, stiffly beaten

Per Muffin:

115.40 Cal (43.70%
from Fat, 13.60% from
Protein, 42.70% from
Carb)

4.18 g Protein
5.97 g Tot Fat
 • 0.54 g Sat Fat
 • 3.79 g Mono Fat
 • 1.29 g Poly Fat
13.15 g Carb
2.96 g Fiber
135.47 mg Sodium
0.00 mg Cholesterol

In a blender or food processor, puree the orange and apple together with the water. Add the vanilla, stevia, xylitol, cinnamon, and olive oil and continue to blend. Pour the mixture into a large bowl and, with a hand mixer, beat in the baking powder, flour, and almonds. Fold in the berries, then the beaten egg whites. Pour into a nonstick muffin pan sprayed with olive oil spray and bake in a preheated 350° F oven for 20 to 30 minutes, until centers spring back when touched.

Makes 12 muffins

Three-Bean Salad

1 16-ounce can green beans,
   rinsed and drained

1 16-ounce can garbanzo
   beans, rinsed and drained

1 16-ounce can butter beans,
   rinsed and drained

½ cup chopped onion

½ cup chopped green pepper

4 tablespoons vinegar

1 tablespoon olive oil

¼ teaspoon onion powder

¼ teaspoon garlic powder

⅛ teaspoon black pepper

Per Serving:

318.17 Cal (16.20%
from Fat, 20.80% from
Protein, 63.00% from
Carb)

17.20 g Protein
5.95 g Tot Fat
  • 0.78 g Sat Fat
  • 3.00 g Mono Fat
  • 1.44 g Poly Fat
52.07 g Carb
13.89 g Fiber
13.73 mg Sodium
0.00 mg Cholesterol

Combine all the ingredients in a bowl, cover, and
allow to marinate in the refrigerator for at least an hour,
gently shaking the bowl several times to mix the seasonings with the vegetables. Serve on a lettuce leaf.

Serves 4

Green Beans à la Française

- 1 pound green beans
- 1 onion, chopped
- 1 16-ounce can tomatoes, chopped but not drained
- ¼ teaspoon basil
- ½ teaspoon salt (or salt substitute to taste)
- ½ teaspoon pepper

Per Serving:

60.86 Cal (3.92% from Fat, 18.20% from Protein, 77.90% from Carb)

3.27 g Protein
0.31 g Tot Fat
 • 0.06 g Sat Fat
 • 0.03 g Mono Fat
 • 0.14 g Poly Fat
14.02 g Carb
5.26 g Fiber
313.87 mg Sodium
0.00 mg Cholesterol

Snap the ends off the beans and add them to a medium saucepan, along with the other ingredients. Cover and bring to a boil. Reduce heat and simmer for about 20 minutes, until tender.

Serves 4

Broiled Fish Fillets

2 4-ounce fish fillets (cod, halibut, bass, or another favorite)

¼ teaspoon salt (or salt substitute to taste)

2 teaspoons olive oil

Parsley

Lemon wedges

Per Serving:

134.40 Cal (44.60% from Fat, 54.50% from Protein, 0.95% from Carb)

17.75 g Protein
6.46 g Tot Fat
• 0.89 g Sat Fat
• 3.96 g Mono Fat
• 1.00 g Poly Fat
0.31 g Carb
0.10 g Fiber
341.06 mg Sodium
27.22 mg Cholesterol

Preheat broiler to high and set the oven rack so the top of the fish will be two inches from the heating element. Dry the fish with paper towels. Season by rubbing with salt or salt substitute and half of the olive oil. Broil for about 2 minutes, brush with additional oil, and broil for another 5 minutes or so. It will be ready when it lightly springs to the touch, yet is still moist. (When in doubt, cut into the fish to see if it is done.) Garnish with parsley and lemon before serving.

Serves 2

Stuft Mushrooms

4 tablespoons spaghetti sauce
(low sodium and sugar, or
homemade from recipe on
page 367)

1 slice sprouted-grain bread

¼ green pepper

1 tablespoon grated Parmesan
cheese

8 ounces large fresh
mushrooms, stems removed

Per Serving:

48.36 Cal (19.50%
from Fat, 21.40% from
Protein, 59.00% from
Carb)

2.75 g Protein
1.11 g Tot Fat
 • 0.40 g Sat Fat
 • 0.28 g Mono Fat
 • 0.25 g Poly Fat
7.58 g Carb
1.12 g Fiber
140.48 mg Sodium
1.29 mg Cholesterol

Blend all the ingredients except the mushrooms in
a blender or food processor. Push the mixture down
with a spoon when the blender/food processor is off
so it will blend smoothly. Stuff the mushroom cavities
with this mixture. Place the mushrooms, caps down,
on an olive oil–sprayed, nonstick cookie sheet and bake
at 450° F for 15 minutes.

Serves 4

Day Nine Menus

▶Breakfast

*Fruit
WHOLE WHEAT WAFFLES
Yogurt, plain, nonfat, sweetened with stevia

▶Lunch

SPLIT PEA SOUP
****Bread

▶Dinner

**Green Salad
GARLIC SHRIMP PASTA
BERRY-YOGURT PARFAIT

Whole Wheat Waffles

- I cup water
- I tablespoon olive oil
- I egg white
- I teaspoon baking powder
- ½ cup unsweetened applesauce
- ½ teaspoon vanilla
- I ¼ cups whole wheat flour

Per Serving:

173.59 Cal (38.50% from Fat, 11.50% from Protein, 49.90% from Carb)

4.99 g Protein
7.41 g Tot Fat
- 1.16 g Sat Fat
- 5.15 g Mono Fat
- 1.16 g Poly Fat
21.58 g Carb
3.24 g Fiber
279.81 mg Sodium
0.00 mg Cholesterol

Put all the ingredients into a blender, except for the flour. Blend. While the blender is running, add the flour a little at a time. Cook on a medium-hot waffle iron, sprayed with a pan spray. These waffles are naturally sweet and crunchy. If you do desire additional sweetening, use a little brown rice syrup, unsweetened applesauce, or the Blueberry Sauce on page 394.

Serves 2

Split Pea Soup

1½ cups uncooked split peas
9 cups water
¼ cup salsa
1 cup chopped onion
3 tablespoons vegetable
   seasoning
1 tablespoon tomato paste

Per Serving:

183.43 Cal (2.99%
from Fat, 27.60% from
Protein, 69.40% from
Carb)

13.60 g Protein
0.05 g Tot Fat
  • 0.09 g Sat Fat
  • 0.13 g Mono Fat
  • 0.28 g Poly Fat
34.24 g Carb
13.32 g Fiber
207.23 mg Sodium
0.00 mg Cholesterol

Soak the peas overnight in a pot. Discard the water, then add 9 cups of fresh water and add the remaining ingredients. Bring to a boil, then simmer until the peas are tender, at least 1 hour. Watch carefully and add more water as needed.

Serves 6

Garlic Shrimp Pasta

2 medium tomatoes
½ cup fresh basil
½ cup fresh parsley
Dash red pepper
1 pound shrimp, fresh or
    frozen
8 ounces fettuccini or linguini
1 tablespoon olive oil
2–3 cloves garlic, minced (or
    more if you are a real garlic
    fan)
¼ cup Parmesan cheese

Per Serving:

345.90 Cal (18.40%
from Fat, 35.90% from
Protein, 45.70% from
Carb)

31.21 g Protein
7.10 g Tot Fat
  • 1.05 g Sat Fat
  • 2.99 g Mono Fat
  • 1.81 g Poly Fat
39.74 g Carb
4.37 g Fiber
190.43 mg Sodium
213.76 mg Cholesterol

Chop the tomatoes, basil, and parsley. Mix with the red pepper and set aside. Shell and devein the shrimp, leaving on the tails if desired. Cook the pasta until just tender (al dente), per package instructions. While the pasta is cooking, heat the olive oil in skillet over medium heat. Add the shrimp and sauté until pink and firm, turning and stirring frequently, about 5 minutes. Add the minced garlic and continue cooking until the garlic is golden brown. Remove from heat. Drain the pasta and toss it together with the shrimp, parsley, basil, chopped tomato, and Parmesan cheese. Serve immediately.

Serves 4

Berry-Yogurt Parfait

3+ drops stevia (to taste)

3 cups yogurt, plain, nonfat

3 tablespoons brown rice
  syrup

1 cup blueberries, fresh or
  frozen

1 cup raspberries, fresh or
  frozen

Per Serving:

94.74 Cal (2.56%
from Fat, 21.40% from
Protein, 76.10% from
Carb)

5.77 g Protein
0.31 g Tot Fat
  • 0.02 g Sat Fat
  • 0.04 g Mono Fat
  • 0.16 g Poly Fat
20.55 g Carb
3.07 g Fiber
39.67 mg Sodium
1.25 mg Cholesterol

Mix the stevia into the yogurt, adding more as
needed for desired sweetness. Mix the brown rice syrup
with the berries. Fill four parfait glasses or wineglasses
with alternating layers of berries and yogurt. For a less
dramatic presentation, you may just top the yogurt
with berries in a bowl.

Serves 4

Day Ten Menus

►Breakfast

FRUIT SALAD WITH YOGURT AND NUTS
****Bread

►Lunch

**Green salad
MISO SOUP
****Bread

►Dinner

**Green salad
MEXICAN SUPPER
Whole wheat tortilla
Salsa
*Fruit

Fruit Salad with Yogurt and Nuts

- 1 apple, cut into chunks
- 1 pear, cut into chunks
- 2 tablespoons raw sunflower seeds
- 2 tablespoons raw pumpkin seeds
- 2 tablespoons raw almonds
- 1 cup plain nonfat yogurt

Per Serving:

215.12 Cal (40.80% from Fat, 9.03% from Protein, 50.20% from Carb)

5.29 g Protein
10.62 g Tot Fat
- 1.31 g Sat Fat
- 4.53 g Mono Fat
- 4.00 g Poly Fat
29.43 g Carb
5.82 g Fiber
4.18 mg Sodium
0.00 mg Cholesterol

Mix the fruit, seeds, and nuts. Stir into the yogurt. May be sweetened with stevia, xylitol, or brown rice syrup.

Serves 2

Miso Soup

3 cups water
1 tablespoon vegetable
    seasoning
½ cup onion, thinly sliced
½ cup firm tofu, cut into
    ¼-inch cubes
3 tablespoons miso paste
1 tablespoon chopped green
    onions

Per Serving:

117.92 Cal (30.00%
from Fat, 28.80% from
Protein, 41.20% from
Carb)

9.63 g Protein
4.45 g Tot Fat
    • 0.64 g Sat Fat
    • 0.98 g Mono Fat
    • 2.50 g Poly Fat
13.76 g Carb
2.45 g Fiber
1074.79 mg Sodium
0.00 mg Cholesterol

Heat the water and vegetable seasoning in a medium saucepan, add the onions, and simmer for 5 minutes. Add the tofu and simmer 1–2 minutes longer. Mix the miso with 2 tablespoons of the liquid and add back to the soup. Stir, garnish with green onions, and serve.

Note: Miso is a Japanese staple made of fermented rice or soybeans. It is strongly flavored and very nutritious. Miso is sold in health food stores and Asian markets. It also contains a lot of sodium, so if you are salt-sensitive, eliminate the vegetable seasoning and cut back the miso paste to 2 tablespoons.

Serves 2

Mexican Supper

2 cups cooked barley
1 pound ground turkey breast
1 zucchini, sliced and
    quartered
1 onion, chopped
1 green pepper, chopped
1 tablespoon olive oil
1 16-ounce can tomatoes,
    drained and chopped
4 tablespoons salsa (or more
    to taste)
½ teaspoon salt (or salt
    substitute to taste)

Per Serving:
333.50 Cal (35.70%
from Fat, 27.80% from
Protein, 36.60% from
Carb)

23.41 g Protein
13.36 g Tot Fat
 • 3.12 g Sat Fat
 • 6.08 g Mono Fat
 • 2.84 g Poly Fat
30.85 Carb
5.22 g Fiber
486.73 mg Sodium
89.59 mg Cholesterol

Cook the barley as directed. Meanwhile, brown the ground turkey and set aside. Sauté the vegetables in the olive oil until tender-crisp. Add the tomatoes, salsa, salt or salt substitute, and ground turkey and cook for 3 minutes. Serve over ½ cup barley per serving and top with extra salsa.

Serves 4

Day Eleven Menus

▶Breakfast

*Fruit
VEGGIE OMELET
****Bread

▶Lunch

OPEN-FACE GOAT CHEESE SANDWICH
*Fruit

▶Dinner

CUCUMBER SALAD
TURKEY CHILI
FRUIT KABOBS

Veggie Omelet

½ cup chopped mushrooms
½ cup chopped onion
1 ½ teaspoons olive oil
   (divided use)
2 whole eggs
4 egg whites
4 teaspoons water
Dash pepper
¼ teaspoon salt (or salt
   substitute to taste)

> **Per Serving:**
>
> 169.99 Cal (50.00% from Fat, 36.00% from Protein, 13.90% from Carb)
>
> 15.13 g Protein
> 9.33 g Tot Fat
> • 2.28 g Sat Fat
> • 4.71 g Mono Fat
> • 1.13 g Poly Fat
> 5.86 g Carb
> 1.01 g Fiber
> 479.68 mg Sodium
> 246.50 mg Cholesterol

Sauté vegetables in ½ teaspoon olive oil until tender-crisp and set aside. Mix the eggs and whites with water, pepper, and salt or salt substitute and beat lightly. Heat a small nonstick skillet over medium heat. Coat the bottom of the pan with ½ teaspoon olive oil. Pour in half of the egg mixture. Gently shake the pan to let uncooked eggs underneath. Slide from the pan, add half the vegetables, fold in half, and serve. Repeat to make second omelet.

Makes 2 omelets

Open-Face Goat Cheese Sandwich

2 teaspoons Dijon mustard
2 slices sprouted-grain bread
½ avocado
2 ounces goat cheese, thinly
   sliced (other cheese is
   optional; look for a low-fat
   variety)
½ cup alfalfa sprouts
1 small tomato, thinly sliced

Per Serving:

258.83 Cal (49.90%
from Fat, 16.90% from
Protein, 33.30% from
Carb)

11.46 g Protein
5.04 g Tot Fat
  • 5.56 g Sat Fat
  • 6.74 g Mono Fat
  • 1.47 g Poly Fat
22.57 g Carb
5.36 g Fiber
393.96 mg Sodium
13.04 mg Cholesterol

Spread the mustard on bread slices (toasted, if desired), then layer as follows: avocado, thin slices of cheese, sprouts, and tomato slices. Eat with care!

Serves 2

Cucumber Salad

- 1 cucumber, peeled and thinly sliced
- ¼ cup vinegar
- 1 teaspoon flaxseed or olive oil
- 1 teaspoon low-sodium soy sauce
- 1 teaspoon sesame seeds
- ½ teaspoon chopped fresh ginger (or ¼ teaspoon powdered ginger)

Per Serving:

45.41 Cal (42.70% from Fat, 9.16% from Protein, 48.20% from Carb)

1.18 g Protein
2.45 g Tot Fat
  • 0.36 g Sat Fat
  • 1.66 g Mono Fat
  • 0.27 g Poly Fat
6.23 g Carb
1.24 g Fiber
91.91 mg Sodium
0.00 mg Cholesterol

Mix all the ingredients, chill at least one hour, and serve.

Serves 2

Turkey Chili

- 1 pound ground turkey breast
- 1 medium yellow onion, chopped
- 1 green pepper, chopped
- 1 tablespoon olive oil
- 2 cups water
- 1 16-ounce can tomatoes, chopped
- 2 tablespoons tomato puree
- 2 tablespoon vegetable seasoning
- ½ teaspoon red chilis (or to taste—very hot)
- 1–2 tablespoons chili powder (to taste)
- 2 chopped green onions

Per Serving:

214.81 Cal (48.10% from Fat, 41.60% from Protein, 10.30% from Carb)

22.94 g Protein
11.81 g Tot Fat
  • 2.79 g Sat Fat
  • 5.37 g Mono Fat
  • 2.37 g Poly Fat
5.69 g Carb
1.30 g Fiber
692.76 mg Sodium
48.76 mg Cholesterol

Sauté the ground turkey, onion, and green pepper in olive oil in a large pot over medium heat. Add the remaining ingredients except the green onions to the pot and simmer until the flavors are thoroughly blended, at least 1 hour. Add more water as needed. Garnish with green onions.

Serves 4

Fruit Kabobs

- 1 apple
- 1 pear
- 1 peach
- 1 cup strawberries
- 4 skewers

> **Per Serving:**
>
> 60.47 Cal (6.01% from Fat, 2.89% from Protein, 91.10% from Carb)
>
> 0.49 g Protein
> 0.45 g Total Fat
> • 0.04 g Sat Fat
> • 0.07 g Mono Fat
> • 0.15 g Poly Fat
> 15.31 g Carb
> 2.74 g Fiber
> 0.38 mg Sodium
> 0.00 mg Cholesterol

Cut the fruit into one-inch cubes; leave the strawberries whole. Arrange attractively on skewers and serve. If peaches and strawberries are not in season, select other types of fruit.

Serves 4

Day Twelve Menus

▶**Breakfast**

APPLE GRANOLA
Soy milk or nonfat milk

▶**Lunch**

PEASANT CABBAGE SOUP
****Bread
*Fruit

▶**Dinner**

ORIENTAL CHICKEN SALAD
****Bread
ASIAN ORANGES

Apple Granola

- ¼ cup plain rye flakes (not instant)
- ¼ cup plain barley flakes (not instant)
- ¼ cup freshly ground flaxseed
- 1 tablespoon raw sesame seeds
- 1 tablespoon raw almonds (or other nuts)
- 1 tablespoon raw pumpkin seeds
- 1 apple, chopped
- 1 tablespoon brown rice syrup

Per Serving:

300.01 Cal (35.30% from Fat, 11.40% from Protein, 53.40% from Carb)

9.27 g Protein
12.78 g Tot Fat
- 1.41 g Sat Fat
- 3.64 g Mono Fat
- 6.52 g Poly Fat
43.54 g Carb
11.71 g Fiber
8.95 mg Sodium
0.00 mg Cholesterol

Mix all the ingredients. Serve with soy milk or non-fat milk.

Serves 2

Peasant Cabbage Soup

8 cups water
½ cup sliced celery
½ onion, chopped
½ small head cabbage,
  chopped coarsely
1 cup cooked barley
1 16-ounce can soybeans,
  rinsed
1 small zucchini, sliced
3 tablespoons tomato paste
2 tablespoons vegetable
  seasoning

> **Per Serving:**
>
> 163.17 Cal (24.60% from Fat, 25.70% from Protein, 49.70% from Carb)
>
> 12.73 g Protein
> 5.41 g Tot Fat
> • 0.77 g Sat Fat
> • 1.19 g Mono Fat
> • 3.02 g Poly Fat
> 24.64 g Carb
> 4.05 g Fiber
> 261.71 mg Sodium
> 0.00 mg Cholesterol

Pour the water into a large pot, then add the remaining ingredients. Simmer until the vegetables are tender, about 20 minutes.

Serves 4

Oriental Chicken Salad

- 1 large chicken breast, cooked, thinly sliced into 1-inch pieces and chilled
- 1 head lettuce (romaine preferred), coarsely chopped
- ½ avocado, sliced
- 1 tomato, chopped
- ½ bunch green onions, chopped
- 1 cup fresh bean sprouts
- ¼ cup sesame seeds

Per Serving:

360.02 cal (63.10% from Fat, 20.80% from Protein, 16.10% from Carb)

19.74 g Protein
26.56 g Tot Fat
   • 3.86 g Sat Fat
   • 14.33 g Mono Fat
   • 6.63 g Poly Fat
15.26 g Carb
6.14 g Fiber
437.73 mg Sodium
34.22 mg Cholesterol

Dressing:
- 1 tablespoon olive oil
- 1 teaspoon sesame oil
- 2 tablespoons lemon juice
- 1 clove garlic, minced
- ¼ teaspoon salt (or salt substitute to taste)
- Pinch black pepper

Combine the salad ingredients except the sesame seeds. Mix the dressing ingredients and toss with the salad. Sprinkle with the sesame seeds.

Serves 2

Asian Oranges

2 oranges
1 lime

> **Per Serving:**
>
> 66.31 Cal (1.60% from Fat, 7.88% from Protein, 90.50% from Carb)
>
> 1.47 g Protein
> 0.13 g Tot Fat
> • 0.02 g Sat Fat
> • 0.02 g Mono Fat
> • 0.03 g Poly Fat
> 16.92 g Carb
> 3.39 mg Sodium
> 0.00 mg Cholesterol

Peel the oranges with a knife, removing most of the white pulp. Slice into ¼-inch rounds. Arrange in overlapping rounds on a plate, squeeze the lime juice over the oranges, and serve chilled. May garnish with mint leaf.

Serves 2

Day Thirteen Menus

►Breakfast

*Fruit
WHEAT BERRY CEREAL
Soy milk or nonfat milk

►Lunch

HUMMUS SANDWICH

►Dinner

**Green salad
ASPARAGUS AND LEEK TART
***Vegetables
*Fruit

Wheat Berry Cereal

2 cups boiling water
A wide-mouthed thermos
⅔ cup wheat berries

> **Per Serving:**
>
> 97.5 Cal (5.31% from Fat, 13.50% from Protein, 81.20% from Carb)
>
> 4.00 g Protein
> 0.7 g Tot Fat
> • (fat breakdown unavailable)
> 24.10 g Carb
> 0.80 g Fiber
> 1.00 mg Sodium
> 0.00 mg Cholesterol

The evening before you plan to eat this, place boiling water in a wide-mouthed thermos with wheat berries. Close the thermos. Allow the mixture to sit overnight, and in the morning the grains will be ready to eat. Serve with soy milk or nonfat milk and flavor with cinnamon, xylitol, or stevia.

Serves 2

Hummus Sandwich

1 cup canned garbanzo beans,
   rinsed and drained
1 tablespoon sesame tahini
Juice of 1 small lemon, about
   ¼ cup
2 cloves minced garlic
¼ teaspoon salt (or salt
   substitute to taste)
1 tablespoon olive oil
½ cup water
2 sprouted-grain pita bread
   rounds
1 tomato, chopped
½ cup lettuce, chopped
1 tablespoon chopped parsley

Per Serving:

271.90 Cal (38.50%
from Fat, 11.90% from
Protein, 49.60% from
Carb)

8.38 g Protein
12.07 g Tot Fat
  • 1.61 g Sat Fat
  • 6.69 g Mono Fat
  • 2.90 g Poly Fat
34.93 g Carb
7.17 g Fiber
383.58 mg Sodium
0.00 mg Cholesterol

In a blender or food processor, mix the garbanzo beans, tahini, lemon juice, garlic, salt or salt substitute, olive oil, and water. If necessary, add more water to thin. Slice a pita in half, open each half, and spread with the hummus. Fill each half with tomatoes and lettuce. Top with parsley.

Note: Tahini is sesame butter. It is sold in health food stores and the ethnic or gourmet sections of many supermarkets.

Asparagus and Leek Tart

½ pound asparagus, trimmed
  and cut into 2-inch pieces
2 leeks, sliced (white part only)
2 tablespoons whole wheat
  flour
8 egg whites, lightly beaten
1 cup nonfat ricotta cheese
¼ cup low-fat, low-sodium
  Swiss cheese, shredded
½ cup nonfat milk
2 teaspoons olive oil
½ cup crumbled sprouted-
  grain bread

Per Serving:
159.44 Cal (25.50% from Fat, 39.90% from Protein, 34.60% from Carb)
13.38 g Protein
3.79 g Tot Fat
• 3.49 g Sat Fat
• 2.58 g Mono Fat
• 0.40 g Poly Fat
11.60 g Carb
1.63 g Fiber
157.33 mg Sodium
6.79 mg Cholesterol

Preheat the oven to 425° F. Boil water in a large pan. Blanch the asparagus for 2–3 minutes. Drain and set aside. In medium pan sprayed with olive oil pan spray, sauté the leeks over medium heat for 4–5 minutes, sprinkle in flour, stir to coat, and transfer the mixture to a bowl. Add the egg whites, ricotta cheese, Swiss cheese, and milk and mix again. Meanwhile, add the olive oil to the bread crumbs, pat flat into the bottom of a pie pan, and toast in the oven for 5–6 minutes or until browned. Cool for 10 minutes. Pour the egg-and-cheese mixture over the browned bread crumbs. Bake until puffy and brown, about 40 minutes. Let stand 10 minutes before slicing.

Serves 6

Day Fourteen Menus

▶Breakfast

*Fruit
YOGURT WITH NUTS AND SEEDS

▶Lunch

GARLIC TOAST
REFRIGERATOR SOUP

▶Dinner

**Green salad
MARINATED CHICKEN BREAST
BREADED EGGPLANT
*Fruit

Yogurt with Nuts and Seeds

1 tablespoon raw almonds

1 tablespoon ground flaxseed

1 tablespoon raw sunflower
seeds

1 tablespoon raw pumpkin
seeds

1 tablespoon sesame seeds

1 cup plain nonfat yogurt

1 teaspoon brown rice
syrup or

2–4 drops stevia

Per Serving:

88.77 Cal (63.20%
from Fat, 14.10% from
Protein, 22.70% from
Carb)

3.32 g Protein
6.63 g Tot Fat
• 0.78 g Sat Fat
• 2.55 g Mono Fat
• 3.01 g Poly Fat
5.35 g Carb
2.14 g Fiber
3.73 mg Sodium
0.00 mg Cholesterol

Mix the nuts and seeds into the yogurt. Sweeten
with brown rice syrup or stevia.

Serves 2

Garlic Toast

1 teaspoon olive oil
½ teaspoon garlic powder
2 teaspoons Parmesan cheese
2 slices sprouted-grain bread

> **Per Serving:**
>
> 111.71 Cal (32.00% from Fat, 14.50% from Protein, 53.50% from Carb)
>
> 4.18 g Protein
> 4.10 g Tot Fat
> • 0.96 g Sat Fat
> • 2.33 g Mono Fat
> • 0.50 g Poly Fat
> 15.43 g Carb
> 2.12 g Fiber
> 194.81 mg Sodium
> 1.64 mg Cholesterol

Mix together the olive oil, garlic powder, and Parmesan cheese. Toast the bread on one side under the broiler. Spread the garlic-cheese-oil mixture on other side and return to the broiler. Watch carefully—this browns very quickly.

Serves 2

Refrigerator Soup

When the refrigerator is bulging with various fresh vegetables that have been partially used, it's time to make refrigerator soup! Fill a pot half full of water, then add the following categories of ingredients, chopped, diced, chunked, etc., according to your personal preference from the list below. (This is a partial list, typical of what you may have on hand.) Season with pepper and vegetable seasoning, and add more water if necessary. Cook for 20–30 minutes, until the vegetables are tender. This freezes well in individual-serving-size containers.

▶ **For Thickness and Bulk**

Barley
Lentils
Split peas
Beans
Pasta
Eggplant
Cabbage
Mushrooms

▶ **For Flavor**

Spaghetti sauce
Salsa
Tomatoes
Onions
Garlic
Garlic and onion powder (and other spices)
Fresh herbs (parsley, basil)
Green pepper
Spinach

Marinated Chicken Breast

I lemon
¼ teaspoon salt (or salt
  substitute to taste)
I clove garlic, minced
2 small or I large chicken
  breast, halved (4 ounces
  each; ½ pound total)
2 tablespoons parsley, chopped

> **Per Serving:**
>
> 136.86 Cal (10.30% from Fat, 79.50% from Protein, 10.30% from Carb)
>
> 26.71 g Protein
> 1.53 g Tot Fat
> • 0.38 g Sat Fat
> • 0.35 g Mono Fat
> • 0.35 g Poly Fat
> 3.46 g Carb
> 0.97 g Fiber
> 80.91 mg Sodium
> 65.77 mg Cholesterol

Mix the juice of one lemon with salt or salt substitute and garlic. Marinate the chicken breasts several hours or overnight in this mixture. Bake in a casserole, uncovered, at 350° F for 45 minutes. Garnish with the parsley.

Serves 2

Breaded Eggplant

½ green pepper

1 small onion

2 rounded tablespoons tomato paste

2 egg whites

½ teaspoon oregano

1 teaspoon basil

2 teaspoons vegetable seasoning

2 tablespoons grated Parmesan cheese

2 slices sprouted-grain bread, crumbled

1 large eggplant, sliced into large, ¼-inch-thick slices

Per Serving:

246.24 Cal (25.50% from Fat, 21.80% from Protein, 52.70% from Carb)

14.34 g Protein
7.44 g Tot Fat
• 3.29 g Sat Fat
• 3.10 g Mono Fat
• 0.67 g Poly Fat
34.64 g Carb
8.02 g Fiber
698.55 mg Sodium
14.97 mg Cholesterol

In a blender, blend the green pepper, onion, tomato paste, egg whites, oregano, basil, vegetable seasoning, and cheese. Pour this mixture over the bread crumbs in a large bowl. Mix thoroughly with a spoon. Arrange the eggplant slices on a nonstick cookie sheet sprayed with olive oil spray. Top each slice with the blended mixture. Bake at 350° F for 30 minutes.

Serves 2

Week Three Shopping List

- ◉ Do you need to replenish any of your staples from last week?

- ◉ Do you have all the items on the shopping list you'll need this week? The amounts listed will feed two people. Several of the recipes serve four and make great leftovers or snacks.

▶Vegetables

Asparagus, 1 pound
Avocado, 1
Broccoli, 1 small bunch
Cabbage, 1 small head
Celery, 1 bunch
Cucumber, 3
Eggplant, 1
Green peppers, 3
**Lettuce, your choice, romaine or Boston preferred (4–5 heads, depending on size, should be enough for your salads for the week)
Mushrooms, 2 pounds
Onions, 7
Onions, green, 1 bunch
Parsley, 2 bunches
Tomatoes, 9
Zucchini, 3
***Vegetables (You will need two side dishes of vegetables per person this week; choose from recommended list.)

►Fruit

Apples, 7 (2 pippin, Granny Smith, or other tart
   variety)
Blueberries (or other berries; frozen okay), 1 cup
Lemons, 3
*Fruit of your choice from acceptable fruit list
   (enough for approximately 10 servings per
   person for the week)

►Canned Foods

Black olives, sliced, 1 small can
Baby lima beans (or frozen or made from dried),
   1 can
Black-eyed peas (or frozen or made from dried),
   1 can
Garbanzo beans (or frozen or made from dried),
   1 can
Green beans (fresh or frozen), 1 can
Kidney beans (or made from dried), 1 can
Pinto beans (or made from dried), 1 can
Ranch salad dressing, low fat, low sugar, 1 small
   bottle
Refried beans (or made from dried), 1 can

►Bakery

Sprouted-grain bread, 1 loaf
Sprouted-grain English muffins, 1 package
Sprouted-grain pita bread, 1 package (or use
   extras from previous week, stored in freezer)
Whole wheat tortillas, small, 1 package (or use
   extras from previous week, stored in freezer)

****See notes on bread. (You will need enough for about seven servings of bread per person for the week.)

▶ Frozen Foods

Blueberries (or fresh), 1 small package
Green beans, 16-ounce package (or canned)

▶ Dried/Packaged Foods

Barley, 1 package (may have leftovers from previous weeks)
Bulgur, 1 package
Quinoa, 1 package

▶ Meat, Eggs, and Dairy

Eggs, 2 dozen
Fish fillets (cod, halibut, or bass), 8 ounces
Cheese, low fat, 2 ounces
Chicken breasts, boneless, 1½ pounds
Cottage cheese, nonfat, 1 pint
Feta cheese, 1 small container (unused portion can be frozen)
Goat cheese, 2 ounces
Milk: soy milk or nonfat milk, small container (or more if used on cereal, in coffee, etc.)
Tofu, firm, 2 1-pound packages
Tuna, water packed, 1 small can
Turkey breast, ground, ½ pound
Yogurt, plain, nonfat, 3 cups

▶ Other

Carob powder, 1 small package
Protein powder, 1 container

Tahini (sesame butter), will have some left from
last week

▶ Staples

(Do you need to replenish anything?)

Almonds, raw
Arrowroot
Baking powder
Brown rice syrup
Cayenne pepper
Chili powder
Cinnamon
Flaxseed oil
Flaxseed, whole
Garlic, fresh and powder
Mayonnaise, low fat, low sugar
Oatmeal, slow cooking
Olive oil
Olive oil pan spray
Onion powder
Oregano
Parmesan cheese
Pepper, black
Pickles, dill
Pumpkin seeds, raw
Salsa
Sesame seeds, raw
Soy sauce, low sodium
Spaghetti sauce, low sugar, low fat (or homemade
from recipe on page 367)
Stevia
Sunflower seeds, raw

Tomato paste
Vegetable seasoning
Vinegar (rice)
Walnuts, raw
Whole wheat flour
Xylitol

Day Fifteen Menus

▶Breakfast

*Fruit
Poached eggs, 2
****Bread

▶Lunch

TUNA MELT
****Vegetables

▶Dinner

**Green salad
RATATOUILLE
QUINOA
*Fruit

Tuna Melt

- I small can water-packed tuna
- ¼ cup low-fat mayonnaise
- I tablespoon chopped green onion
- I tablespoon pickle, chopped
- I tablespoon finely chopped celery
- 2 slices sprouted-grain bread, lightly toasted
- I ounce low-fat cheese, thinly sliced
- 2 tomato slices

Per Serving:

317.54 Cal (30.30% from Fat, 35.30% from Protein, 34.50% from Carb)

28.18 g Protein
10.74 g Tot Fat
- 2.56 g Sat Fat
- 2.76 g Mono Fat
- 4.60 g Poly Fat
27.54 g Carb
2.76 g Fiber
792.57 mg Sodium
46.55 mg Cholesterol

Mix the tuna with the next four ingredients. Spread on the toast and top with the cheese. Place under the broiler until the cheese is melted thoroughly and bubbles. Top with a fresh tomato slice.

Serves 2

Ratatouille

- 1 tablespoon olive oil
- 1 onion, cut in chunks
- 1 green pepper, cut in chunks
- 2 zucchini, cut in chunks
- 1 eggplant, peeled and cut in chunks
- 1 cup mushrooms
- ½ teaspoon salt (or salt substitute to taste)
- 1 16-ounce can tomatoes, chopped and drained

Per Serving:

101.55 Cal (30.90% from Fat, 12.20% from Protein, 56.90% from Carb)

3.50 g Protein
3.93 g Tot Fat
  • 0.55 g Sat Fat
  • 2.54 g Mono Fat
  • 0.52 g Poly Fat
16.27 g Carb
5.39 g Fiber
312.50 mg Sodium
0.00 mg Cholesterol

In a large skillet, heat the olive oil, then add the vegetables in the following order, cooking and stirring for about 3 minutes between each addition: onion, green pepper, zucchini, eggplant, and mushrooms. Add the salt and tomatoes and stir until hot and the mixture begins to dry. Serve over hot quinoa (½ cup quinoa per person, recipe follows).

Serves 4

Quinoa

2 cups water
1 cup quinoa

Per Serving:

105.97 Cal (13.70%
from Fat, 13.80% from
Protein, 72.50% from
Carb)

3.71 g Protein
1.64 g Tot Fat
• 0.17 g Sat Fat
• 0.43 g Mono Fat
• 0.66 g Poly Fat
19.52 g Carb
1.67 g Fiber
8.32 mg Sodium
0.00 mg Cholesterol

Rinse the quinoa in a medium saucepan, then add 2 cups fresh water. Bring to a boil, reduce heat, and simmer for about 15 minutes, until the water is absorbed and the grains have turned from white to transparent. Quinoa, which is native to South America, provides very high-quality protein. Reheat leftover quinoa, add fruit, milk, and, if desired, a healthy sweetener, and eat as a breakfast cereal.

Serves 6 (½-cup servings)

Day Sixteen Menus

▶ Breakfast

*Fruit
SCRAMBLED TOFU WITH ONIONS
****Bread

▶ Lunch

FALAFEL
TAHINI SAUCE
*Bread (pita preferred)

▶ Dinner

**Green salad
CHICKEN WITH TERIYAKI SAUCE
MUSHROOM PILAF
BAKED APPLES

Scrambled Tofu with Onions

¾ cup chopped onions
1 teaspoon olive oil
½ container firm tofu
1 teaspoon vegetable
   seasoning (or salt substitute
   to taste)
¼ teaspoon pepper

Per Serving:

160.85 Cal (48.00% from Fat, 31.30% from Protein, 20.70% from Carb)

13.84 g Protein
9.42 g Tot Fat
  • 1.34 g Sat Fat
  • 3.24 g Mono Fat
  • 4.22 g Poly Fat
9.15 g Carb
3.01 g Fiber
53.26 mg Sodium
0.00 mg Cholesterol

In a medium skillet over medium heat, sauté the chopped onions with the olive oil until tender. Add the tofu, crumbled up. Sprinkle with vegetable seasoning or salt substitute and pepper to taste. Blend well and cook on low heat for 3–4 minutes.

Serves 2

Falafel

- ½ cup bulgur
- 1 cup boiling water
- 2 cups canned garbanzo beans, rinsed and drained
- 3 cloves garlic, minced
- ¼ cup lemon juice
- ½ teaspoon salt (or salt substitute to taste)
- ¼ teaspoon Tabasco sauce
- 3 egg whites
- ½ cup dry sprouted-grain bread crumbs
- 1 teaspoon olive oil
- 6 sprouted-grain pita bread rounds
- 2 tomatoes, thinly sliced
- 1 cucumber, thinly sliced
- 1½ cups lettuce, chopped

Per Serving:

368.69 Cal (9.51% from Fat, 15.80% from Protein, 74.70% from Carb)

15.16 g Protein
4.07 g Tot Fat
- 0.62 g Sat Fat
- 1.22 g Mono Fat
- 1.35 g Poly Fat
71.86 g Carb
11.27 g Fiber
888.12 mg Sodium
0.00 mg Cholesterol

Soak the bulgur in the boiling water for 20 minutes, then drain well in a colander. In a blender or food processor combine the garbanzo beans, garlic, lemon juice, salt, and Tabasco sauce. In a large bowl beat the egg whites, then mix in the bread crumbs, pureed garbanzo mixture, drained bulgur, and the olive oil. Shape the mixture into 12 thin patties. On a nonstick, medium-hot griddle sprayed with olive oil spray, brown the patties for 3–5 minutes on each side. Serve immediately in the pita pockets with the vegetables and Tahini Sauce (1 tablespoon for each pita, recipe follows). Falafel makes a great snack and also freezes well.

Serves 6

Tahini Sauce

3 tablespoons sesame tahini
½ teaspoon olive oil
2 tablespoons water (or more)
1 clove garlic, minced
2 teaspoons lemon juice
Dash of cayenne pepper

Per Serving:

8.71 Cal (71.30% from
Fat, 7.30% from Protein,
21.40% from Carb)

0.17 g Protein
0.74 g Tot Fat
 • 0.10 g Sat Fat
 • 0.41 g Mono Fat
 • 0.19 g Poly Fat
0.50 g Carb
0.09 g Fiber
0.80 mg Sodium
0.00 mg Cholesterol

In a small bowl, stir all the ingredients until thoroughly mixed, adding a little extra water if needed.
Serve with Falafel.

Makes 6 tablespoons

Chicken with Teriyaki Sauce

2 chicken breasts, 4 ounces each

¾ cup water

2 tablespoons low-sodium soy sauce

½ teaspoon vinegar (rice vinegar preferred)

1 clove garlic, minced

Per Serving:

135.45 Cal (9.96% from Fat, 84.20% from Protein, 5.88% from Carb)

27.09 g Protein
1.43 g Tot Fat
  • 0.37 g Sat Fat
  • 0.34 g Mono Fat
  • 0.33 g Poly Fat
1.89 g Carb
0.16 g Fiber
607.82 mg Sodium
65.77 mg Cholesterol

Brown the chicken breasts in a medium skillet over medium heat for 3–4 minutes on each side. Add 2 tablespoons of water plus 1 teaspoon of the soy sauce, cover, reduce heat, and continue cooking for about 10 minutes until cooked through. Meanwhile, cook the remaining ingredients in a small saucepan over low heat for 10 minutes. Pour the sauce over the chicken before serving.

Serves 2

Mushroom Pilaf

1 teaspoon olive oil
1½ cups finely chopped
   mushrooms
1 cup bulgur
2 teaspoons vegetable
   seasoning
¼ teaspoon pepper
2 cups water
2 green onions, thinly sliced

Per Serving:

136.77 Cal (10.30% from Fat, 14.00% from Protein, 75.80% from Carb)

5.20 g Protein
1.70 g Tot Fat
• 0.25 g Sat Fat
• 0.89 g Mono Fat
• 0.33 g Poly Fat
28.24 g Carb
6.76 g Fiber
50.62 mg Sodium
0.00 mg Cholesterol

Heat the olive oil over medium-high heat in a medium saucepan. Add the mushrooms and cook, stirring often, for 5 minutes. Add the bulgur, seasonings, and water and bring to a boil, then reduce heat to a simmer, cover pan, and cook for 20 minutes. The pilaf is done when all the liquid is absorbed. Fluff with a fork, garnish with green onions, and serve.

Serves 4

Baked Apples

2 large baking apples (pippin,
   Granny Smith, or other tart
   apples)
1 teaspoon cinnamon
1 tablespoon brown rice syrup
2 teaspoons lemon juice

Per Serving:
79.75 Cal (5.02% from Fat, 1.39% from Protein, 93.60% from Carb)
0.31 g Protein
0.50 g Tot Fat
• 0.08 g Sat Fat
• 0.03 g Mono Fat
• 0.14 g Poly Fat
20.86 g Carb
4.10 g Fiber
0.35 mg Sodium
0.00 mg Cholesterol

Wash the apples but do not peel them. Cut out the center core from the top down, leaving about ¼ inch uncut on the very bottom to hold the sweeteners. Mix the cinnamon, brown rice syrup, and lemon juice together. Pour half of the mixture into each apple center. Place the apples in a nonstick baking dish. Bake at 300° F for 45 minutes to 1 hour. May be served with Cream Sauce from page 474. This recipe may be doubled, as the leftovers make a nice topping for cereal or yogurt.

Serves 2

Day Seventeen Menus

▶Breakfast

*Fruit
HOT CAROB CEREAL
Soy milk or nonfat milk

▶Lunch

TOSTADAS
*Fruit

▶Dinner

**Green salad
VEGELOAF
MUSHROOM GRAVY
***Vegetables

Hot Carob Cereal

- 2¼ cups water
- 1 cup oatmeal (not instant)
- 1 tablespoon unsweetened carob powder
- ½ teaspoon cinnamon
- 1 tablespoon xylitol

Per Serving:

154.23 Cal (17.00% from Fat, 16.30% from Protein, 66.70% from Carb)

6.98 g Protein
3.23 g Tot Fat
- 0.58 g Sat Fat
- 1.05 g Mono Fat
- 1.22 g Poly Fat
28.49 g Carb
7.31 g Fiber
11.26 mg Sodium
0.00 mg Cholesterol

Bring the water to a boil. Stir in the oatmeal, carob, and cinnamon. Cook for 3 minutes. Remove from heat and stir in the xylitol. Let stand with lid on for 1 minute. Delicious as is, or may be served with soy milk or nonfat milk.

Serves 2

Tostadas

½ cup refried beans (canned
   or made from dried pinto
   beans)

3 tablespoons salsa (mild or
   hot, to taste)

2 whole wheat tortillas

1 tomato, chopped

2 tablespoons chopped onion

1 cup chopped lettuce

Per Serving:

196.64 Cal (15.50%
from Fat, 15.60% from
Protein, 68.80% from
Carb)

7.89 g Protein
3.49 g Tot Fat
   • 0.92 g Sat Fat
   • 1.61 g Mono Fat
   • 0.62 g Poly Fat
34.79 g Carb
6.43 g Fiber
457.35 mg Sodium
5.04 mg Cholesterol

Heat the beans with the salsa in a small saucepan. Bake the tortillas in 350° F oven until crisp, about 8 minutes, turning after 5 minutes. Spread ¼ cup bean mixture on each tortilla, and top with chopped tomatoes, onion, and lettuce. Serve with extra salsa.

Serves 2

Vegeloaf

4 slices sprouted-grain bread
2 cups green beans (canned or frozen)
1 cup water
¼ cup walnut pieces
1 egg white
2 tablespoons tomato paste
¾ cup cooked barley
2 tablespoons vegetable seasoning
½ cup mushrooms
2 cloves garlic

Per Serving:
197.38 Cal (25.40% from Fat, 15.70% from Protein, 58.80% from Carb)
8.25 g Protein
5.94 g Tot Fat
• 0.60 g Sat Fat
• 1.51 g Mono Fat
• 3.36 g Poly Fat
30.91 g Carb
5.92 g Fiber
183.46 mg Sodium
0.00 mg Cholesterol

Toast the bread, then process it in a blender or food processor to fine crumbs and set aside. Rinse and drain the beans and puree in a blender with the water. Add the remaining ingredients, except the bread crumbs, and blend. Pour the mixture into a bowl over the bread crumbs and stir until evenly moist. Pour into a nonstick loaf pan sprayed with olive oil spray, and bake at 300° F for 45 minutes. Serve with Mushroom Gravy (recipe follows).

Serves 4

Mushroom Gravy

¾ cup chopped onions
1 teaspoon olive oil
1 cup sliced mushrooms
½ teaspoon salt (or salt
  substitute to taste)
¼ teaspoon black pepper
1 tablespoon arrowroot
1 cup water

Per Serving:

27.28 Cal (38.30%
from Fat, 11.00% from
Protein, 50.80% from
Carb)

0.81 g Protein
1.25 g Tot Fat
 • 0.17 g Sat Fat
 • 0.84 g Mono Fat
 • 0.15 g Poly Fat
3.74 g Carb
0.81 g Fiber
298.64 mg Sodium
0.00 mg Cholesterol

In a small saucepan, brown the onions in the olive oil for 5 minutes, then add the mushrooms and continue sautéing for another 2 minutes. Add the salt, pepper, and arrowroot to the water. Stir into the mushrooms and onions. Cook gently until thickened (it will only take a minute or so), stirring constantly. Serve over Vegeloaf. Also makes a nice gravy for grains.

Serves 4

Day Eighteen Menus

▶ Breakfast

BREAKFAST SMOOTHIE
****Bread

▶ Lunch

PERSONAL PIZZAS
*Fruit

▶ Dinner

TACO SALAD
GUACAMOLE
WHOLE WHEAT TORTILLA CHIPS

Breakfast Smoothie

1 apple (or other fruit)
1 cup fresh or frozen berries
   (or other fruit)
¼ cup flaxseed, freshly ground
2 scoops protein powder
1 cup soy milk (or water)
1 cup ice

> **Per Serving:**
>
> 200–300 Cal (variable, depending on type of protein powder)
>
> 15–30+ g Protein (depending on type of protein powder used)
> 9.41 g Tot Fat
> • 0.93 g Sat Fat
> • 1.76 g Mono Fat
> • 5.59 g Poly Fat
> 27.54 g Carb
> 12.03 g Fiber
> 24.84 mg Sodium
> 0.00 mg Cholesterol

Mix all the ingredients in a blender and blend until smooth. Adjust soy milk and ice to obtain the desired thickness. This is a great, well-balanced breakfast you can easily drink on the go.

Serves 2

Personal Pizzas

2 sprouted-grain English
  muffins, halved
4 tablespoons spaghetti sauce
  (or more to taste)
¼ green pepper, thinly sliced
4 mushrooms, thinly sliced
5 teaspoons grated Parmesan
  cheese

Per Serving:

186.54 Cal (16.50%
from Fat, 17.00% from
Protein, 66.50% from
Carb)

7.89 g Protein
3.39 g Tot Fat
  • 1.40 g Sat Fat
  • 0.83 g Mono Fat
  • 0.78 g Poly Fat
30.81 g Carb
2.51 g Fiber
522.24 mg Sodium
4.92 mg Cholesterol

Top each English muffin half with 1 tablespoon spaghetti sauce, green pepper, and 1 sliced mushroom. Sprinkle 1¼ teaspoons of the grated cheese evenly over the top. Place the muffins on a cookie sheet. Bake at 350° F for 10–15 minutes.

Serves 2

Taco Salad

½ pound ground turkey breast
1 teaspoon olive oil
1½ teaspoons chili powder, divided use
3 cups lettuce (romaine preferred) torn into bite-size pieces
¼ cup onion, thinly sliced
1 tomato, coarsely chopped
¼ cup black olives, sliced
½ cup kidney beans
3 tablespoons fat-free, sugar-free ranch dressing
1 ounce cheese, low fat, grated

Per Serving:

412.19 Cal (35.90% from Fat, 42.10% from Protein, 21.90% from Carb)

43.58 g Protein
16.51 g Tot Fat
  • 3.49 g Sat Fat
  • 4.53 g Mono Fat
  • 2.39 g Poly Fat
22.69 g Carb
6.90 g Fiber
683.86 mg Sodium
96.59 mg Cholesterol

Brown the ground turkey in the olive oil in a medium skillet over medium-high heat, adding 1 teaspoon chili powder. Drain and set aside. Combine the salad ingredients except the dressing and cheese in a large bowl. Mix the ranch dressing with ½ teaspoon chili powder and toss with the salad, along with the meat mixture. Top with cheese.

Serves 2

Guacamole

1 ripe avocado
½ small tomato, chopped
1 green onion, thinly sliced
Juice of ½ lemon
¼ teaspoon salt (or salt
   substitute to taste)
1 tablespoon salsa

Per Serving:

168.66 Cal (74.00%
from Fat, 5.49% from
Protein, 20.50% from
Carb)

2.53 g Protein
15.18 g Tot Fat
   • 2.27 g Sat Fat
   • 9.72 g Mono Fat
   • 1.84 g Poly Fat
9.45 g Carb
5.18 g Fiber
346.20 mg Sodium
0.00 mg Cholesterol

Mash the avocado with a fork in a small bowl. Add the remaining ingredients. Serve with Whole Wheat Tortilla Chips (recipe follows) and extra salsa.

Serves 2

Whole Wheat Tortilla Chips

2 whole wheat tortillas

Per Serving:

104.00 Cal (19.90% from Fat, 10.80% from Protein, 69.30% from Carb)

2.78 g Protein
2.27 g Tot Fat
- 0.56 g Sat Fat
- 1.21 g Mono Fat
- 0.34 g Poly Fat

17.79 g Carb
1.06 g Fiber
152.96 mg Sodium
0.00 mg Cholesterol

Cut the tortillas into eighths. Place on a cookie sheet and heat in a 350° F oven until crisp, about 8 minutes. Turn after 5 minutes and watch carefully so they do not burn. Serve with Guacamole and salsa.

Serves 2

Day Nineteen Menus

▶Breakfast

*Fruit
MEXICAN SCRAMBLED EGGS
****Bread

▶Lunch

**Green salad
QUICK MULTI-BEAN SOUP
****Bread

▶Dinner

**Green salad
ASPARAGUS CHICKEN
CURRIED QUINOA

Mexican Scrambled Eggs

1 small onion, chopped
½ green pepper, chopped
1 teaspoon olive oil
2 eggs
4 egg whites
1 tablespoon water
¼ teaspoon pepper
¼ teaspoon salt (or salt substitute to taste)
3 tablespoons salsa

Per Serving:

157.20 Cal (47.50% from Fat, 38.50% from Protein, 14.00% from Carb)

14.93 g Protein
8.19 g Tot Fat
• 2.12 g Sat Fat
• 3.88 g Mono Fat
• 1.04 g Poly Fat
5.43 g Carb
1.05 g Fiber
583.84 mg Sodium
246.50 mg Cholesterol

Brown the onions and green pepper in the olive oil in a medium skillet over medium-high heat for about 5 minutes. Lightly beat the eggs, egg whites, water, pepper, and salt or salt substitute. Pour into the skillet over the onions and peppers and continue to cook, stirring, until the eggs are set. Serve with salsa.

Serves 2

Quick Multi-Bean Soup

5 cups water
½ cup garbanzo beans (canned or cooked from dry)
½ cup baby lima beans (canned or cooked from dry)
½ cup black-eyed peas (canned or cooked from dry)
1 medium zucchini, sliced
1 cup chopped celery
2 cups chopped cabbage
2 tablespoons tomato paste
1 tablespoon vegetable seasoning

Per Serving:

104.36 Cal (5.95% from Fat, 18.80% from Protein, 75.20% from Carb)

5.39 g Protein
0.76 g Tot Fat
 • 0.12 g Sat Fat
 • 0.11 g Mono Fat
 • 0.34 g Poly Fat
21.52 g Carb
5.68 g Fiber
279.68 mg Sodium
0.00 mg Cholesterol

Put the water in a large pot and add the cooked beans and vegetables. Bring to a boil and cook for 20 minutes, then add the tomato paste and seasoning. Cook 10 more minutes.

Serves 4

Asparagus Chicken

- 1 lemon
- 1 onion, chopped
- 2 cloves garlic, minced
- 1 teaspoon olive oil
- 3 cups asparagus spears, cut into 1-inch pieces
- 1 cup sliced mushrooms
- 1 pound skinless, boneless chicken breasts, sliced into 2-inch strips
- ¾ cup water
- ½ teaspoon salt (or salt substitute to taste)
- ¼ teaspoon pepper
- 3 tablespoons parsley, chopped

Per Serving:

234.09 Cal (21.30% from Fat, 65.30% from Protein, 13.50% from Carb)

38.24 g Protein
5.53 g Tot Fat
 • 1.36 g Sat Fat
 • 2.26 g Mono Fat
 • 1.11 g Poly Fat
7.89 g Carb
2.97 g Fiber
384.99 mg Sodium
96.39 mg Cholesterol

Grate lemon and set aside peel. Halve lemon and juice. Sauté the onion and garlic in the olive oil for about 3 minutes. Add the asparagus and mushrooms and cook for 3 more minutes. Remove from the pan and set aside. Add the chicken to the pan and cook until lightly browned, about 3 minutes. Return the vegetables to the pan along with the chicken, and add the lemon juice and peel, water, salt or salt substitute, and pepper. Stir and let simmer for 10 minutes, or until heated and the chicken is cooked through. Sprinkle with parsley before serving.

Serves 4

Curried Quinoa

1 cup quinoa
2 cups water
1 teaspoon curry powder

Per Serving:

105.97 Cal (13.70% from Fat, 13.80% from Protein, 72.50% from Carb)

3.71 g Protein
1.64 g Tot Fat
 • 0.17 g Sat Fat
 • 0.43 g Mono Fat
 • 0.66 g Poly Fat
19.52 g Carb
1.67 g Fiber
8.32 mg Sodium
0.00 mg Cholesterol

Rinse the quinoa in a medium saucepan. Add 2 cups fresh water and the curry powder. Bring to a boil, reduce heat, and simmer for about 15 minutes, until the water is absorbed and the grains have turned from white to transparent.

Serves 6 (½-cup servings)

Day Twenty Menus

►Breakfast

Yogurt, plain, nonfat (sweetened with stevia)
*Fruit (may add to yogurt)
Oatmeal
Soy milk or nonfat milk

►Lunch

GREEK SALAD
****Bread

►Dinner

BROCCOLI SALAD
TOFU STEAKS
BARLEY PILAF
POACHED APPLES WITH NUTS and CREAM
SAUCE

Greek Salad

3 cups lettuce (romaine preferred), torn into bite-size pieces

½ cucumber, sliced

¼ cup onion, thinly sliced

1 tomato, coarsely chopped

¼ cup black olives, sliced

1 tablespoon crumbled feta cheese

Dressing:

1 tablespoon olive oil

2 tablespoons vinegar

1 clove garlic, minced

¼ teaspoon salt (or salt substitute to taste)

¼ teaspoon black pepper

Per Serving:

143.20 Cal (58.70% from Fat, 9.77% from Protein, 31.60% from Carb)

3.81 g Protein
10.15 g Tot Fat
 • 1.95 g Sat Fat
 • 6.58 g Mono Fat
 • 1.02 g Poly Fat
12.29 g Carb
4.02 g Fiber
510.89 mg Sodium
4.17 mg Cholesterol

Combine the salad ingredients in a large bowl. Mix the dressing ingredients in a small bowl, then toss with the salad.

Serves 2

Broccoli Salad

1 tablespoon olive oil
1 tablespoon vinegar (balsamic preferred)
¼ teaspoon salt (or salt substitute to taste)
⅛ teaspoon pepper
1 cup broccoli spears, coarsely chopped
2 tablespoons onion, chopped

Per Serving:

64.86 Cal (90.90% from Fat, 0.78% from Protein, 8.31% from Carb)

0.13 g Protein
6.77 g Tot Fat
  • 0.92 g Sat Fat
  • 4.98 g Mono Fat
  • 0.57 g Poly Fat
1.39 g Carb
0.22 g Fiber
295.16 mg Sodium
0.00 mg Cholesterol

Mix the oil and vinegar with salt and pepper. Combine the broccoli and onions in a small bowl and toss with the dressing. Let the salad marinate for 1 hour before serving.

Serves 2

Tofu Steaks

1 pound extra-firm tofu
4 teaspoons low-sodium soy
    sauce

Per Serving:

167.25 Cal (48.70% from Fat, 39.70% from Protein, 11.60% from Carb)

18.17 g Protein
9.89 g Tot Fat
  • 1.43 g Sat Fat
  • 2.18 g Mono Fat
  • 5.58 g Poly Fat
5.31 g Carb
2.65 g Fiber
192.94 mg Sodium
0.00 mg Cholesterol

Slice the tofu lengthwise into four slices. Sprinkle each slice with 1 teaspoon soy sauce. Heat a large nonstick skillet over medium heat. Spray with olive oil spray and add the tofu steaks, two at a time. Cook for 3–5 minutes on each side, until brown. This is good with Mushroom Gravy, recipe on page 456.

Serves 4

Barley Pilaf

1 tablespoon olive oil
1 medium onion, chopped
½ pound mushrooms, sliced
1 cup pearl barley
2 cups water
½ teaspoon salt (or salt
   substitute to taste)

Per Serving:

221.91 Cal (16.40% from Fat, 10.80% from Protein, 72.80% from Carb)

6.20 g Protein
4.20 g Tot Fat
   • 0.61 g Sat Fat
   • 2.56 g Mono Fat
   • 0.66 g Poly Fat
41.93 g Carb
8.57 g Fiber
305.19 mg Sodium
0.00 mg Cholesterol

Preheat the oven to 350° F. Heat the olive oil in a medium oven-proof skillet with a lid. Add the onions and mushrooms and cook for 5 minutes. Add the barley, stirring to coat. Meanwhile, bring the water to a boil. Add to the skillet with the vegetables and barley, along with the salt or salt substitute. Cover and cook in 350° F oven for 30 minutes. (May transfer to a covered casserole if skillet has no lid.) Add a little water if the pilaf becomes too dry.

Serves 4

Poached Apples with Nuts

3 apples, chopped
½ cup water
½ teaspoon cinnamon (or to
   taste)
1 tablespoon xylitol or
   3–4 drops stevia (to taste)
¼ cup chopped walnuts

Per Serving:

104.80 Cal (37.50%
from Fat, 7.32% from
Protein, 55.20% from
Carb)

2.10 g Protein
4.77 g Tot Fat
  • 0.34 g Sat Fat
  • 1.01 g Mono Fat
  • 3.03 g Poly Fat
15.81 g Carb
3.14 g Fiber
1.04 mg Sodium
0.00 mg Cholesterol

Place the chopped apples in a medium saucepan. Cover with the water. Add the cinnamon and sweetener. Cook the apples in water until they are tender yet still firm. Place in individual bowls, sprinkle with the chopped nuts, and top with Cream Sauce (recipe follows). These apples are also nice on cereal, waffles, pancakes, or yogurt.

Serves 4

Cream Sauce

1 pint nonfat cottage cheese
1 teaspoon vanilla
1–2 tablespoons soy milk or
   nonfat milk
2–3 drops stevia (or more to
   taste)

> **Per Cup:**
>
> 130.16 Cal (5.18% from Fat, 84.60% from Protein, 10.20% from Carb)
>
> 25.15 g Protein
> 0.68 g Tot Fat
> • 0.40 g Sat Fat
> • 0.17 g Mono Fat
> • 0.05 g Poly Fat
> 3.03 g Carb
> 0.05 g Fiber
> 19.21 mg Sodium
> 9.72 mg Cholesterol

Place the ingredients in a blender or food processor and process until smooth, adding soy milk or nonfat milk to desired consistency and stevia to taste. Serve 1 tablespoon over poached fruit. Keeps well in the refrigerator. Delicious over baked or poached fruit and other desserts.

Makes 2 cups

Day Twenty-one Menus

▶Breakfast

*Fruit
APPLE-OAT GRIDDLE CAKES

▶Lunch

*Green salad
BROILED GOAT CHEESE MELT

▶Dinner

TABOULI
FISH AND SALSA BAKE
*Fruit

Apple-Oat Griddle Cakes

½ cup whole wheat flour
½ tablespoon baking powder
½ teaspoon cinnamon
1 egg
2–3 drops stevia
⅓ cup soy milk or nonfat milk
½ cup grated apple
½ cup cooked oatmeal
1 tablespoon olive oil

Per Serving:

250.36 Cal (31.90%
from Fat, 16.00% from
Protein, 52.10% from
Carb)

10.32 g Protein
9.15 g Tot Fat
  • 1.65 g Sat Fat
  • 4.76 g Mono Fat
  • 1.69 g Poly Fat
33.62 g Carb
5.87 g Fiber
530.03 mg Sodium
82.17 mg Cholesterol

Sift the dry ingredients together. Beat the egg, then blend in the stevia, milk, apple, oats, and olive oil. Add dry the ingredients and mix well. Pour ¼ cup of this batter onto a medium-high griddle sprayed with olive oil spray. Turn as bubbles appear on the surface, then brown on the other side.

Serves 2–3; makes 6–7 pancakes

Broiled Goat Cheese Melt

2 slices sprouted-grain bread
2 ounces goat cheese, thinly
   sliced
½ tomato, thinly sliced

Per Serving:

164.31 Cal (39.00%
from Fat, 20.80% from
Protein, 40.20% from
Carb)

8.79 g Protein
7.32 g Tot Fat
• 4.41 g Sat Fat
• 1.86 g Mono Fat
• 0.49 g Poly Fat
16.95 g Carb
2.41 g Fiber
262.08 mg Sodium
13.04 mg Cholesterol

Toast one side of the bread under the broiler. Place thin slices of goat cheese on the untoasted side and return to the broiler. Watch carefully and remove when the cheese bubbles. Top with slices of tomato.

Serves 2

Tabouli

2 cups boiling water
1 cup bulgur
2 tablespoons olive oil
4 tablespoons lemon juice
½ teaspoon salt (or salt
   substitute to taste)
⅛ teaspoon ground pepper
1 cup fresh parsley, chopped
2 large tomatoes, chopped
1 cucumber, chopped
½ onion, chopped

> **Per Serving:**
>
> 199.48 Cal (31.40% from Fat, 10.10% from Protein, 58.50% from Carb)
>
> 5.36 g Protein
> 7.44 g Tot Fat
> • 1.04 g Sat Fat
> • 5.08 g Mono Fat
> • 0.82 g Poly Fat
> 31.16 g Carb
> 7.63 g Fiber
> 314.39 mg Sodium
> 0.00 mg Cholesterol

Pour the boiling water over the bulgur, stir, and let stand for 30 minutes. Drain in a strainer, squeezing out excess moisture. Place in a large bowl. Mix the olive oil, lemon juice, salt or salt substitute, and pepper and stir into the bulgur. Add the chopped parsley and vegetables and mix well. Chill at least two hours before serving.

Serves 4

Fish and Salsa Bake

- 2 4-ounce cod or halibut fillets
- 2 teaspoons olive oil
- ¼ teaspoon each onion and garlic powder
- ½ cup mild salsa

Per Serving:

131.61 Cal (36.00% from Fat, 50.20% from Protein, 13.80% from Carb)

16.46 g Protein
5.25 g Tot Fat
- 0.74 g Sat Fat
- 3.42 g Mono Fat
- 0.66 g Poly Fat
4.51 g Carb
1.09 g Fiber
328.41 mg Sodium
37.55 mg Cholesterol

Brush the fish with olive oil. Sprinkle with the onion and garlic powder. Place the fish in a baking dish sprayed with olive oil spray and cover with the salsa. Bake for 15–20 minutes just until fish is flaky.

Serves 2

Resources

Medical Clinics and Physician Referrals

Whitaker Wellness Institute
4321 Birch Street
Newport Beach, CA 92660
(800) 488-1500
www.whitakerwellness.com
Dr. Whitaker's medical clinic specializes in one-week programs that include:

- *One-week residential program*
- *Medical consultations*
- *Comprehensive medical testing*
- *Seminars on the latest in medical research and natural therapies*
- *Personalized exercise programs*
- *Nutritional consultations*
- *Stress management instruction*
- *Individualized nutritional supplementation*
- *Specific therapies for various health conditions, including diabetes, hypertension, and heart disease*

American College for Advancement in Medicine
P.O. Box 3427
Laguna Hills, CA 92654
(800) 532-3688
www.acam.org
This is a professional organization of alternative health medical doctors and osteopathic physicians, many of whom utilize the therapies discussed in this book. A majority of them administer chelation therapy. To receive a list of such physicians in your area, send a self-addressed, stamped envelope (two stamps).

American Association of Naturopathic Physicians
8201 Greensboro Drive,
Suite 300
McLean, VA 22102
(703) 610-9037
www.aanp.org
Naturopathic physicians are licensed professionals who have attended four-year graduate level naturopathic medical school. Their education covers the same basic sciences as an M.D. or D.O. but they are also

schooled in nutritional and other nontoxic approaches. Contact for local practitioners.

American Preventive Medical Association
P.O. Box 458
Great Falls, VA 22066
(800) 230-APMA
This political action group is involved in lobbying for legislation that allows medical freedom. It offers a directory of practitioners, books, and other resources on alternative medicine.

Resources for Specific Therapies

Nutritional Supplements
Healthy Directions, Inc.
P.O. Box 6000
Kearneysville, WV 25430
(800) 722-8008
www.drwhitaker.com
Dr. Whitaker's line of high-quality nutritional supplements is distributed by Healthy Directions. It includes the supplements for reversing diabetes discussed in this book, such as the Forward multivitamin/mineral supplement and Glucose Essentials. Healthy Directions is also one of the few sources for the inexpensive topical pain reliever Penetran+Plus.

Enhanced External Counterpulsation (EECP™)
Vasomedical, Inc.
180 Linden Avenue

Westbury, NY 11590
(800) 455-3327
www.naturalbypass.com
Vasomedical, Inc., provides information on EECP™ and a list of clinics offering the therapy. If you would like to consider EECP treatment at the Whitaker Wellness Institute Medical Clinic, please call (800) 826-1550 ext. 183.

Hyperbaric Medicine Education and Research Institute
P.O. Box 9653
Newport Beach, CA 92658
(949) 852-9855
The Hyperbaric Medicine Education and Research Institute provides information on hyperbaric oxygen therapy and offers education programs for physicians. It also has a listing of chamber locations throughout the country.

Mail-Order Sources of Food Items
Healthy Sweeteners

Stevia
Wisdom of the Ancients
2546 West Birchwood Avenue, Suite 104
Mesa, AZ 85202
(800) 899-9908
www.wisdomherbs.com
www.steviaplus.com

NOW
395 South Glen Ellyn Road
Bloomingdale, IL 60108
(800) 469-5552
www.nowfoods.com

Body Ecology
1266 West Paces Ferry Road,
Suite 505
Atlanta, GA 30327
(800) 4-STEVIA or (404)
266-1366
www.bodyecologydiet.com

Xylitol
Advantage International
61 West 74th Street, Suite 6B
New York, NY 10023
(917) 441-1038
www.advantageintl.qupg.com
www.xerix.com/cavityfree

Brown Rice Syrup
Mother's Market
225 E. 17th Street
Costa Mesa, CA 92627
(800) 595-MOMS or (949)
631-4741

Healthy Salt Substitutes

Vegetable Broth Seasoning
Dr. Bernard Jensen's Broth or
Vegetable Seasoning
535 Stevens Avenue West
Solana Beach, CA 92075
(800) 755-4027 or (858)
755-4027

Cardia Salt
Whitaker Wellness Institute
Vitamin and Book Store
4301 Birch Street
Newport Beach, CA 92660
(800) 810-6655

Whitaker Wellness Health & Nutrition Bar

Whitaker Wellness Institute
Vitamin and Book Store
4301 Birch Street
Newport Beach, CA 92660
(800) 810-6655

Additional Information and Suggested Reading

Glycemic Index of Foods
www.mendosa.com
Medical writer Rick Mendosa's
Web site contains extensive lists
of the glycemic indexes of specific foods. He also has links to
many excellent articles explaining the glycemic index.

Cooking with Stevia
The Stevia Cookbook, by Ray
Sahalien, M.D., and Donna
Gates. Garden City Park, N.Y.:
Avery Publishing Group, 1999.

Magnets
The Pain Relief Breakthrough,
by Julian Whitaker, M.D. New
York: Little, Brown, 1999.

Hypertension and Heart Disease

Reversing Hypertension, by Julian Whitaker, M.D. New York: Warner Books, 2000.

Reversing Heart Disease, by Julian Whitaker, M.D. New York: Warner Books, 1985; revision 2001.

General Health

Health & Healing, Dr. Whitaker's monthly newsletter, informs half a million households every month about a variety of aspects of health and cutting-edge alternative therapies. Subscriptions are available from Phillips Publishing Company, (800) 539-8219.

Dr. Whitaker's Web site, drwhitaker.com, provides up-to-date research and patient-proven solutions to the most common health problems that plague us. New articles, drug alerts, supplement recommendations, and recipes are updated frequently, and details about the programs offered at the Whitaker Wellness Institute are available.

Dr. Whitaker's Guide to Natural Healing, by Julian Whitaker, M.D. Rocklin, Calif.: Prima Publishing, 1995.

Encyclopedia of Natural Medicine, by Michael Murray, N.D., and Joseph Pizzorno, N.D. Rocklin, Calif.: Prima Publishing, 1998.

Encyclopedia of Nutritional Supplements, by Michael Murray, N.D. Rocklin, Calif.: Prima Publishing, 1996.

The Healing Power of Herbs, by Michael Murray, N.D. Rocklin, Calif.: Prima Publishing, 1995.

Notes

Chapter 1

[1] American Diabetes Association. Diabetes facts and figures, 1999; http://www.diabetes.org/ada/facts/asp.

[2] Schatz, DA, et al. Prevention of insulin-dependent diabetes mellitus: An overview of three trials. *Cleveland Clinic Journal of Medicine* 63(5): 270–74, 1996.

[3] Yoon, JW. Isolation of a virus from the pancreas of a child with ketoacidosis. *New England Journal of Medicine* 300: 1173–79, 1979.

[4] Head, KA. Type-1 diabetes: Prevention of the disease and its complications. *Alternative Medicine Review* 2(4): 256–81, 1997.

[5] Leslie, RDG, et al. Early environmental events as a cause of IDDM. *Diabetes* 43: 843–50, 1994.

[6] Srikanta, S. Islet-cell antibodies and beta-cell function in monozygotic triplets and twins initially discordant for type 1 diabetes mellitus. *New England Journal of Medicine* 308: 322–25, 1983.

[7] Murray, M, and Pizzorno, J. *Encyclopedia of Natural Medicine.* Rocklin, Calif.: Prima Publishing, 1998.

[8] Sweeney, JS. Dietary factors that influence the dextrose tolerance test. *Archives of Internal Medicine* 40: 818–30, 1927.

[9] Siperstein, M. Diabetes diagnoses grounded on GTT are wrong most of the time. *Family Practice News* 9(20): 1, Oct. 15, 1979.

[10] Diabetes facts and figures, the dangerous toll of diabetes; http://www.diabetes.org/ada/facts.asp.

Chapter 2

[1] Ignorance about insulin resistance linked with poor disease control. *Cardiology Review* 17(suppl. 1): 1–2, 2000.

[2] Reaven, GM. Role of insulin resistance in human disease. *Diabetes* 37: 1595–1607, 1988.

[3] Reaven, GM. *Syndrome X: Overcoming the Silent Killer That Can Give You a Heart Attack.* New York: Simon & Schuster, 2000.

[4] Ibid.

[5] DECODE study group. Glucose tolerance and mortality: Comparison of WHO and American Diabetes Association diagnostic criteria. *Lancet* 354: 617–21, 1999.

[6] Bland, JS. *Nutritional Management of the Underlying Causes of Chronic Disease.* Gig Harbor, Wash.: The Institute for Functional Medicine, 2000.

[7] Neel, JF. The "thrifty genotype" in 1998. *Nutrition Review* 57(5): S2–S9, 1999.

[8] Rich-Edwards, JW, et al. Birthweight and the risk for type 2 diabetes mellitus in adult women. *Annals of Internal Medicine* 130: 278–84, 1999.

[9] Mayer-Davis, EJ. Intensity and amount of physical activity in relation to insulin sensitivity. *Journal of the American Medical Association* 279(9): 669–74, 1998.

[10] Hu, FB, et al. Walking compared with vigorous physical activity and risk of type 2 diabetes in women: A prospective study. *Journal of the American Medical Association* 282(15): 1433–1439, 1999.

[11] Eaton, SB, et al. Paleolithic nutrition, a consideration of its nature and current implications. *New England Journal of Medicine* 312(5): 283–89, 1985.

Chapter 3

[1] Davidson, JK. *Clinical Diabetes Mellitus: A Problem-Oriented Approach.* 3rd. ed. New York: Thieme Medical Publishers, Inc., 2000.

[2] Diabetes Control and Complications Trial Reseach Group. The effects of intensive treatment of diabetes on the development and progression of insulin-dependent diabetes mellitus. *New England Journal of Medicine* 329(14): 977–86, 1993.

[3] UK Prospective Diabetes Study Group. Intensive blood-glucose control with sulphonylureas or insulin compared with conventional treatment and risk of complications in patients with type 2 diabetes (UKPDS 33). *Lancet* 352(9131): 837–53, 1998.

[4] UK Prospective Diabetes Study Group. Tight blood pressure control and risk of macrovascular and microvascular complications in type 2 diabetes (UKPDS 38). *British Medical Journal* 317(7160): 703–13, 1998.

[5] Gaede, P, et al. Intensified multifactorial intervention in patients with type 2 diabetes mellitus and microalbuminaria: The Steno type 2 randomized study. *Lancet* 353: 617–22, Feb. 20, 1999.

[6] Emanuele, N, et al. Effect of intensive glycemic control on fibrinogen, lipids, and lipoproteins. *Archives of Internal Medicine* 158: 2485–90, 1998.

[7] Goldstein, DE. How much do you know about glycated hemoglobin testing? *Clinical Diabetes*, July/August 1995: 60–64.

Chapter 4

[1] Davidson, JK. *Clinical Diabetes Mellitus: A Problem-Oriented Approach.* 3rd ed. New York: Thieme Medical Publishers, Inc., 2000.

[2] Cryer, PE. Glucose counterregulation, hypoglycemia, and intensive insulin therapy in diabetes mellitus. *New England Journal of Medicine* 313: 232–41, 1985.

[3] Somogyi, M. *Bulletin of the St. Louis Jewish Hospital Medical Staff,* Oct. 1949.

[4] Somogyi, M. *Bulletin of the St. Louis Jewish Hospital Medical Staff,* May 1951.

[5] Campbell, P., et al. Pathogenesis of the dawn phenomenon in patients with insulin-dependent diabetes mellitus. *New England Journal of Medicine* 312: 1473–79, 1985.

[6] Coustan, DR. A randomized clinical trial of the insulin pump vs intensive conventional therapy in diabetic pregnancies. *Journal of the American Medical Association* 255: 631–36, 1986.

[7] Knatterud, GL, et al. Effects of hypoglycemic agents on vascular complications in patients with adult-onset diabetes. *Journal of the American Medical Association* 240: 37–42, 1978.

[8] *USGDP Data Book.* USGDP Coordinating Center, Baltimore, Md., 1971.

[9] UK Prospective Diabetes Study Group. Intensive blood-glucose control with sulphonylureas or insulin compared with conventional treatment and risk of complications in patients with type 2 diabetes (UKPDS 33). *Lancet* 352(9131): 837–53, 1998.

[10] UK Prospective Diabetes Study Group. Tight blood pressure control and risk of macrovascular and microvascular complications in type 2 diabetes (UKPDS 38). *British Medical Journal* 317(7160): 703–13, 1998.

[11] Davidson, JK. *Clinical Diabetes Mellitus.*

[12] Ilkova, H, et al. Induction of long-term glycemic control in newly diagnosed type 2 diabetic patients by transient intensive insulin treatment. *Diabetes Care* 20: 1353–56, 1997.

Chapter 5

[1] Warner, R, et al. *Off Diabetes Pills: A Diabetic's Guide to Longer Life*. Washington, D.C.: Public Citizen's Health Research Group, 1978.

[2] Public Citizen's Health Research Group. Risk of serious low blood sugar with antidiabetic drugs. *Worst Pills Best Pills News* 2(12): 46, Dec. 1996.

[3] University Group Diabetes Program. A study of the effects of hypoglycemic agents on vascular complications in patients with adult-onset diabetes. 11. Mortality results. *Diabetes* 19 (suppl.): 814, 1970.

[4] University Group Diabetes Program. *Journal of the American Medical Association* 218: 1400–1410, 1971.

[5] Goodman, J. *Cleveland Plain Dealer*, Feb. 18, 1975.

[6] Carter, JR, et al. *Cleveland Plain Dealer*, April 10, 1975.

[7] Davidson, JK. *Clinical Diabetes Mellitus: A Problem-Oriented Approach*. 3rd. ed. New York: Thieme Medical Publishers, Inc., 2000.

[8] Schor, S. The University Group Diabetes Program: A statistician looks at the mortality results. *Journal of the American Medical Association* 217: 1671–75, 1971.

[9] Cornfield, J. The University Group Diabetes Program: A further study of the mortality finding. *Journal of the American Medical Association* 217: 1676–87, 1971.

[10] Biometric Society. Report of the committee for assessment of biometric aspects of controlled trials of the hypoglycemic agents. *Journal of the American Medical Association* 231: 583–608, 1975.

[11] Chalmers, TC, ed. Settling the UGDP controversy. *Journal of the American Medical Association* 231: 624–25, 1975.

[12] *Physicians' Desk Reference*. Montvale, N.J.: Medical Economics, 2000.

[13] UK Prospective Diabetes Study Group. Intensive blood-glucose control with sulphonylureas or insulin compared with conventional treatment and risk of conventional treatment and risk of complications in patients with type 2 diabetes (UKPDS 33). *Lancet* 352(9131): 832–53, 1998.

[14] Goldstein, BJ. Treatment of type 2 diabetes: Efficacy of thiazolidinediones as monotherapy. *Consultant* (suppl.): S21–S27, Nov. 1999.

[15] Willman, D. Fear grows over delay in removing Rezulin. *Los Angeles Times*, March 10, 2000.

[16] Public Citizen's Health Research Group. The new diabetes drug rosiglitazone (Avandia) rejected by European regulators. *Worst Pills Best Pills News* 5(12): 93–94, Dec. 1999.

[17] Public Citizen's Health Research Group. Acarbose (Precose) for diabetes no substitute for diet and exercise. *Worst Pills Best Pills News* 2(4): 14, April 1996.

[18] Public Citizen's Health Research Group. Liver toxicity with the diabetes drug acarbose (Precose). *Worst Pills Best Pills News* 4(6): 41–42, June 1998.

[19] Berger, M. Oral agents in the treatment of diabetes mellitus. In JK Davidson, *Clinical Diabetes Mellitus: A Problem-Oriented Approach*, p. 268.

[20] Davidson, JK. *International Diabetic Foundation Bulletin* 20(19): 99–108.

[21] Turner, RC, et al. Glycemic control with diet, sulfonylurea, metformin, or insulin in patients with type 2 diabetes mellitus. *Journal of the American Medical Association* 281(21): 2005–12, June 2, 1999.

Chapter 6

[1] Samsum, WD. The use of high carbohydrate diets in the treatment of diabetes mellitus. *Journal of the American Medical Association* 86: 78–181, Jan. 16, 1926.

[2] Rabinowitch, IM. Experiences with a high carbohydrate–low calorie diet for the treatment of diabetes mellitus. *Canadian Medical Association Journal* 23: 489–98, 1930.

[3] Rabinowitch, IM. Effects of the high carbohydrate–low calorie diet upon carbohydrate tolerance in diabetes mellitus. *Canadian Medical Association Journal* 33: 136–44, 1935.

[4] Meyer, KA, et al. Carbohydrates, dietary fiber, and incident type 2 diabetes in older women. *American Journal of Clinical Nutrition* 71(4): 921–30, April 2000.

[5] Williams, DE, et al. Frequent salad vegetable consumption is associated with a reduction in the risk of diabetes mellitus. *Journal of Clinical Epidemiology* 52(4): 329–35, 1999.

[6] Miranda, PM, and DL Horwitz. High-fiber diets in the treatment of diabetes mellitus. *Annals of Internal Medicine* 88: 482–86, 1978.

[7] Anderson, JW, et al. Beneficial effects of a high carbohydrate, high fiber diet on hyperglycemic diabetic men. *American Journal of Clinical Nutrition* 29: 895–99, 1976.

[8] Chandalia, M, et al. Beneficial effects of high dietary fiber intake in patients with type 2 diabetes mellitus. *New England Journal of Medicine* 342(19): 1392–98, 2000.

[9] Jarvi, AE, et al. Improved glycemic control and lipid profile and normalized fibri-nolytic activity on a low-glycemic index diet in type 2 diabetic patients. *Diabetes Care* 22(1): 10–18, 1999.

[10] High sugar intake ups heart risk. Reuters Health Information, Inc. http://www.reutershealth.com, June 22, 1998.

[11] Werman, MJ, et al. The chronic effect of dietary fructose on glycation and collagen cross-linking in rats. *American Journal of Clinical Nutrition* 66: 219, 1977.

[12] Jacobson, MF. Liquid candy: How soft drinks are harming Americans' health. Center for Science in the Public Interest, http://www.cspinet.org/sodapop/liquid_candy.htm.

[13] CSPI Reports. Sample quotes from cancer experts' letters on Acesulfame testing. http://www.cspinet.org/reports/asekquot.html.

[14] Renaud, S, et al. Wine, alcohol, platelets and the French paradox for coronary heart disease. *Lancet* 339: 1523–26, 1992.

[15] Facchini, F, et al. Light-to-moderate alcohol intake is associated with enhanced insulin sensitivity. *Diabetes Care* 17(2): 115–18, 1994.

Chapter 7

[1] Rose, WC. Amino acid requirements of man. *Journal of Biological Chemistry* 217: 997–1004, 1955.

[2] Mitch, WE, et al. The effect of a keto acid–amino acid supplement to a restricted diet on the progression of chronic renal failure. *New England Journal of Medicine* 311: 623–29, 1984.

[3] Johnson, NE. Effect of level of protein intake on urinary and fecal calcium and calcium retention of young adult males. *Journal of Nutrition* 100: 1425–30, 1970.

[4] Himsworth, HR. The dietetic factor determining the glucose tolerance and sensitivity to insulin of healthy men. *Clinical Science* 2: 67–94, 1935.

[5] Ascherio, A, and WC. Willett. Health effects of trans fatty acids. *American Journal of Clinical Nutrition* 66(suppl. 4): S1006–S1010, Oct. 1997.

Chapter 8

[1] Goodyear, LJ, and BB Kahn. Excercise, glucose transport, and insulin sensitivity. *Annual Review of Medicine* 49: 235–61, 1998.

[2] Klachko, DM, et al. Blood glucose levels during walking in normal and diabetic subjects. *Diabetes* 21: 89–100, 1972.

[3] Kirwan, JP, et al. Regular exercise enhances insulin activation of IRS-1-associated PI3-kinase in human skeletal muscle. *Journal of Applied Physiology* 88(2): 797–803, Feb. 2000.

[4] Pedersen, O. Increased insulin receptors after exercise in patients with insulin-dependent diabetes mellitus. *New England Journal of Medicine* 302: 886–92, 1980.

[5] Soman, VR, et al. Increased insulin sensitivity and insulin binding to monocytes after physical training. *New England Journal of Medicine* 301: 1200–04, 1979.

[6] Uusitupa, M. The Finnish Diabetes Prevention Study. *British Journal of Nutrition* 83(suppl. 1): S137–S142, March 2000.

[7] Increasing evidence suggests that exercise is protective against the development of type 2 diabetes mellitus. http:www.diabetes.org/am99/abshtml/a100607.html.

[8] Austin, MA. Epidemiology of hypertriglyceridemia and cardiovascular disease. *American Journal of Cardiology* 83(9B): 2290–96, May 13, 1999.

[9] Poor prognosis for diabetics unable to exercise. Reuters Health Information, Inc. http://www.reutershealth.com, Jan. 11, 1999.

[10] Peterson, L. *Cardiovascular Rehabilitation: A Comprehensive Approach.* New York: Macmillan, 1983.

[11] Ornish, D, et al. Can lifestyle changes reverse coronary heart disease? The lifestyle heart trial. *Lancet* 336: 129–33, 1990.

Chapter 9

[1] Goodwin, JS, et al. Battling quackery: Attitudes about micronutrient supplements in American academic medicine. *Archives of Internal Medicine* 158: 2187–91, 1998.

[2] Graci, S. *The Power of Superfoods.* Scarborough, Ontario: Prentice Hall Canada, Inc., 1997.

[3] Stampfer, MJ, et al. Vitamin E consumption and the risk of coronary disease in women. *New England Journal of Medicine* 328: 1444–48, 1993.

[4] Rimm, EB. Vitamin E consumption and the risk of coronary disease in men. *New England Journal of Medicine* 328: 1450–55, 1993.

[5] Sano, M, et al. A controlled trial of selegiline, alpha-tocopherol, or both as treatment for Alzheimer's disease. The Alzheimer's Disease Cooperative Study. *New England Journal of Medicine* 336(17): 1216–22, April 24, 1997.

[6] Lazarou, J, et al. Incidence of adverse drug reactions in hospitalized patients. *Journal of the American Medical Association* 279(15): 1200–1205, 1998.

[7] Eisenberg, DM, et al. Unconventional medicine in the United States: Prevalence, cost and patterns of use. *New England Journal of Medicine* 328(4): 246–52, Jan. 28, 1993.

[8] Eisenberg, DM, et al. Trends in alternative medicine use in the United States, 1990–1997: Results of a follow-up national survey. *Journal of the American Medical Association* 280(18): 1569–75, Nov. 11, 1998.

[9] Alternative treatments popular among diabetics. Reuters Health Information, Inc. http://www.reutershealth.com, June 23, 1999.

[10] Mooradian, AD, et al. Micronutrient status in diabetes mellitus. *American Journal of Clinical Nutrition* 45: 877–95, 1987.

[11] Mooradian, AG, et al. Selected vitamins and minerals in diabetes. *Diabetes Care* 17(5): 464–79, May 1994.

[12] Shepherd, PR, et al. Glucose transporters and insulin action: Implications for insulin resistance and diabetes mellitus. *New England Journal of Medicine* 341(4): 248–57, 1999.

[13] Borden, G, et al. Effects of vanadyl sulfate on carbohydrate and lipid metabolism in patients with non-insulin-dependent diabetes mellitus. *Metabolism* 45(9): 1130–35, Sept. 1996.

[14] Goldfine, AB, et al. Clinical trials of vanadium compounds in human diabetes mellitus. *Canadian Journal of Physiology and Pharmacology* 72 (suppl. 3): 11, 1994.

[15] Mertz, W. Effects and metabolism of glucose tolerance factor. *Nutrition Review* 33: 1929, 1975.

[16] Anderson, RA, et al. Elevated intakes of supplemental chromium improve glucose and insulin variables in individuals with type 2 diabetes. *Diabetes* 46(11): 1786–91, Nov. 1997.

[17] Kaats, GR, et al. A randomized, double-masked, placebo-controlled study of the effects of chromium picolinate supplementation on body composition: A replication and extension of a previous study. *Current Therapeutic Research* 59(6): 379–88, June 1998.

[18] Stearns, DM, et al. A prediction of chromium (III) accumulation in humans from chromium dietary supplements. *FASEB Journal* 9: 1649–55, 1995.

[19] Shils, ME, et al. *Modern Nutrition in Health and Disease.* Malvern, Pa.: Lean & Febiger, 1994.

[20] Mather, HM. Hypomagnesaemia in diabetes. *Acta Clinica Chemica* 95: 235–42, 1979.

[21] McNair, P, et al. Hypomagnesemia, a risk factor in diabetic retinopathy. *Diabetes* 27(11): 1075–77, Nov. 1978.

[22] Engstrom, JE, et al. Vitamin C intake and mortality among a sample of the United States population. *Epidemiology* 3: 194–202, 1992.

[23] Cunningham, JJ, et al. Vitamin C: An aldose reductase inhibitor that normalizes erythrocyte sorbitol in insulin-dependent diabetes mellitus. *Journal of the American College of Nutrition* 4: 344–350, 1994.

[24] Mooradian, A, et al. Selected vitamins and minerals in diabetes. *Diabetes Care* 17(5): 464–79, 1994.

[25] Ceriello, A, et al. Vitamin E reduction of protein glycosylation in diabetics. *Diabetes Care* 14: 68–72, 1991.

[26] Murray, M, and J. Pizzorno. *Encyclopedia of Natural Medicine.* Rocklin, Calif.: Prima Publishing, 1998.

[27] Devaraj, S, and I. Jialal. Low-density lipoprotein postsecretory modification, monocyte function, and circulating adhesion molecules in type 2 diabetic patients with and without macrovascular complications: The effect of alphatocopherol supplementation. *Circulation* 102(2): 191–96, July 11, 2000.

[28] Estrada, DE, et al. Stimulation of glucose uptake by the natural coenzyme a-lipoic acid/thioctic acid. *Experimental and Clinical Endocrinology and Diabetes* 45: 1798–1804, 1996.

[29] Jacob, S, et al. Oral adminisration of RAC-a-lipoic acid modulates insulin sensitivity in patients with type-2 diabetes mellitus: A placebo-controlled pilot trial. *Free Radical Biology and Medicine* 27(3/4): 309–14, 1999.

[30] Ruhnau, KJ, et al. Effects of 3-week oral treatment with the antioxidant thioctic acid (alpha-lipoic acid) in symptomatic diabetic polyneuropathy. *Diabetic Medicine* 16(2): 1040–43, Dec. 1999.

[31] Packer, L, et al. Alpha-lipoic acid as a biological antioxidant. *Free Radical Biology and Medicine* 19(2): 227–50, Aug. 1995.

[32] Vague, PH, et al. Nicotinamide may extend remission phase in insulin dependent diabetes. *Lancet* 1: 619–20, 1987.

[33] Elliot, RB, et al. Prevention of diabetes in normal school children. *Diabetes Research and Clinical Practice* 14: S85, 1991.

[34] Mandrup-Poulsen, T, et al. Nicotinamide in the prevention of insulin dependent diabetes mellitus. *Diabetes/Metabolism Reviews* 9: 295–309, 1993.

[35] Elam, MB, et al. Effect of niacin on lipid and lipoprotein levels and glycemic control in patients with diabetes and peripheral arterial disease: The ADMIT study: A randomized trial.

Arterial Disease Multiple Intervention Trial. *Journal of the American Medical Association* 284(10): 1263–70, Sept. 13, 2000.

[36] Murray, M, and J Pizzorno. *Encyclopedia of Natural Medicine*. Rocklin, Calif.: Prima Publishing, 1998.

[37] Coggeshall, JC, et al. Biotin status and plasma glucose in diabetics. *Annals of the New York Academy of Science* 447: 389–92, 1995.

[38] Coelinagh-Bennick, HJT, et al. Improvement of oral glucose tolerance in gestational diabetes. *British Medical Journal* 3: 13–15, 1975.

[39] Connor, WE, et al. Reduction of plasma lipids, lipoproteins, and apoproteins by dietary fish oils in patients with hypertriglyceridemia. *New England Journal of Medicine* 312: 1210–16, 1985.

[40] Luo, J, et al. Moderate intake of n-3 fatty acids for 2 months had no detrimental effects on glucose metabolism and could ameliorate the lipid profile in type 2 diabetic men. Results of a controlled study. *Diabetes Care* 21(5): 717–24, May 1998.

[41] Giron, MD, et al. Increased diaphragm expression of GLUT4 in control and streptozotocin-diabetic rats by fish oil-supplemented diets. *Lipids* 34(8): 801–7, Aug. 1999.

[42] Keen, H, et al. Treatment of diabetic neuropathy with gamma-linolenic acid. *Diabetes Care* 16(1): 8, 1993.

[43] Shimizu, K. Suppression of glucose absorption by some fractions extracted from *Gymnema sylvestre* leaves. *Journal of Veterinary Medical Science* 59(4): 245–51, April 1997.

[44] Shanmugasundaram, ERB, et al. Use of *Gymnema sylvestre* leaf extract in the control of blood glucose in insulin-dependent diabetes mellitus. *Journal of Ethnopharmacology* 30: 281–94, 1990.

[45] Baskaran, K, et al. Antidiabetic effect of a leaf extract from *Gymnema sylvestre* in noninsulin-dependent diabetes mellitus patients. *Journal of Ethnopharmacology* 30: 295–305, 1990.

[46] Ikeda, Y. The clinical study on the water extract of leaves of *Lagestroemia speciosa L.* for mild cases of diabetes mellitus. Unpublished, 1998.

[47] Murray, M. *The Healing Power of Herbs.* Rocklin, Calif.: Prima Publishing, 1995.

[48] Srivastava, Y, et al. Antidiabetic and adaptogenic properties of *Momordica charantia* extract: An experimental and clinical evaluation. *Phytotherapy Research* 7: 285–89, 1993.

[49] Welihinda, J, et al. Effect of *Momordica charantia* on the glucose tolerance in maturity onset diabetes. *Journal of Ethnopharmacology* 17: 277–82, 1986.

[50] Brancati, FL, et al. Body weight patterns from 20 to 49 years of age and subsequent risk for diabetes mellitus. *Archives of Internal Medicine* 159: 957–63, May 10, 1999.

[51] McCarty, MF, et al. Pyruvate and hydroxycitrate/carnitine may synergize to promote reverse electron transport in hepatocyte mitochondria, effectively "uncoupling" the oxidation of fatty acids. *Medical Hypotheses* 52(5): 407–16, 1999.

Chapter 10

[1] Callsen, ME. Presented at the 44th Annual Meeting of the American Diabetes Association with a synopsis in *Cardiovascular News,* Feb. 1985.

[2] Williams, G. *Medical Tribune,* September 17, 1986, p. 8.

[3] Hadley, HW, et al. A topically applied quaternary ammonium compound exhibits analgesic effects for orthopedic pain. *Alternative Medicine Review* 3(5): 361–66, 1998.

[4] Magnetic foot pads reduce pain in 90 percent of diabetic patients with neuropathy. Reuters Health Information, Inc. http://www.reutershealth.com, Jan. 25, 1999.

[5] Olszewer, E, et al. EDTA chelation therapy: A retrospective study of 2,870 patients. *Journal of Advancement in Medicine* 2(1/2): 197–211, spring/summer 1990.

[6] Neubauer, RA, et al. *Hyperbaric Oxygen Therapy.* New York: Avery, 1998.

[7] Lawson, WE, et al. Efficacy of enhanced external counterpulsation in the treatment of angina pectoris. *American Journal of Cardiology* 70: 859–62, Oct. 1, 1992.

[8] Multiple Risk Factor Intervention Trial Research Group. *Journal of the American Medical Association* 248(12): 1465–77, 1984.

[9] Kempner, W. Treatment of hypertension vascular disease with rice diet. *American Journal of Medicine* 4: 545–77, 1948.

Chapter 12

[1] Walker, KZ, et al. Effects of regular walking on cardiovascular risk factors and body composition in normoglycemic women and women with type 2 diabetes. *Diabetes Care* 22(4): 555–61, April 1999.

[2] Eriksson, JG. Exercise and the treatment of type 2 diabetes mellitus: An update. *Sports Medicine* 27(6): 381–91, June 1999.

[3] Anderson, RE, et al. Effects of lifestyle activity vs structured aerobic exercise in obese women: A randomized trial.

Journal of the American Medical Association 281(4): 335–40, Jan. 27, 1999.

[4] Dustman, RE, et al. Aerobic exercise training and improved neuropsychological function of older individuals. *Neurobiology of Aging* 5(1): 35–42, spring 1984.

[5] Dunn, AL, et al. Comparison of lifestyle and structured interventions to increase physical activity and cardiorespiratory fitness. *Journal of the American Medical Association* 281(4): 327–34, Jan. 27, 1999.

Chapter 13

[1] U.S. Department of Agriculture, Agricultural Research Service. USDA Nutrient Database for Standard Reference, Release 13, 1999. Nutrient Data Laboratory Home Page, http://www.nal.usda.gov/fnic/foodcomp.

[2] Netzer, CT. *The Complete Book of Food Counts.* New York: Dell, 2000.

Index

About the Author

JULIAN WHITAKER, M.D., a medical practitioner for more than thirty years, treats thousands of patients a year at his Whitaker Wellness Institute in Newport Beach, California. Dr. Whitaker is the editor of *Health & Healing*, one of the nation's leading health newsletters, as well as a founder and past president of the American Preventive Medical Association. He is the author of *Reversing Hypertension* and *Reversing Heart Disease*. For more information, visit www.DrWhitaker.com.